ANTIBIOTICS

ACTIONS, ORIGINS, RESISTANCE

ANTIBIOTICS

ACTIONS, ORIGINS, RESISTANCE

by

Christopher Walsh

Harvard Medical School, Boston, Massachusetts

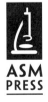

**ASM
PRESS**

WASHINGTON, D.C.

Cover illustration is adapted from a poster, "Mechanisms of antibiotic action and resistance," by C. Walsh, J. Trauger, P. Courvalin, and J. Davies (*Trends in Microbiology*, volume 9, 2001, with permission from Elsevier Science).

Library of Congress Cataloging-in-Publication Data

Walsh, Christopher.
    Antibiotics : actions, origins, resistance / by Christopher Walsh.
      p. ; cm.
   Includes bibliographical references and index.
    ISBN 1-55581-254-6
   1. Antibiotics.   2. Drug resistance in microorganisms.
    [DNLM: 1. Antibiotics—pharmacology.   2. Drug Resistance, Bacterial.
   QV 350 W223a 2003]   I. Title.

RM267 .W357 2003
615′.329—dc21

                           2002152389

Address editorial correspondence to: ASM Press, 1752 N St., N.W., Washington, DC 20036-2904, U.S.A.

Send orders to: ASM Press, P.O. Box 605, Herndon, VA 20172, U.S.A.
Phone: 800-546-2416; 703-661-1593
Fax: 703-661-1501
Email: books@asmusa.org
Online: www.asmpress.org

Dedicated to

Diana
Allison
Thomas

Contents

Preface

THIS BOOK HAS DEVELOPED FROM FOUR SUSTAINED, CONVERGENT INTERESTS IN MY RESEARCH GROUP: enzyme inhibitors; bacterial cell wall biosynthetic pathways; the mechanism of action of antibiotics and the development of resistance mechanisms; and the biosynthesis of polyketide and nonribosomal peptide natural products.

The basic premise of the approach is that one can understand and categorize antibiotic action, both historically and prospectively, by analysis of how these small molecules interfere selectively with one or more processes central to the survival of bacterial cells. Most of the attention in this book is on natural products with antibiotic activity elaborated by microbes to act as chemical weapons on neighboring bacteria, but synthetic chemicals with antibiotic activity are also examined. Thousands of molecules have been reported to have antibiotic activity, but only a few structural classes have had an impact in human infectious disease. The focus of this text is on those classes of antibiotics. This book is, then, not meant to be encyclopedic, nor a compendium of pharmacologic information, nor a microbiologic survey of pathogens and how to treat them. Authoritative texts already exist on those aspects of antimicrobial agents.

The current major classes of antibiotics act on only a small set of targets: bacterial cell wall biosynthesis, bacterial protein synthesis, DNA replication and repair, and the folate coenzyme-dependent pathway for thymidine biosynthesis. The first section of the book examines how antibiotics block specific proteins acting in these essential bacterial processes and how the molecular structure of the small-molecule drugs enables their antibiotic activity.

The middle section of the book takes up the development of bacterial resistance to antibiotics, starting with the molecular logic that microbial producers of antibiotics use for self-protection. The three major routes of resistance in antibiotic producers—destruction of the antibiotic, active extrusion of antibiotics by transmembrane pumps, and modification of target structures to antibiotic insensitivity—are seen to be the major mechanisms of resistance in bacterial pathogens.

The third part of the text takes up the molecular logic of antibiotic biosynthesis, starting with regulatory networks that control gene transcription of secondary metabolites in streptomycetes, those prolific producers of antibiotics. Polyketide and nonribosomal peptide antibiotics are manufactured on multimodular "assembly lines" that resemble fatty acid synthase machinery. The modular assembly line strategy enables wide variation of structure in these classes of antibacterial agents and offers the prospect of directed combinatorial biosynthesis.

The last section of the book examines the prospects for broadening the base of bacterial targets and also where new antibiotics are likely to emerge. Bacterial genomic sequencing has moved antibacterial research from a target-poor to a target-rich arena. New antibiotics are likely to arise both from synthetic chemical efforts, perhaps via combinatorial chemistry efforts, and also from natural products, by combinatorial biosynthetic variants.

I am indebted to many members of my research group, over the past 5 years in particular, for many discussions and ideas about antibiotic action, biosynthesis, and resistance. I thank John Trauger for his design and execution of artwork on targets in bacterial cells that led to the book cover art and the chapter opener figures. I thank Gary Marshall, Raymond Chen, Hiten Patel, Steve Bruner, Mike Burkart, Susan Clugston, Rahul Kohli, Heather Losey, and Lusong Luo for their many contributions to artwork creation, design, and implementation, as well as the correction of numerous inconsistencies and errors along the way. I acknowledge the help and input of Tanya Schneider, Sarah O'Connor, and particularly Lusong Luo for efforts in literature citations. My special thanks go to Gary Marshall for his tremendous diligence and attention to the text and especially the bulk of the final artwork of the book.

CHRISTOPHER WALSH
January 2003

Introduction to Antibiotics

I N THIS INTRODUCTORY SECTION THE SCOPE and focus of the book are set, with attention to antibiotics, from both natural and synthetic sources, that have a substantial role in the treatment of human bacterial diseases. The origins of natural antibiotics are noted, along with self-protection strategies in producer organisms and the development of resistance in previously susceptible bacteria. The inevitable progression of bacteria exposed to antibiotics to develop resistance ensures the need for continual cycles of discovery and development of new antibiotics.

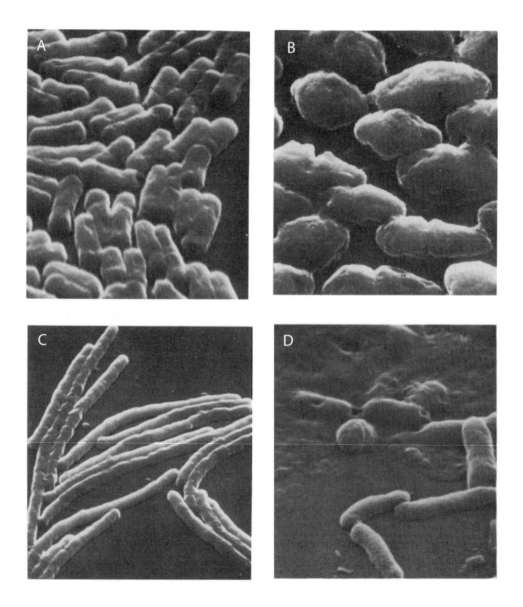

The effect of β-lactam antibiotics on bacterial cells. (A) Untreated rod-shaped *Escherichia coli* cells; (B–D) Cells after treatment with various β-lactam antibiotics, showing lysed debris, central wall lesions, and a spheroplast. (Panels A–C from Greenwood and O'Grady [1973], and panel D from Greenwood and O'Grady [1969], with permission.)

chapter 1

Antibiotics: Initial Concepts

What are antibiotics and where do they come from?

Antibiotics are molecules that stop microbes, both bacteria and fungi, from growing or kill them outright. As diagrammed in **Fig. 1.1**, antibiotics that stop bacteria from growing are bacteriostatic, exemplified by the drug chloramphenicol. Antibiotics that cause bacterial cell death are bactericidal; they lower the bacterial count, as shown for penicillin. Some antibiotics can display bacteriostatic activity in some circumstances and bactericidal activity in others, where sufficient damage to one or more cell pathways or structures occurs such that a net bactericidal response is triggered.

Antibiotics, agents "against life," can either be natural products or man-made synthetic chemicals, designed to block some crucial process in microbial cells selectively. Most of the antibiotics introduced into human clinical use to treat infectious disease in the past 60 years have been natural products, elaborated by one microorganism in a particular habitat and set of environmental conditions to affect neighboring microbes, either to regulate their growth or to trigger their elimination. Antibiotic natural products are produced by both bacteria and fungi, with the major group of antibiotic-producing bacteria being the actinomycetes. Antimicrobial drugs can be antibacterial or antifungal. There are almost no therapeutically useful agents that are effective as both antibacterial and antifungal agents, because of different molecular and cellular targets and microbial cell penetration issues. The focus of this book will be on antibacterial agents only, in part because of the greater number and diversity of therapeutic antibacterial drugs, the greater incidence of serious pathogenic bacterial infections, and finally the lack of space to cover both topics adequately in one volume.

While most of the major classes of antibiotics in therapeutic use are natural products or semisynthetic derivatives thereof, as we shall note in chapter 2, there are three classes of man-made, synthetic antibiotics in clinical use: the sulfa

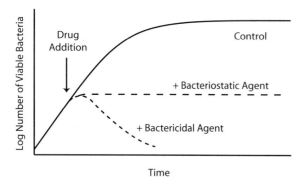

Figure 1.1 Effects of bacteriostatic versus bactericidal antibiotics on a logarithmically growing bacterial culture. (From Scholar and Pratt [2000], with permission.)

drugs, introduced in the 1930s; the quinolones, introduced in the 1960s; and an oxazolidinone, approved in the United States in 2000. We will examine their discovery and development in parallel with those of natural antibiotics. The purpose and origin of the synthetic antibiotics is clear: they emanate from medicinal chemistry/infectious disease programs in pharmaceutical research laboratories.

The existence and clinical development of both synthetic and natural product antibiotics reflect a dichotomy in antibiotic discovery programs in the 20th century. At one end of the spectrum was the medicinal chemistry view and the classical "magic bullet" approach that pure compounds could be made with therapeutic specificity and utility. The early introduction of the sulfa drugs as antibacterials, still in use six decades later, was an early triumph for this approach (Amyes, 2001). From a separate track came the isolation of penicillin, a natural product, as a potent antibacterial agent. This led to recognition of the paradigm that microbes wage war against each other with antibiotics, setting off decades of intensive screening of microbial cultures for new antibiotic classes and leading to the discovery and successful clinical development of penicillins and cephalosporins, tetracyclines, streptomycins and later generations of aminoglycosides, chloramphenicol, rifamycins, glycopeptides, and the erythromycin class of macrolide antibiotics.

The two paradigms of antibiotic discovery have converged with the introduction of later generations of semisynthetic variants of both β-lactam antibiotics and macrolides, in which chemistry is used to engineer some desired new property, such as oral bioavailability, increased stability, broader spectrum of activity, or efficacy against resistant microbes.

Different classes of antibiotics revealed distinct targets in bacteria

The availability of different structural classes of antibiotics, synthetic, natural, and semisynthetic, allowed identification of bacteriostatic and bactericidal targets in bacteria (see Gale, 1981; Russell and Chopra, 1996), as will be addressed in the next chapter in more detail. When a new antibiotic molecule was detected in a microbial culture broth or a screen in a synthetic medicinal chemistry program, it was possible to compare it against benchmark antibiotics with known mechanisms of action. A novel mechanism suggested a new target that could be delineated through biochemical analysis. In turn, knowledge of the targets and mechanisms of action of major antibacterial drug classes also gave a range of assays that would allow categorization of newly discovered antibacterials by mechanism of action, e.g., against cell wall biosynthesis or as inhibitors of protein biosynthesis.

The evaluation of new antibacterial molecules typically follows a hierarchical procedure. First, a new compound is tested against a panel of bacterial strains, many of them pathogens arising from clinical isolates, and many of those possessing resistance to prior generations of antibiotics. If a new antibiotic candidate shows sufficient potency against marker strains, then the molecule may be evaluated in animals inoculated to have high levels of infections with specific strains of bacteria in particular tissues (e.g., bacterial infections of blood, or bacteremias) to see if the candidate molecule is protective and/or curative. The new antibiotic may then be compared against standard antibiotics used against such bacterial infections, with both antibiotic-sensitive and antibiotic-resistant strains of pathogens. If the new molecule passes those tests, it may well be on its way as a development candidate.

When do microbes make antibiotics and how do they manage self-protection?

Natural products with antibiotic activities are almost all products of secondary metabolic pathways, pathways dispensable under many growth conditions and secondary to the primary routes and life-sustaining functions of metabolism while microorganisms are in active growth phases. But when antibiotic producers enter stationary phases and face competition for space and/or nutrients, they turn on the genes that encode the antibiotic molecules and use them to regulate the growth of, or perhaps more actively wage chemical war on, their neighbors. The antibiotic producers then have a selective advantage for growth, including access to nutrients from their dying neighbors, and will have selective pressure to maintain the antibiotic-producing pathways and to turn them on in times of need. We will examine the signals and communication machinery between (quorum sensing) and within bacteria (two-component regulatory pathways) known to turn on antibiotic pathways.

Bacteria and fungi that make antibiotics need self-protection or autoimmunity mechanisms to protect themselves from the lethal chemical weapons they are producing. They employ a variety of strategies, as we shall note in detail in chapter 7. Common among them is the tightly coupled export of the mature antibiotic from the producing cell into the external medium to keep intracellular concentrations low in the producing organism. Some antibiotics, such as the aminoglycoside streptomycin and the macrolide oleandomycin, are exported while still inactive and one step away from the final enzymatic maturation, which happens extracellularly. Other antibiotic producers alter the structure of their own cell walls, modify the peptidyltransferase component of the protein synthesis machinery on the bacterial ribosomes, or produce desensitizing structural mutations in DNA replication enzymes to provide protection from self-destruction.

It has been argued that mechanisms for self-protection must have coevolved with antibiotic biosynthetic pathways, and the self-protection and antibiotic biosynthetic genes are very often clustered together and coregulated.

How does resistance develop?

In the hundreds of millions of years that antibiotics have been produced by some subsets of bacteria and fungi to act on their neighbors, evolutionary pressure has been at work for the bacteria under attack to devise resistance mechanisms to survive. Analogously, in the 70 years of the antibiotic era in the treatment of human infectious disease, pathogenic bacteria have developed relentlessly with clinically significant resistances to one class of antibiotic after another (Amyes, 2001; Levy, 1998). The large numbers of bacterial cells in a population and the short generation times facilitate the development of mutants. Bacterial DNA replication machinery may produce one error in 10^7; in replication of a 3×10^6-bp genome containing about 3,000 genes, that is 0.3 errors per generation. If there are 10^{11} bacteria in a population, e.g., in a patient being treated for a systemic blood-borne bacterial infection, then there may be 1,000 mutant variants. If the mutations are randomly distributed throughout the bacterial genome then 1,000 genes, one out of every three, will have a mutation. If one of these confers a selective advantage for survival, e.g., in the presence of a given antibiotic, then the resistant bacterium will be selected for, grow up as its neighbors perish, and take over the culture. This can happen in a matter of days in patients being treated with antibiotics. By this logic, development of resistance in bacterial populations is highly probable. The more widely used the antibiotic, the more probable the resistance, unless multiple mutations are required. As noted in **Table 1.1**, from the first sulfonamide antibiotics introduced in the 1930s, through the cephalosporins and semisynthetic penicillins introduced in the 1960s, clinically significant antibiotic resistance has followed one to three decades later. People in the United States fill about 80 million prescriptions for antibiotics annually, involving about 12,500 tons of drugs per year. In the

Table 1.1 Evolution of resistance to antibiotics

Antibiotic	Year deployed	Resistance observed
Sulfonamides	1930s	1940s
Penicillin	1943	1946
Streptomycin	1943	1959
Chloramphenicol	1947	1959
Tetracycline	1948	1953
Erythromycin	1952	1988
Vancomycin	1956	1988
Methicillin	1960	1961
Ampicillin	1961	1973
Cephalosporins	1960s	late 1960s

From Palumbi (2001), with permission.

roughly 50 years of the antibiotic era, an estimated one million tons of antibiotics have been produced and disseminated, including those for animal and agricultural uses, suggesting a significant reservoir for the rise of resistant bacteria.

The second requirement, beyond the statistical likelihood of selection, for bacterial resistance to antibiotics is the availability of mechanisms. We shall note that for natural product antibiotics, most of the various resistance mechanisms in pathogenic bacteria that cause human disease seem to be acquired resistance determinants and machinery from antibiotic-producing bacteria. The intrinsic self-protection devices of the antibiotic producers have been acquired by the pathogens under pressure to adapt or die. One potential advantage that may accrue to synthetic antibacterials is that they have not been in the biosphere for eons already and so there may not be reservoirs of intrinsic resistance mechanisms that can be rapidly acquired by target pathogens. However, existing enzymes have undergone rounds of mutation to yield resistance to sulfonamides and trimethoprim (see chapter 6). Efflux mechanisms, for example, are important in nullifying quinolone antibacterial drugs.

The continuing need for new antibiotics: where will they come from?

The infectious disease experience of the last half century is that the introduction of a new class of antibiotic, if efficacious and safe, leads to widespread use and in turn to development of resistance, for the molecular reasons cited above (elaborated in chapter 17). To combat such resistance, medicinal chemists have used the resistant pathogens as targets to test modifications of existing antibiotics for expanded-spectrum molecules that have regained potency against the resistant microbes. Among the β-lactam antibiotics, this has resulted in multiple iterations of penicillin structures and up to four generations of cephalosporins, each representing chemical modifications introduced either to extend the spectrum or to combat spreading resistance. In the macrolide antibiotics, erythromycin has been followed by the expanded-spectrum agents azithromycin and clarithromycin and the ketolides, broad-spectrum agents that have just entered the marketplace. These examples are the product of tinkering with natural product antibiotic structures for incremental change.

A second way to view the challenge (Palumbi, 2001) is to look at the cascade of antibiotics used to treat staphylococcal infections over the past half century (Fig. 1.2). Penicillin was almost universally effective upon its introduction in 1946. By 1961 the semisynthetic ampicillin was required to deal with β-lactamase enzymatic activity in staphylococcal infections. For methicillin-resistant *Staphylococcus aureus* (MRSA), vancomycin was the drug of choice by 1986. In the continuing saga, the oxazolidinone linezolid (Zyvox), introduced in 1999, showed indications of activity against multidrug-resistant staphylococci.

Two contemporary parallel approaches for identifying new molecules active against resistant pathogenic bacteria are the continued screening of microbial broths for new antibiotics and the development of large synthetic libraries from combinatorial chemical approaches. After six decades of intensive screening there may be diminishing returns from conventional screening approaches, but new efforts to find novel antibiotic biosynthetic genes from the vast bulk of microbes

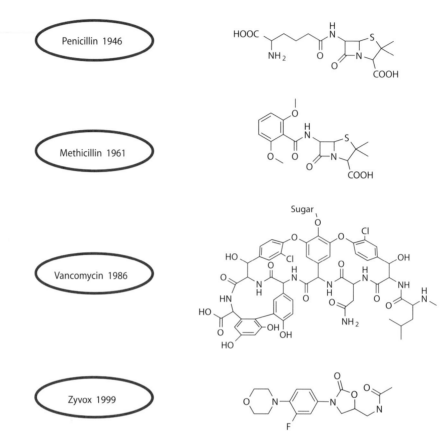

Figure 1.2 Progression of antibiotics required for efficacy in staphylococcal infections. (Adapted from Palumbi [2001], with permission.)

not yet culturable and approaches to combinatorial biosynthesis of antibiotics may improve the yield of novel antibiotic structures from nature. Both of these approaches build on observations that many of the genes that encode metabolic pathways for antibiotics are clustered together and so can be cloned and manipulated as contiguous units of DNA. Synthetic chemical libraries continue to be expanded, with increases in functional group and architectural complexity, and may become the dominant source for hits representing novel structural scaffolds that can be optimized.

In the next section we will review the major validated targets in bacteria against which the main classes of antibiotics have been found to act. In the last section of the book we will delineate efforts to find and validate new targets for antibiotics arising from the availability of fully sequenced genomes of almost five dozen bacterial species.

Approach and organization of this text

This book addresses the questions raised in the above sections. It examines the origins of antibiotics that have been of major consequence in human infectious disease treatment, the mechanisms of action of these antibiotics, the modes of major resistance development, and finally the strategies for cycles of new and replacement antibiotics.

After this introductory chapter, section II (chapters 2 to 6) encompasses the major antibiotic classes and the killing targets in bacteria that have become validated by these antibacterial drugs, most notably cell wall biosynthesis, protein biosynthesis, DNA replication and repair, and folate and RNA biogenesis.

Section III (chapters 7 to 10) takes up mechanisms of antibiotic resistance. This section starts with analysis of the self-protection mechanisms of antibiotic-producing strains. Then the three strategies of resistance—destruction of the antibiotic, action of efflux pumps, and modification of antibiotic target structures—are examined.

Section IV (chapters 11 to 14) deals with the molecular logic of antibiotic biosynthesis. The first chapter in this section discusses both quorum-signaling molecules that function between bacteria and two-component regulatory systems that transduce information from the exterior for selective gene activation to turn on antibiotic biosynthesis pathways in response to environmental cues. Then the assembly-line logic for creation of such polyketide antibiotics as tetracyclines and erythromycins is delineated and compared with the parallel assembly-line logic for making nonribosomal peptide antibiotics such as penicillins, vancomycin, and bacitracin. Knowledge of how these assembly lines work is a prelude to metabolic engineering for new molecules.

Section V (chapters 15 to 17) provides a concluding discussion of contemporary strategies for finding and producing novel antibiotics both by reexamination of established targets and by the bacterial genomics efforts that have validated many new gene products as antibacterial targets. The final chapter deals with the need for policies to extend the useful lifetimes of existing and new antibiotics.

Validated Targets and Major Antibiotic Classes

IN THIS SECTION OF THE BOOK, CHAPTERS 2 TO 6, we examine the major classes of antibacterial drugs that have proven useful in the treatment of clinical infectious diseases of humans. Antibiotics are grouped into classes according to their targets at the bacterial cell surface or inside the cell. Four major targets are examined. (i) Bacterial cell wall biosynthesis (chapter 3) is inhibited by β-lactam antibiotics and the vancomycin class of glycopeptides. (ii) Bacterial ribosomes are selectively blocked at the 30S subunits by aminoglycosides and tetracyclines and at the 50S subunits by the macrolide family of antibiotics (chapter 4). (iii) The quinolone family of antibacterial drugs, exemplified by ciprofloxacin, act to block bacterial DNA replication by derailing catalytic intermediates in the reactions catalyzed by DNA topoisomerases (chapter 5). (iv) The folate coenzyme biosynthetic pathway, essential for providing monomer units for DNA synthesis, is blocked by sulfa drugs and trimethoprim (chapter 6), while cationic peptides disrupt membrane integrity.

Antibacterial Drugs

Natural Products

Amoxicillin

Erythromycin A

Tetracycline

Vancomycin

Synthetic Molecules

Sulfamethoxazole

Trimethoprim

Ciprofloxacin

Linezolid

Structures of naturally and synthetically derived antibacterials.

chapter 2

Introduction to Major Antibiotic Classes and Modes of Action

Major classes of antibiotics in human clinical use

While hundreds to thousands of natural product structures have been isolated in screens for new antibiotics, only a small number of structural types have proven efficacious and safe enough to be taken through clinical development and approved for human clinical use to treat bacterial diseases. The major antibacterial drugs in current human use can be categorized in multiple ways.

One is by economic impact as shown in **Table 2.1** for the year 1997. The cephalosporin class of β-lactam antibiotics had the largest sales, while classical penicillin forms of the β-lactams were represented largely by amoxicillin (Amoxil). The combination of β-lactamase inhibitors with β-lactams in amoxicillin-potassium clavulanate (Augmentin), imipenem-cilastatin (Primaxin), and ampicillin-sulbactum (Unasyn) rounds out the β-lactam class at about $6 billion in sales for that year. The two expanded-spectrum macrolide antibiotics of the erythromycin class, clarithromycin (Biaxin) and azithromycin (Zithromax), amounted to almost $2 billion in sales. The third major class, the quinolones, was represented by the $1 billion drug ciprofloxacin. These three categories of drugs block cell wall biosynthesis, protein biosynthesis, and the DNA replication enzyme DNA gyrase, respectively. A somewhat broader cut of the antibiotic market, this time for the year 1995 (see **Table 2.2**), indicates three other classes of antibacterial drugs with over $400 million in sales in that year: tetracyclines, aminoglycosides, and glycopeptides. The antitubercular drug rifampin and the carbapenem version of the β-lactam imipenem are also listed. Representative brand names are indicated, as well as infections for which these drugs have been utilized and where clinically significant resistance had been detected. These classes of antibiotics are taken up in detail in this and later sections of the book, with discussions of mechanisms of action, modes of resistance development, and prospects for development of new versions to overcome resistance. Global sales of these antibiotics approached $24 billion by 2000.

Table 2.1 Antibiotic sales in 1997

Drug	$ millions
Cephalosporins	
Rocephin (Roche)	933
Ceftin (GlaxoWellcome)	640
Ceclor (Lilly)	542
Fortaz (GlaxoWellcome)	449
Claforan (Hofmann LaRoche)	335
Macrolides	
Biaxin (Abbott)	1,150
Zithromax (Pfizer)	619
β-Lactamase inhibitors	
Augmentin (GlaxoSmithKline)	1,354
Primaxin (Merck)	555
Unasyn (Pfizer)	619
Penicillins	
Amoxil (GlaxoSmithKline)	406
Quinolones	
Ciprofloxacin (Bayer)	1,290

A second method of categorizing antibiotics is by the bacterial diseases they are prescribed to treat (Anonymous, 1999; Levy, 1998). **Table 2.3** lists some common infections, broken into two columns based on whether the causative agents are gram-positive versus gram-negative bacteria. The Gram-staining status reflects differences in cell wall complexity (chapter 3) and is a broad index for antibiotic susceptibility. The gram-negative organisms have an intact outer membrane permeability barrier, while gram-positive organisms do not, and in general, such antibiotics as vancomycin can block gram-positive but not gram-

Table 2.2 Antibiotic market in 1995

Class	Worldwide sales ($ millions)	Representative drugs	Infections that have developed resistance
Cephalosporins	8,446	Cefaclor, cefuroxime	Bronchitis, pneumonia, meningitis
Penicillins	4,413	Amoxicillin, ampicillin	Pneumonia, septicemia, bronchitis
Fluoroquinolones	3,309	Ciprofloxacin, ofloxacin	Toxic shock syndrome, meningitis
Macrolides	2,927	Clarithromycin, erythromycin	Toxic shock syndrome, meningitis
Tetracyclines	744	Minocycline	Urinary tract infections, pelvic inflammatory disease
Aminoglycosides	729	Gentamicin	Intestinal infections, septicemia
Glycopeptides	462	Vancomycin	Intestinal infections
All other systemic antibiotics	1,873	Imipenem, rifampin	Bronchitis, tuberculosis

Table 2.3 Bacteria that are common causes of infections

Infections	Gram-negative pathogens	Gram-positive pathogens
Burns	*Pseudomonas aeruginosa*	*Staphylococcus aureus*
Skin infections		*S. aureus*
Throat		*Streptococcus pyogenes*
Otitis media	*Haemophilus influenzae*	*Streptococcus pneumoniae*
Pneumonia	*H. influenzae*	*S. pneumoniae*
Endocarditis		*S. aureus, Enterococcus faecalis*
Septicemia	*Escherichia coli*	*S. aureus, S. pyogenes*
Gastrointestinal tract	*Salmonella enterica* serovar Typhimurium *Helicobacter pylori, E. coli, Shigella dysenteriae*	
Urinary tract	*E. coli*	*Enterococcus* sp.

Adapted from Table 1.1 of Scholar and Pratt (2000), with permission.

negative bacterial growth for that reason, as explained in detail in the subsequent chapters of this section. After the staining test, gram-positive bacteria show up as purple/black while gram-negative organisms show red colors. **Color Plate 2.1A** shows a photograph of a gram-positive *Streptococcus pneumoniae* isolated from the cerebrospinal fluid of a meningitis patient. **Color Plate 2.1B** shows a Gram stain of an *Escherichia coli* culture, with the typical red appearance of gram-negative bacteria.

The gram-positive streptococci are important pathogens in pneumonia, meningitis, and middle ear infections, while the gram-positive staphylococci and enterococci are problematic pathogens in postsurgical infections. The gram-positive *Mycobacterium tuberculosis* still causes millions of deaths annually. The historical scourges of plague and cholera are caused by two gram-negative bacteria, *Yersinia pestis* and *Vibrio cholerae*, respectively, while *E. coli*, *Salmonella*,

Color Plate 2.1 Gram stains of gram-positive *Streptococcus pneumoniae* (A) and gram-negative *E. coli* (B). (From Elliot et al., 1997.)

A

B

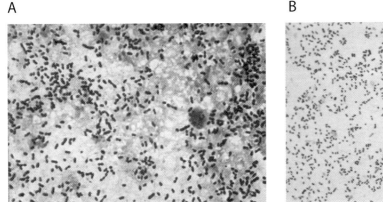
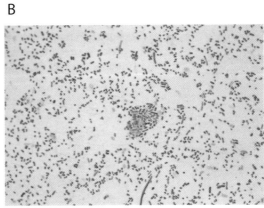

and *Shigella* strains are common causes of diarrheal diseases. The gram-negative *Pseudomonas aeruginosa* is often described as an opportunistic pathogen, causing disease in settings where the patient may have compromised immunity and/or some underlying disease such as cystic fibrosis. We shall note that *P. aeruginosa* has many facets that contribute to decreased susceptibility to many classes of antibacterial drugs, making it a difficult pathogen to treat.

This volume will not focus on the clinical pharmacology of existing antimicrobial drugs or the regimens used in infectious disease therapies. Two excellent texts for thorough and up-to-date coverage on those key aspects of antibiotics are *The Antimicrobial Drugs* (2nd edition), by Scholar and Pratt (2000), and *Antimicrobial Chemotherapy*, edited by Greenwood (2000). The latter book has a section dedicated to the treatment of bacterial infections in different tissues, e.g., respiratory tract infections, urinary tract infections, skin and soft tissue infections, bacteremias, endocarditis, and tuberculosis.

Some bacterial infections such as pneumonia are most often acquired in community settings, as are plague, cholera, and diarrheal diseases, while others may be acquired during hospital stays, so-called nosocomial infections. The staphylococci and enterococci that cause infections in postsurgical patients fall into the latter category, and since they exist in environments where antibiotics are in constant use, many staphylococcal and enterococcal strains are antibiotic resistant and are especially problematic bacteria (Lowy, 1998). Staphylococci with resistance to penicillins and in particular to methicillin can occur with high incidence (40% infection rate with methicillin-resistant *S. aureus* [MRSA] and 50% with methicillin-resistant *S. epidermidis* [MRSE] in some clinical wards). These pathogens have high mortality rates (25 to 63%) in hospital infections of the blood (bacteremias). In the late 1990s enterococci accounted for up to 12% of hospital infections in some U.S. cities, with >15% incidence of vancomycin resistance. Vancomycin-resistant enterococcal (VRE) infections produced mortality rates of 42 to 81%.

A typical first-line approach for antibiotic treatment, as published in *The Medical Letter* (Anonymous, 2001), is summarized in **Table 2.4**.

Table 2.4 intersects with the data of Tables 2.1 and 2.2 on the use of cephalosporins, macrolides, quinolones, aminoglycosides, and vancomycin. It also notes the trimethoprim-sulfamethoxazole combination, fosfomycin, and the antitubercular drug cocktail, all of which will be evaluated further in the chapters of this section. A more extensive list of antibiotic recommendations for bacterial diseases and likely causative agents can be found in Table 1-3 of Scholar and Pratt (2000), and their Table 1-5 includes antibiotics recommended in surgical prophylaxis based on clean versus contaminated surgical sites.

Many other antibiotics are used in specific situations and against particular pathogens, for example, bacitracin used topically against skin infections and tetracyclines for Helicobacter, *V. cholerae*, and brucella-derived infections. Some of the disease-causing pathogens are shown in **Fig. 2.1**, which highlights their distinct morphology.

Each of the antibiotic classes displayed in Table 2.5 has been shown by accrued experience to be more useful against certain bacterial pathogens than others in different clinical situations. The constraints are probably a mixture of both antibiotic levels and penetration efficacy and the intrinsic sensitivity of the

Table 2.4 Summary of typical first-line approach for antibiotic treatment

Infection	Likely pathogen	Reasonable first-choice therapy
Community-acquired pneumonia	*Streptococcus pneumoniae*	For hospitalized patients: broad-spectrum or "fourth-generation" cephalosporin; for ambulatory patients: an orally available macrolide or fluoroquinolone
Hospital-acquired pneumonia	Gram-negative bacterium or *Staphylococcus*	For *Pseudomonas aeruginosa*: broad-spectrum or "fourth-generation" cephalosporin, imipenem, and aminoglycoside; for MRSA: vancomycin
Meningitis	*S. pneumoniae* or *Neisseria meningitidis*	Broad-spectrum cephalosporin + vancomycin + rifampin
Sepsis syndrome	Gram-negative bacilli but also gram-positive cocci such as MRSA	Cephalosporin + aminoglycoside; vancomycin
Urinary tract infections	Gram-negative bacterium such as *E. coli*	Sulfamethoxazole + trimethoprim; fluoroquinolones; fosfomycin
Tuberculosis	*Mycobacterium tuberculosis*	Isoniazid + rifampin + pyrizinamide + ethambutol

Figure 2.1 Electron microscopic view of some bacterial pathogens. (Courtesy Visuals Unlimited; all © D. M. Phillips except panel A © M. Abbey.)

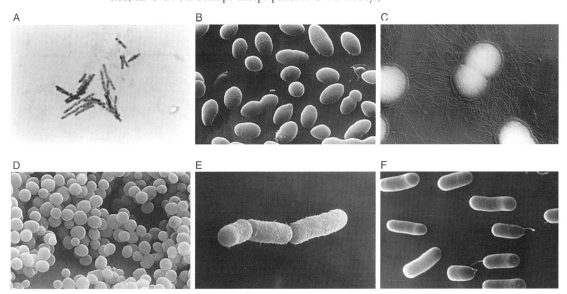

antibiotic target in the recipient bacteria. The β-lactam antibiotics have progressed through several stages of optimization of the five-ring penicillins and up to four iterations of the six-ring cephalosporins to combat emergence of strains resistant to the prior generations of these classes of antibiotics. Similarly, in the macrolide antibiotics, both the original erythromycins and the successors, clarithromycin and azithromycin, are on the market. Structures of some of the penicillins and cephalosporins currently in wide use are in **Table 2.5**, as is that of the combination of amoxicillin and clavulanate, sold under the trade name Augmentin. The narrow-spectrum (erythromycin) and expanded-spectrum (azithromycin and clarithromycin) members of the macrolide polyketide antibiotics are widely used. Fluoroquinolones and aminoglycosides are also represented, along with the glycopeptide antibiotics vancomycin and teicoplanin. The trimethoprim-sulfamethoxazole combination, among the oldest antibiotics, is still on the market decades after its clinical introduction.

Validated targets in bacteria for antibiotics

The mechanisms of action of most antibacterial drugs were worked out after the discovery that the molecules had effects on bacterial growth, either slowing growth dramatically (bacteriostatic) or killing the bacteria (bactericidal). Molecules of clear therapeutic utility and potential were then examined for the molecular basis of their antibacterial properties, their selectivity, and their associated toxicity. Four major targets in bacterial pathogens have emerged from decades of study on mechanism of antibiotic action (**Fig. 2.2**): cell wall biosynthesis; protein biosynthesis; DNA replication and repair; and folate coenzyme biosynthesis. Each of these targets and the mechanisms of the major classes of antibiotics that interdict one or more steps in these pathways will be discussed in detail in chapters 3 to 7. Figure 2.2 serves as a master control diagram for chapters 3 to 10, and those chapters will focus on and illustrate distinct pathways of antibiotic action and antibiotic resistance.

Table 2.5 Major antibiotics: structural classes, targets, and resistance mechanisms

Antibiotic	Target	Resistance mechanism
Cell wall		
β-Lactams	Transpeptidases/transglycosylases (PBPs[1])	β-Lactamases, PBP mutants
Vancomycin	D-Ala-D-Ala termini of	Reprogramming of D-Ala-D-Ala
Teicoplanin	peptidoglycan and of lipid II	to D-Ala-D-Lac or D-Ala-D-Ser
Protein synthesis		
Erythromycins	Peptidyltransferase/ribosome	rRNA methylation/efflux
Tetracyclines	Peptidyltransferase	Drug efflux
Aminoglycosides	Peptidyltransferase	Drug modification
Oxazolidinones	Peptidyltransferase	Unknown
DNA replication/repair		
Fluoroquinolones	DNA gyrase	Gyrase mutations

[1]PBP, penicillin-binding protein.

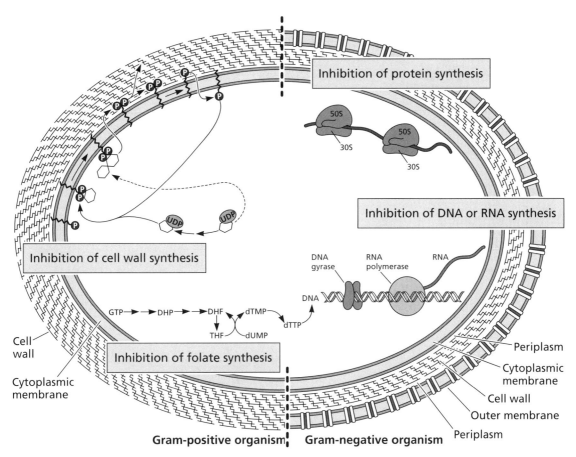

Figure 2.2 Major targets for antibacterial action. (Adapted from a poster on Mechanisms of Antibiotic Action and Resistance, C. Walsh, J. Trauger, P. Courvalin, and J. Davies [2001], *Trends in Microbiology, The Lancet Infectious Disease, Current Opinion in Microbiology, Trends in Molecular Medicine.*)

One guiding precept for selectively killing bacteria while sparing the human host taking the antibiotic would be for the antibiotic to act against a target present in bacteria but not found in animals and humans. This precept holds for two of the established targets, the enzymes of bacterial cell wall biosynthesis and the folic acid biosynthetic pathway enzymes, which do not have counterparts in humans. The other two major targets for antibacterial drugs, protein biosynthesis and DNA replication and repair machinery, clearly have human counterparts, but there are enough differences structurally between the prokaryotic and eukaryotic DNA and protein synthesis machinery that selective inhibition is achievable.

The cell wall biosynthetic processes and protein biosynthesis on the ribosome historically have been the site of action of the largest number of antibiotics, perhaps because of the many enzymatic steps, which offer multiple opportunities for disrupting these key attributes of a healthy bacterial cell. Genomic sequencing of the major bacterial pathogens is essentially complete, and efforts to delineate essential genes or virulence-enhancing genes are well under way, as noted in chapter 15, offering a new molecular and genetic approach to validated novel targets that have not been targeted by existing natural product antibiotics. Those will be prime candidates for synthetic library-based screens to develop effective new antibiotics.

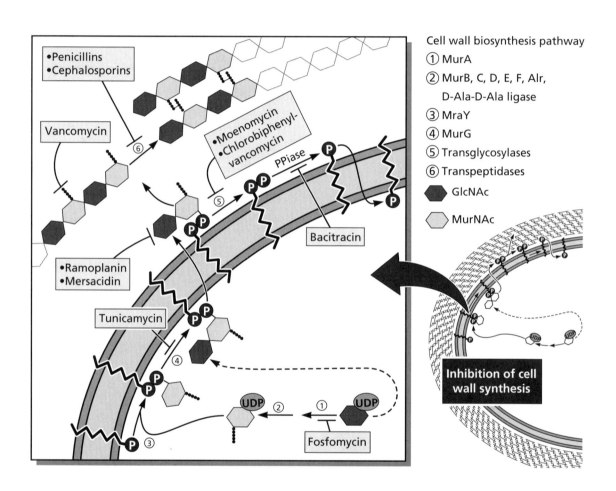

Antibiotics that act on cell wall biosynthesis.

chapter 3

Antibiotics That Act on Cell Wall Biosynthesis

This chapter deals with antibiotics that interdict any of the several steps in bacterial cell wall assembly, from biogenesis of the dedicated monomers to the specialized assembly, membrane translocation, and extracellular cross-linking and strengthening of the exoskeletal peptidoglycan layers. The figure on the facing page shows a blowup of a section of Fig. 2.2 and emphasizes the reactions of cell wall biosynthesis and the antibiotics that block them.

Similarities and differences in gram-negative and gram-positive cell wall structure affect susceptibility to antibiotics

Bacteria such as *Escherichia coli*, *Salmonella*, *Pseudomonas*, and *Yersinia* are negative in Gram staining, while staphylococci, streptococci, and enterococci are gram positive. The difference in retention of the stain, crystal violet in an ethanol solution, depends on the extent to which the outer membrane of bacteria is intact and a significant permeability barrier (gram-negative organisms) or is incomplete and fragmentary (gram-positive organisms) (**Fig. 3.1A**) (Lee and Schneewind, 2001; Navarre and Schneewind, 1999; Nikaido, 1994). Gram-negative and gram-positive bacteria both have a peptidoglycan (PG) layer as part of their cell wall structure. The PG layer is generally substantially thicker and multilayered in the gram-positive bacteria (Fig. 3.1A). The PG, with orthogonal glycan and peptide strands (**Fig. 3.1B**), undergoes enzymatic cross-linking of the glycan strands, by transglycosylase action, and of the peptide strands, by transpeptidase action (**Fig. 3.1C**). The peptide cross-links introduce covalent connectivity to the meshwork, impart mechanical strength, and provide the major structural barrier to osmotic pressure forces that could kill the bacteria. Many of the antibiotics that affect bacterial cell walls inhibit enzymes or sequester substrates involved in PG assembly and cross-linking, as we will note in the subsequent sections of this chapter.

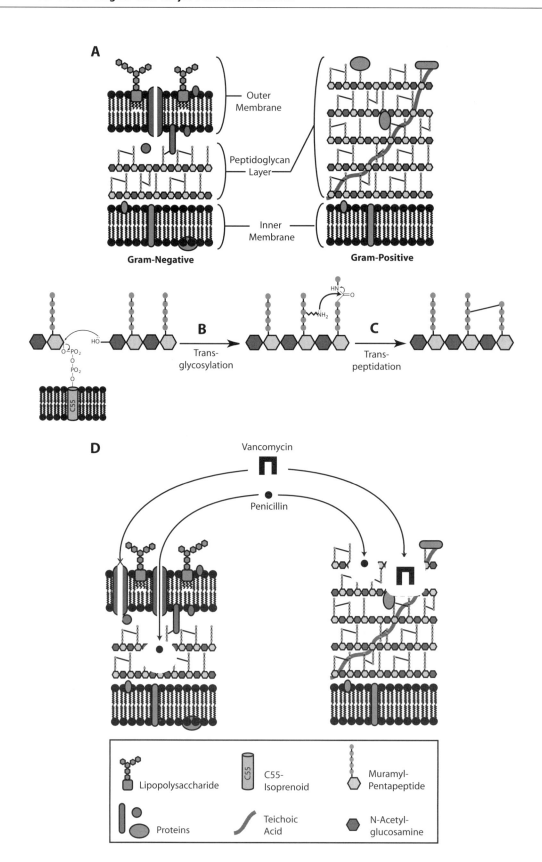

Table 3.1 Proteins covalently linked to peptidoglycan

Functional category	Example protein	Mechanism
Protection from immune system	M-family proteins	Antigenic shift, antiphagocytic
	Proteins A	Antigenic shift, antiphagocytic
	C5a peptidases	Destroy chemoattractant
Structural	Lipoproteins	Link to outer membrane
	Fimbriae	Assemble to form filaments
Infection/virulence	MSCRAMMs	Bind components of extracellular matrix
	Invasins	Bind to β1-integrin, tissue invasion
	Internalin	Facilitate host cell invasion
Nutrient acquisition	Glycosidases	Cleave saccharides
	Peptidases	Cleave peptides
	Nucleotidases	Cleave oligonucleotides?
Bacterial cell adhesion	Aggregation substance	Bind to enterococcal binding substance
	Surface exclusion protein	Prevent mating between bacteria with identical plasmid by unknown mechanism

The thick PG layer of gram-positive bacteria has been described as a surface organelle, for display of carbohydrates and proteins, while the outer membrane is the equivalent surface organelle in gram-negative organisms (Lee and Schneewind, 2001). Both gram-negative and gram-positive bacteria have proteins that are covalently linked to peptide chains of the PG layer (**Table 3.1**) (Braun and Hantke, 1974). Some of these outer membrane proteins act as adhesions for specific proteins on vertebrate cell membranes, such as the protein invasin from *Yersinia pseudotuberculosis*, which binds to β1-integrin proteins displayed on host cells, an interaction required for bacterial penetration into intestinal lymphoid tissue (Isberg and Leong, 1990). Surface proteins tethered to the thick PG layer of gram-positive bacteria are connected during biosynthesis by the action of the enzyme sortase, discussed in chapter 15 as a potential antibacterial target. The outer membrane of gram-negative bacteria is asymmetric in its lipid composition, with phospholipids in the inner leaflet and lipid A as the predominant lipid in the outer leaflet (Raetz, 1987), with variable O-antigen chains covalently attached and facing the external environment as highly antigenic surface carbohydrates (Fig. 3.1A). The thick PG layer in gram-positive bacteria also has polymers of teichoic acids (Fig. 3.1A) associated with it. The surface carbohydrates and proteins can serve many roles, including protection against host-cell killing, providing specific ligands for attachment to biotic and abiotic surfaces, and facilitating interconversion between singe cell (planktonic) forms and biofilm communities of bacteria.

Figure 3.1 Cell wall structures of gram-positive and gram-negative bacteria: (A) differences in outer membrane permeability barriers; (B) peptidoglycan elongation by transglycosylase action; (C) peptidoglycan cross-linking by transpeptidase action; (D) penetration of antibiotics to the cytoplasmic membrane in gram-positive bacteria.

Gram-positive bacteria are susceptible to some antibiotics that do not work or work poorly (e.g., against pseudomonads) against gram-negative baceria, and this difference is related to the ability of antibiotics to be blocked by the limiting pore sizes of the porin proteins (Fig. 3.1A and D) (Koebnik et al., 2000) of the gram-negative organisms' outer membranes. There is no such barrier to diffusion in gram-positive bacteria. Vancomycin, for example, cannot penetrate the outer membrane and so is effective as an antibiotic only against gram-positive pathogens. In gram-negative bacteria the space between the inner and outer membranes is the periplasmic space (**Fig. 3.1D**). In addition to the strands of the PG layer, the periplasm has hydrolytic enzymes to convert oligomeric and polymeric nucleotides, peptides, and saccharides to monomers that are then bound by periplasmic carrier proteins, presented to membrane transport proteins, and internalized. There are also protein chaperones to help proteins being secreted to the outer membrane to fold and transit the periplasmic space.

Each of these cell wall structures is a potential target for interruption by antibiotics. Distinct features of outer membranes even among gram-negative bacteria can lead to differences in permeability to antibiotics. For example, *Pseudomonas aeruginosa* outer membranes show about 100-fold lower permeability to cephalosporins such as cephaloridine (Nikaido, 1998) than other gram-negative bacteria, in part because of porins with small pores to reduce inward passage of the antibiotics into the periplasmic space.

The distinctive appearances of the cell walls of gram-negative and gram-positive bacteria can be discerned in both transmission electron micrographs and in scanning electron micrographs. In **Fig. 3.2A and B**, cell wall schematics are mirrored by the photograph of the gram-positive *Arthrobacter crystallopoietes* (**Fig. 3.2C**) and of the gram-negative *Leucothrix mucor* (**Fig. 3D**). The scanning micrographs of the gram-positive *Bacillus subtilis* (**Fig. 3.2E**) and of the gram-negative *E. coli* (**Fig. 3.2F**) show different surface textures.

Three phases of peptidoglycan enzymatic assembly: cytoplasmic, membrane-associated, and extracytoplasmic

Enzymes in the cytoplasmic phase of the Mur pathway: MurA-F

As bacteria grow and divide, PG layer(s) have to be laid down both transversely and laterally (for septum formation) (Holtje, 1998). The PG unit that is added to the expanding PG layers is a disaccharyl pentapeptide, presented at the membrane surface while attached to a C_{55} (undecaprenyl) lipid (lipid II) in phosphodiester linkage that gets cleaved in the enzymatic transglycosylation step (**Fig. 3.3**). The lipid, sugars, and pentapeptide moieties are each provided by enzymes committed to PG assembly. The PG layer is also known as murein (from the Greek for "wall") and the genes for the early steps in assembly are named *murA-G* (van Heijenoort, 2001a).

The cytoplasmic phase of murein assembly is accomplished by the six enzymes MurA-F, starting from the nucleotide diphosphosugar UDP-*N*-acetylglucosamine (UDP-GlcNAc) and proceeding to the UDP-muramyl pentapeptide, UDP-muramyl-L-Ala-D-γ-Glu-*meso*-diaminopimelate-D-Ala-D-Ala (**Fig. 3.4**). The UDP-GlcNAc is itself made by a bifunctional enzyme, GlmU

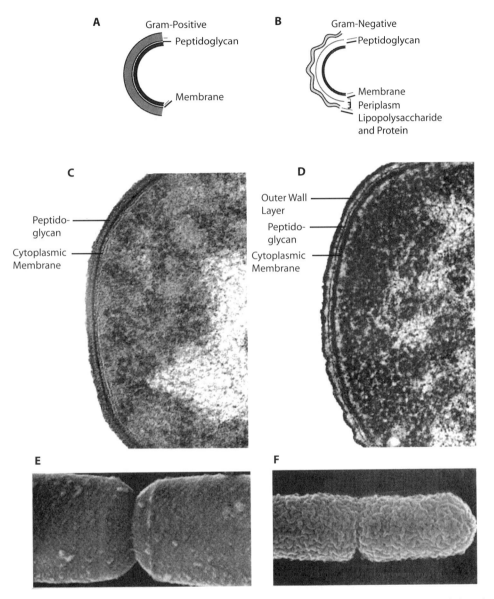

Figure 3.2 Cell walls of bacteria. (A and B) Schematic diagrams of gram-positive (A) and gram-negative (B) cell walls. (C and D) Electron micrographs showing the cell walls of a gram-positive bacterium, *Arthrobacter crystallopoietes* (C), and a gram-negative bacterium, *Leucothrix mucor* (D). (E and F) Scanning electron micrographs of gram-positive (*Bacillus subtilis*) (E) and gram-negative (*Escherichia coli*) (F) bacteria. Note the surface texture in the cells shown in panels E and F. A single cell of *B. subtilis* or *E. coli* is about 1 μm in diameter.

(Gehring et al., 1996; Mengin-Lecreulx and van Heijenoort, 1994), that acetylates glucosamine-1P and then uridylylates it.

The conversion of the GlcNAc to the muramyl moiety involves construction of the 3′-*O*-lactyl ether of the GlcNAc residue and is accomplished by two enzymes, MurA and MurB (**Fig. 3.5A**). MurA uses phosphoenolpyruvate (PEP) as cosubstrate and installs the 3′-*O*-enolpyruvyl ether linkage by an unusual

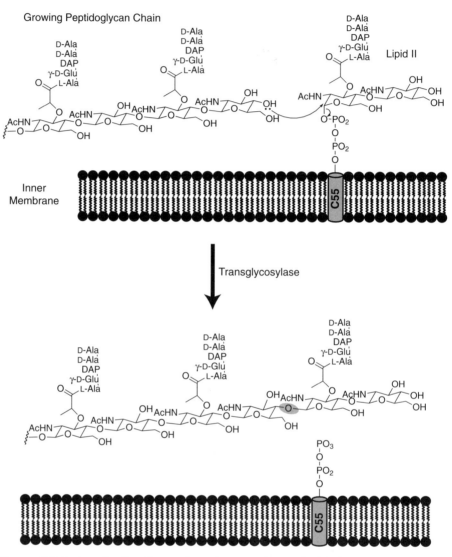

Figure 3.3 Action of cell wall transglycosylases on the C_{55}-lipid-linked *N*-acetyl-muramyl (MurNAc) pentapeptide substrate.

Figure 3.4 Assembly of UDP-MurNAc pentapeptide by the six enzymes MurA-F.

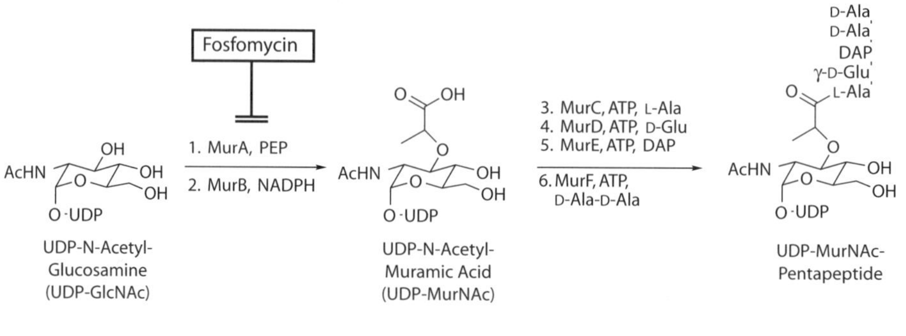

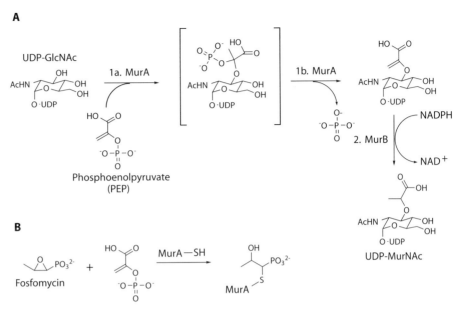

Figure 3.5 (A) Sequential action of MurA and MurB to convert UDP-*N*-acetyl-glucosamine (GlcNAc) to UDP-*N*-MurNAc. (B) Inactivation of MurA by the antibiotic fosfomycin.

addition/elimination sequence, where the 3' oxygen of the GlcNAc is added into the PEP double bond, regio- and stereospecifically at C_2, and C_3 transiently becomes a methyl group (Cassidy and Kahan, 1973; Walsh et al., 1996a). The second step is enzyme-catalyzed elimination of H^+ and P_i to generate the enol ether. MurB is an NADPH-oxidizing flavoprotein that adds a hydride to C_3 and protonates C_2 to generate the lactyl ether and produce UDP-muramic acid (Benson et al., 1993). The carboxylate of the lactyl ether is the locus for subsequent peptide chain building by MurC, D, E, and F.

The X-ray structures of MurA and MurB have been determined (Benson et al., 1995; Schonbrunn et al., 1996; Skarzynski et al., 1996) and corroborate the above mechanistic observations architecturally. MurA is the target of the antibiotic fosfomycin (see Table 2.1 for its recommended use in treating urinary tract infections), a simple three-carbon epoxy propyl phosphonate metabolite from streptomycetes (Seto, 1997) that acts as an inactivating analog of PEP (**Fig. 3.5B**). There is an active-site cysteine in MurA, Cys-115 in the *E. coli* MurA, whose thiolate side chain opens the reactive epoxide of bound fosfomycin, producing a stable covalent tether, blocking the active site and preventing subsequent catalytic turnover. An X-ray structure of the fosfomycin-inactivated MurA has been determined (Skarzynski et al., 1998), which should be an aid to design of successors to fosfomycin. Thiazolidinone inhibitors of MurB have recently been reported (Andres et al., 2000).

MurC, D, and E carry out homologous reactions and belong to the same superfamily (van Heijenoort, 2001a), as they sequentially make amide bonds adding L-Ala, D-Glu, and *meso*-DAP (lysine instead of DAP in some gram-positive bacteria) to the growing UDP-muramyl chain, resulting in the UDP-muramyl tripeptide (**Fig. 3.6**) at the end of the MurE step. MurD makes the

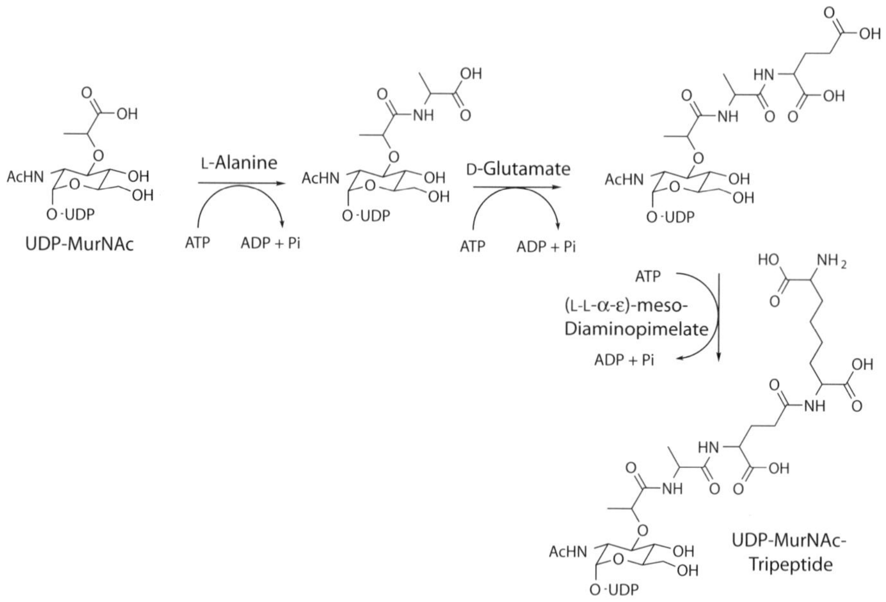

Figure 3.6 Conversion of UDP-MurNAc to UDP-MurNAc tripeptide by action of MurC, D, and E.

γ-glutamyl isopeptide bond rather than the standard peptide bond to the α-carboxylate of D-Glu. ATP is the cosubstrate cleaved by each of these three enzymes, to ADP and P_i, with the intermediacy of acyl phosphates as the donors in the amide-forming steps to each of the three amino acids (**Fig. 3.7A**). For example, the UDP-muramyl phosphate is the presumed mixed anhydride intermediate generated in the active site of MurC and captured by L-Ala (**Fig. 3.7B**). X-ray structures of several of these amino acid ligases are available (van Heijenoort, 2001b) to enable structure-based inhibitor design, and nanomolar inhibitors of both MurC (Marmor et al., 2001) and MurD have been described (Gegnas et al., 1998).

MurF completes the pentapeptidyl chain by adding the D-Ala-D-Ala dipeptide as a unit, again cleaving ATP to ADP and P_i, and presumably involving the UDP-muramyl tripeptidyl-phosphoric anhydride as intermediate (**Fig. 3.7C**). This concludes the classically defined cytoplasmic phase of PG assembly. Aminoalkylphosphinate inhibitors of MurF are weak (K_i values of 200 to 700 μM) but might be starting points for optimization (Miller et al., 1998) of more-potent drug candidates. Teichmann et al. (2001) have noted that the whole collection of Mur pathway enzymes may have arisen by gene self-duplication.

Enzymes that convert L-Ala to D-Ala-D-Ala: racemase and D-D-ligase

The D-Ala-D-Ala cosubstrate for MurF is in turn provided by a pair of enzymes acting sequentially: the first is alanine racemase, the second D-alanyl-D-alanine ligase (**Fig. 3.8A**). The racemase is a pyridoxal phosphate-dependent catalyst, taking the normal cellular metabolite L-alanine and equilibrating its configuration to make D-Ala with an equilibrium constant of 1 (Walsh, 1988). The D,D-ligase is the fifth enzyme in the Mur pathway to spend an ATP to make an amide

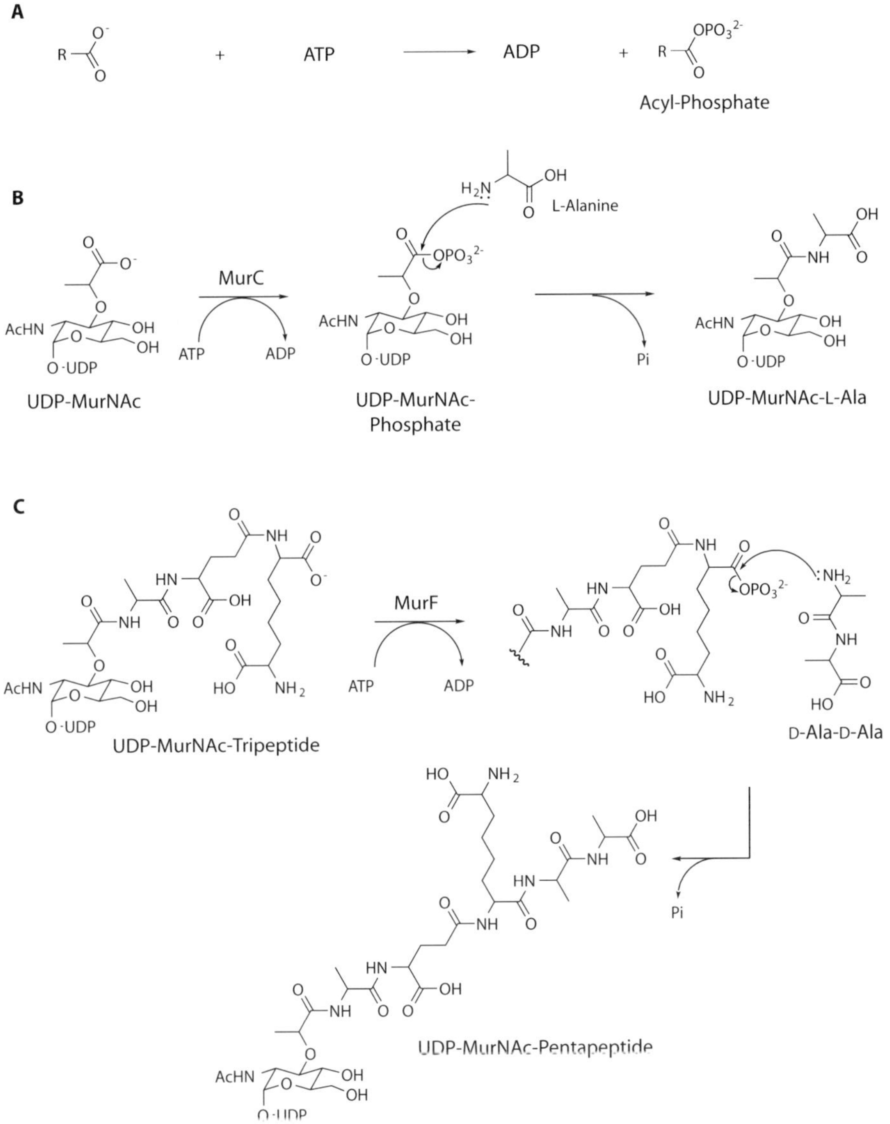

Figure 3.7 (A) Aminoacyl-phosphate generation. (B) MurC example with UDP-MurNAc-P as a bound intermediate attacked by the amino group of cosubstrate L-Ala. (C) UDP-tripeptidyl acyl-P intermediate in MurF catalysis: attack by D-Ala-D-Ala.

bond, with cleavage to ADP and an acyl phosphate, in this instance D-alanyl-PO_3, to be captured by the second D-alanine (**Fig. 3.8B**). X-ray structures are available for both the racemase and the ligase (Fan et al., 1994; Shaw et al., 1997). The racemase is inhibited by a phosphonate analog of L- and D-Ala, Ala-PO_3, which had promise as an antibiotic (reviewed in Bugg and Walsh, 1992; Neuhaus and Hammes, 1981), but a high frequency of mutation of the transporter systems for uptake of Ala-P rendered bacteria resistant. The D-Ala-D-Ala ligase and the racemase both are inhibited by cycloserine (Neuhaus and Hammes, 1981), a natural product, but the activity is weak and relatively unselective,

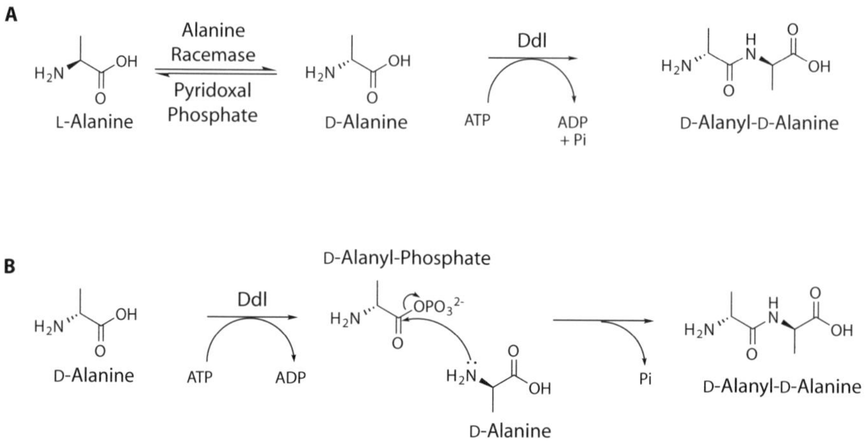

Figure 3.8 (A) Sequential action of alanine racemase and D-Ala-D-Ala ligase (Ddl) to generate D-Ala-D-Ala. (B) D-Ala-P intermediate in Ddl catalysis.

creating toxicity. These examples suggest that all eight enzymes noted above are in principle good targets for new antibiotic development. We will return to the D,D-ligase story when we discuss vancomycin resistance in chapter 10 and observe that glycopeptide antibiotic resistance centers around D,D-ligase specificity.

Enzymes that provide D-glutamate and *meso*-DAP for MurD and MurE

The pathways to D-glutamate have been reviewed recently (van Heijenoort, 2001b) and involve either a glutamate racemase encoded by the *murI* gene or a D-amino acid transaminase pathway. In bacteria using the MurI route, *murI* is an essential gene, and the racemase has been well characterized structurally and mechanistically as a cofactor-independent racemase acting by a two-base mechanism. No useful inhibitors with antibacterial activity have been described. In gram-positive bacteria such as bacilli that use D-alanine as the donor to α-ketoglutarate, the transaminase is pyridoxal phosphate (PLP) dependent; the structure is known but no antibacterial leads have been described.

The biosynthesis of *meso*-DAP in gram-negative bacteria is a multistep pathway, well characterized mechanistically and structurally with recent X-ray structures of almost every enzyme in the pathway (Born and Blanchard, 1999), but to date no inhibitors that are effective antibacterial agents have been found by design or screening.

Lipid attachment and addition of the second sugar: the lipid I and lipid II intermediates and actions of ramoplanin and bacitracin

The membrane-associated stage two of murein assembly starts with the enzyme MraY, which transfers the muramyl pentapeptide from its UDP water-soluble anchor to an unusual membrane component, the C_{55} undecaprenyl phosphate on the cytoplasmic surface of the membrane. The C_{55} lipid phosphate oxygen attacks the pyrophosphate linkage of the UDP moiety, releases UMP, and produces a new pyrophosphate bridge between the membrane-anchored C_{55} lipid and the muramyl pentapeptide (**Fig. 3.9A**). This is the first lipid intermediate, known as lipid I. MraY has also been called translocase, but there is no direct experimental evidence that the pentapeptidyl chain is translocated at this step; indeed, the subsequent conversion of lipid I to lipid II described below utilizes a cytoplasmic cosubstrate, UDP-GlcNAc, consistent with the active site of MraY and MurG being accessible to the cytoplasmic face of the membrane. Natural

Figure 3.9 (A) Enzymatic formation of the lipid I and lipid II intermediates in the membrane phase of peptidoglycan assembly. (B) Nucleoside-peptide inhibitors of MraY.

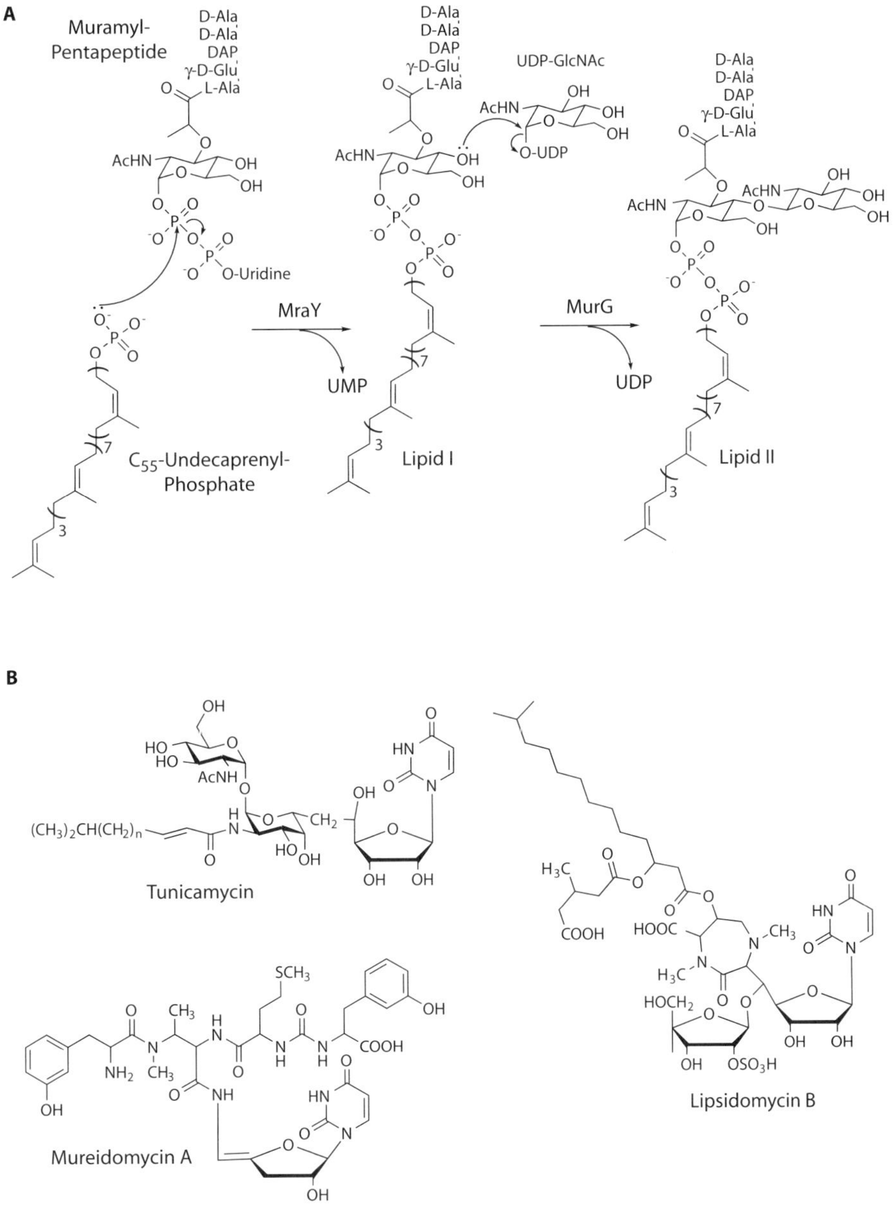

products that inhibit MraY action include mureidomycins A to F (**Fig. 3.9B**) (Lee and Hecker, 1999), liposidomycins, and tunicamycin, all uridyl peptide antibiotics that are thought to compete with the UDP-muramyl pentapeptide substrate for MraY. While tunicamycin also inhibits the eukaryotic biosynthesis of dolichol-PP-GlcNAc in glycoprotein biosynthesis, the liposidomycins and mureidomycins are selective for inhibition of the prokaryotic MraY (Lee and Hecker, 1999). They may offer starting points for semisynthetic antibiotic development.

At this point the second sugar is added to the C_4-OH of the muramyl group of lipid I by the enzyme MurG via UDP-GlcNAc as cosubstrate. The product is the lipid-disaccharyl pentapeptide known as lipid II (Fig. 3.9A). The MurG glycosyltransferase, associated with the membrane but not deeply buried in it, has been solubilized, purified, and crystallized (Ha et al., 2000). Because the substrates and products of MurG have been difficult to obtain in quantities, recent progress in synthesis of reasonable quantities of substrate and substrate analogs has facilitated both assay and screening for inhibitors (Ha et al., 1999; Liu et al., 2001; Men et al., 1998) and, as noted below, suggests a mechanism of action of the lipoglycopeptide antibiotic ramoplanin.

The translocation and extracellular reactions to complete PG unit synthesis and assembly

Subsequent to its formation by MurG, lipid II is translocated from the internal face of the cytoplasmic membrane to the periplasmic/external face. No definitive evidence for or identification of a translocase protein is yet available. Once facing outside and presumably anchored at the membrane surface by the C_{55} lipid tail, the disaccharyl pentapeptide unit is substrate for transglycosylases and transpeptidases that are also membrane bound (Fig. 3.3). There are multiple transglycosylases (four known in the *E. coli* genome and two in the *Staphylococcus aureus* and *Streptococcus pneumoniae* genomes) and multiple transpeptidases. Some of them are bifunctional with discrete transglycosylase and transpeptidase domains (Spratt, 1994), and members of this subset are of particular importance as killing targets of β-lactam antibiotics, as will be noted below. The transglycosylase activities cleave the muramyl-C_1-O-PO_3 bond by attack of the 4'-OH of a terminal GlcNAc moiety of an elongating glycan chain in a PG layer onto the PG unit to be incorporated (Fig. 3.3), releasing the C_{55} lipid pyrophosphate. For the C_{55} lipid carrier to cycle back to the cytoplasmic face of the membrane, the pyrophosphate linkage of the C_{55} lipid pyrophosphate must be hydrolyzed to the starting C_{55} lipid phosphate by a membrane-bound phosphatase. The C_{55} lipid phosphate can then be available for another round of lipid I synthesis, conversion to lipid II, and translocation (**Fig. 3.10**).

This lipid carrier cycle is susceptible at several points to inhibition by antibiotics. The cyclic lipodepsipeptide ramoplanin (**Fig. 3.11A**) has been shown in in vitro studies (Lo et al., 2000) to complex with both lipid I and lipid II. Sequestration of these lipo-sugar-pentapeptides away from transglycosylases could block subsequent enzymatic maturation of the PG units. The three-dimensional structure of this cyclic 17-residue nonribosomal depsipeptide has

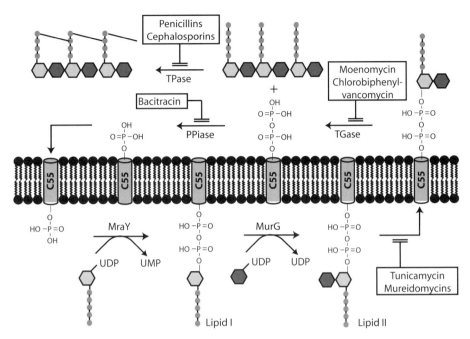

Figure 3.10 The lipid carrier cycle in peptidoglycan assembly. TGase, transglycosylase; PPiase, pyrophosphatase.

been determined by nuclear magnetic resonance (NMR) imaging (Kurz and Guba, 1996) and resembles that of the lantibiotic peptide mersacidin (**Fig. 3.11B**) (McCafferty et al., 1999; Prasch et al., 1997) which also complexes with lipid II, in 1:1 stoichiometry and thereby inhibits PG biosynthesis (Brotz et al., 1998). The molecular details of complexation of mersacidin with lipid II are not yet known, while progress has been made with ramoplanin (Cudic and Otvos, 2002; Cudic et al., 2002). Mersacidin and a related peptide antibiotic, actigardin (Zimmermann and Jung, 1997), are ribosomally synthesized as inactive precursor peptides, which are then posttranslationally cross-linked by four methyl lanthionine thioether bridges and finally proteolyzed to release a signal peptide (see chapter 6). The resultant peptide is globular, highly constrained, and thought to interact with the sugar-pyrophosphate and lipid moieties of lipid II. It has been reported (Breukink et al., 1999) that the lantibiotic nisin Z also complexes with lipid II as well as being a pore former. The large size (1.8 to 4.6 kDa) of lantibiotics restricts their passage across the outer membranes of gram-negative organisms; they are primarily active at killing gram-positive bacteria (Sahl and Bierbaum, 1998).

The nonribosomal decapeptide antibiotic bacitracin (**Fig. 3.12**) also interdicts the C_{55} lipid carrier cycle, at the stage of the C_{55} lipid phosphate (Brotz et al., 1998), with a cation-dependent complexation between the thiazoline ring at residue 2 of bacitracin and the phosphate moiety of the C_{55}-O-PO$_3$ likely.

In the steady state there has to be a balance between PG polymerases and PG hydrolases to allow orderly insertion of new PG units into existing walls during PG enlargement as bacteria grow and to initiate septum formation at cell division (Holtje, 1998). As will be noted below, the cell wall transpeptidases (PG

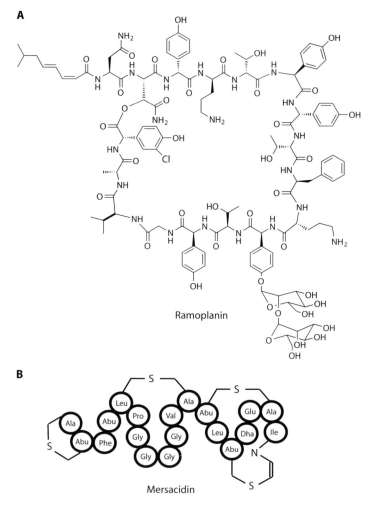

Figure 3.11 Structures of two antibiotics that form stoichiol metric complexes with lipid II: (A) ramoplanin; (B) mersacidin.

polymerases) are covalently acylated by penicillins and were identified historically as penicillin-binding proteins (PBPs). Complexes between the high-molecular-weight PBP1B, a lytic transglycosylase, MltA, and a scaffolding protein, MipA, have been described from *E. coli* and are thought to be fragments of a larger protein machine involved in the growth of the PG meshwork, also known as the sacculus (Holtje, 1998). Such a complex is proposed to contain PBP2 and PBP3 for transpeptidase and endopeptidase action in PG chain growth, with attachments to both the outer membrane (MltA) and the inner membrane (PBP1B) (**Fig. 3.13**).

β-Lactam antibiotics; penems, cephems, carbapenems, and the plethora of PBPs

The most celebrated of the antibiotics that kill bacteria by blocking the crucial transpeptidations that lead to mechanically strong PG through the covalent

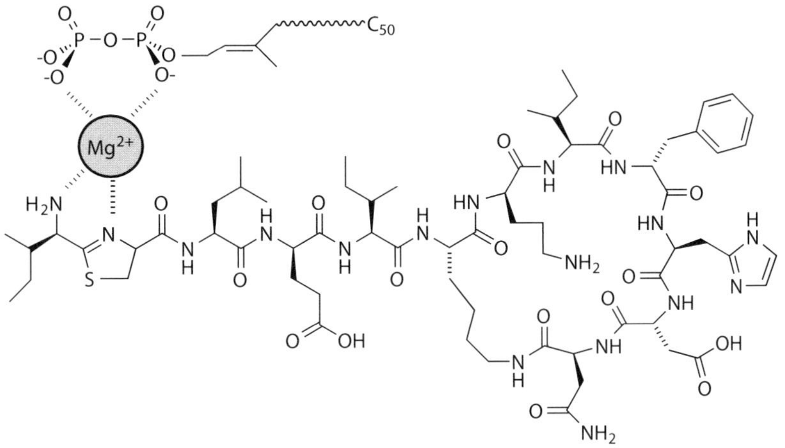

Figure 3.12 Bacitracin and a model for complexation of the C_{55} lipid phosphate to block the lipid cycle.

cross-links of peptide strands are the β-lactam antibiotics (**Fig. 3.14**). These include the penicillins, where the chemical warhead, the four-membered β-lactam ring, is fused to a five-membered sulfur ring system, and the cephalosporins, where the β-lactam is fused to a sulfur-containing ring-expanded system. Penicillins are converted enzymatically to the cephalosporins by a ring expandase enzyme, as we shall note in chapter 13. Both are fungal secondary metabolites, with *Penicillium chrysogenum* an important producer organism for the penicillin two-ring system and *Acremonium chrysogenum* for the cephalosporin nucleus (O'Sullivan and Ball, 1983). The antibacterial drug imipenem is a slight variant of a naturally occurring carbapenem, thienamycin (Fig. 3.14), and is administered along with an inhibitor of a renal dipeptidase, cilastatin, to enhance the carbapenem in vivo lifetime by blockade of β-lactam hydrolysis. Thienamycin was first isolated from the bacterium *Streptomyces cattleya* (Kahan et al., 1979), and the epimeric side chain alcohol olivanic acid has been isolated from *S. flavogriseus*. The simplest carbapenem is the unsubstituted bis ring system with the 2,3-double bond, produced by the plant-pathogenic *Erwinia* bacteria (see chapter 11) (Bycroft et al., 1988). Two other variants of β-lactam natural products are known: the monobactams, represented by nocardicins and the synthetic aztreonam, and the clavams, represented by clavulanate, not in

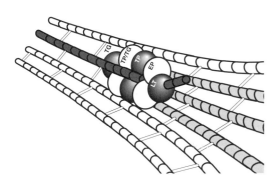

Figure 3.13 Schematic of a multienzyme complex involved in traveling along the peptidoglycan scaffold during elongation. TG, transglycosylase; TP, transpeptidase; TP/TG, bifunctional transpeptidase/transglycosylase; EP, endopeptidase; LT, lytic transglycosylase. (Adapted from Holtje [1998], with permission.)

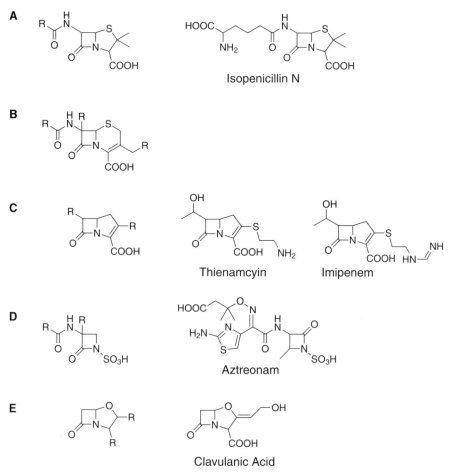

Figure 3.14 β-Lactam antibiotics: (A) penicillins, (B) cephalosporins, (C) carbapenems, (D) monobactams, and (E) clavams.

itself an antibiotic but a mechanism-based inactivator of β-lactamases (discussed in chapter 8).

To understand how penicillins inactivate the PG-cross-linking transpeptidases requires a brief analysis of the catalytic mechanism followed by all the transpeptidase isoforms. As the name of this enzyme family implies, the cross-linking steps are transpeptidations with no net peptide bonds being formed. One Lys-D-Ala or DAP-D-Ala isopeptide bond is formed and one D-Ala-D-Ala peptide bond is cleaved in each catalytic cycle, releasing free D-Ala (**Fig. 3.15**), which is recycled to the cytoplasm or oxidized at the cytoplasmic membrane. There is no requirement for energy input, in accord with the fact that these enzymes work outside the cell on the periplasmic face of the membrane where ATP and other energy sources are not routinely available. The transpeptidases are all variants of active-site "serine" hydrolases, with an active-site serine as nucleophile and another side chain that functions as a general base (Bush and Mobashery, 1998). The first half-reaction involves attack of the active-site serine on the amide bond joining the D-Ala$_4$ to D-Ala$_5$. The tetrahedral adduct collapses to an acyl-O-Ser

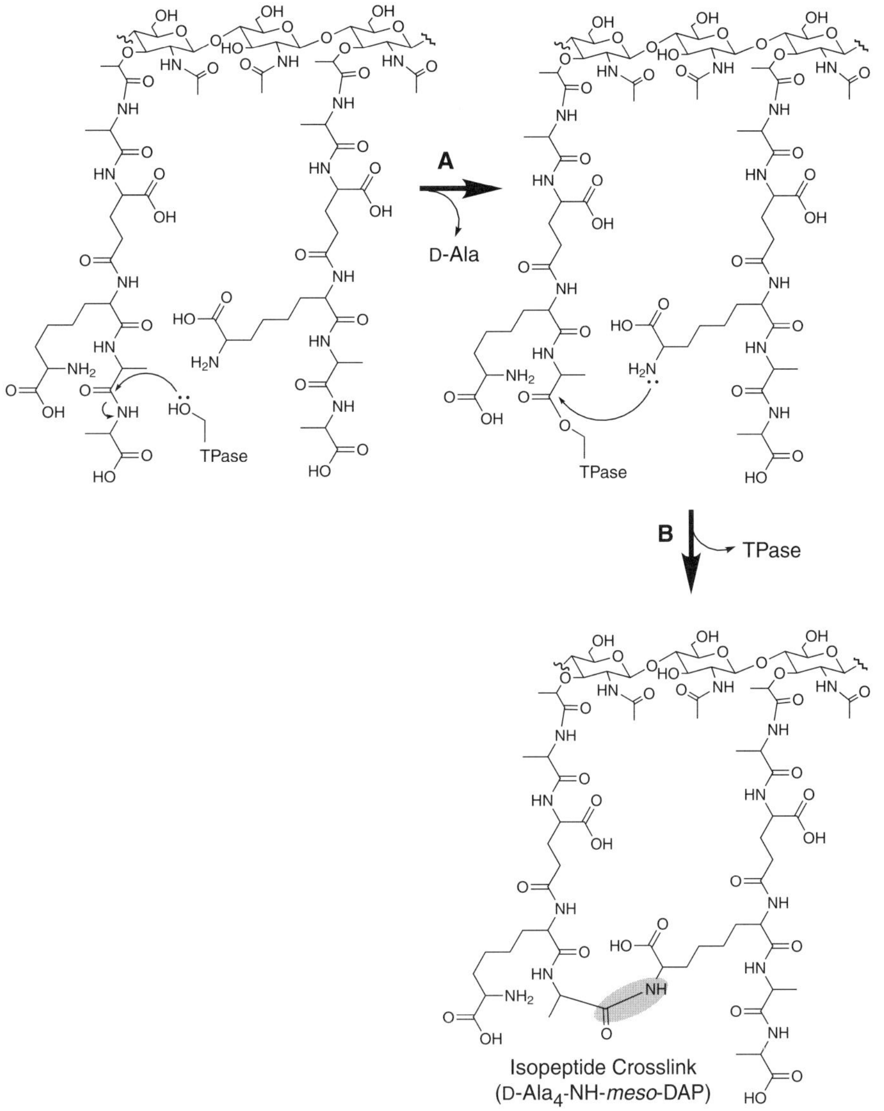

Figure 3.15 Mechanism of the PG transpeptidation reaction to create the DAP-D-Ala iso-peptide bond: acyl enzyme intermediate in transpeptidase action. (A) Acyl enzyme formation; (B) acyl enzyme deacylation and capture by the amine nucleophile of a neighboring chain.

enzyme with release of D-Ala$_5$ as the free amino acid. The acyl-O-transpeptidase intermediate has the glycan-tetrapeptidyl moiety as the transiently tethered acyl group (Fig. 3.15A). In most "serine" enzyme family members, a water molecule is productively bound in the active site and acyl transfer to water ensues, with regeneration of the starting form of the enzyme for another catalytic cycle. This is the fate in the PBP forms that act as D-,D-carboxypeptidases. But in these transpeptidases, water is excluded and the only kinetically competent nucleophile is the amine group of C$_6$ of DAP$_3$ or Lys$_3$ of an adjacent PG chain. Acyl transfer to this nucleophile in the second half-reaction (Fig. 3.15B) completes the catalytic cycle, regenerating free enzyme as the isopeptide bond introduces a meshwork-strengthening cross-link. The X-ray structures for several transpeptidase catalytic domains have been solved (Knox, 1995; Knox et al., 1996; Pares et al., 1996) and support this mechanistic view. In some gram-positive bacteria such as *S. aureus*, the cross-link between peptide chains does not occur directly via the ε-NH$_2$ of a Lys or DAP side chain but involves peptide cross-bridges. Such a pentaglycine bridge (Gly$_5$) is built up on the Lys before cross-linking occurs in *S. aureus*. The transpeptidation is then between the NH$_2$ group of Gly$_5$ and the D-Ala$_4$ carbonyl on an adjacent peptide chain.

The transpeptidases commit suicide when they start a catalytic cycle with β-lactam antibiotics as substrates, mistaking them for a yet to be cross-linked PG chain terminating in D-Ala-D-Ala. The active-site serine adds into the strained four-ring lactam carbonyl (**Fig. 3.16**) and generates an acyl enzyme intermediate in which the β-lactam ring has opened. Now the enzyme gets stuck in mid-catalytic cycle. These transpeptidases are designed to exclude water from intercepting the normal acyl enzyme intermediates and, analogously, the penicilloyl enzyme forms are very slow to hydrolyze (half-lives of many hours to days). The enzyme piles up as the covalent penicilloyl enzyme and is effectively dead until slow hydrolysis allows it to recover. As we shall note in chapter 8, the long lifetimes of these structurally variant acyl enzyme intermediates account for β-lactam killing of bacteria.

With radioactive penicillins or cephalosporins it is easy to demonstrate long-lived covalently labeled acyl transpeptidases by sodium dodecyl sulfate gel electrophoresis, which resolves denatured proteins by size. Bacteria typically show multiple radiolabeled protein bands (**Fig. 3.17**), of which there are four in *S. pneumoniae* and up to eight in *E. coli* (Denome et al., 1999; Spratt, 1977). This approach gave the first historical evidence of multiple transpeptidases and established the full catalytic inventory of these enzyme families. It was then possible to identify each labeled PBP and prove their enzymatic activity after the penicilloyl enzymes finally hydrolyzed. Low-molecular-weight PBPs tend to be N-acyl-D-Ala$_4$-D-Ala$_5$ carboxypeptidases, hydrolases that generate un-cross-linkable tetrapeptide stems, while the high-molecular-weight PBPs (PBP1A, B, and C) are bifunctional transglycosylases/transpeptidases (Holtje, 1998; Schiffer and Holtje, 1999). Mutational analysis could determine which PBPs represented major targets to particular antibiotics and pinpoint their physiologic roles in PG maturation and assembly (for a recent example in *S. pneumoniae*, see Paik et al., 1999). Different lactam antibiotics can induce characteristic changes in phenotype, such as long chains or rounded appearances, reflecting preferential blockade of a subset of PBPs (Greenwood, 2000). Mutations to penicillin resis-

Figure 3.16 Reaction of penicillin as a suicide substrate for PG transpeptidases.

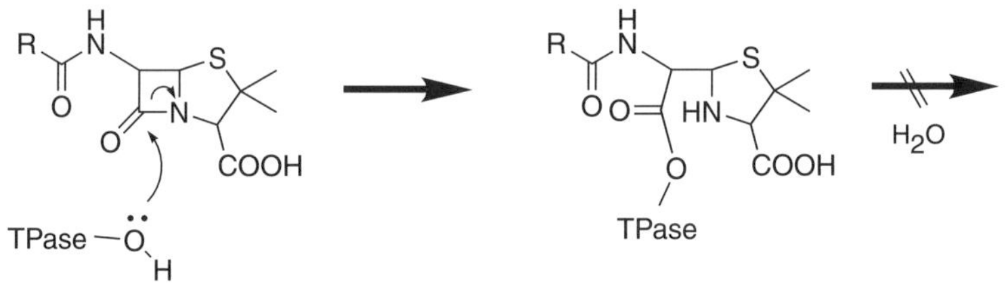

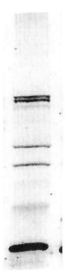

Figure 3.17 Multiple penicillin-binding proteins in *E. coli*: autoradiographs of ¹⁴C-penicilloyl-proteins of *E. coli* separated on denaturing gel electrophoresis. (From Dougherty et al. [1996], with permission.)

tance could also be correlated with decreased affinity of a given PBP to a particular β-lactam antibiotic, and this helped further define the physiologic role of PBPs.

In *E. coli* both the bifunctional transpeptidase/transglycosylase PBP1A and 1B forms, when inhibited, e.g., by acylation with the cephalosporin cephaloridine, lead to spheroplast formation and rapid lysis. They are clearly prime killing targets for β-lactam antibiotics. Selective inhibition of PBP2 by acylation with low concentrations of the penicillin mecillinam produces spherical forms, relative osmotic stability, and slow lysis. Penicillin G at low concentrations acylates PBP3 first, generating chains of bacteria in filaments. It is not clear if PBP3 has much significance as a target for lactam antibiotics. At higher levels of penicillin G, PBP1 isoforms are acylated and lysis occurs. A quantitative estimate from radiolabeled penicillin binding yields about 2,500 PBP molecules per *E. coli* cell (Dougherty et al., 1996), with about 220 PBP1A and 125 PBP1B molecules as major killing targets and about 1,500 (two-thirds of the total) low-molecular-weight PBP4 7, which are not killing targets (Scholar and Pratt, 2000).

How the acylation and inhibition of PBPs by β-lactam antibiotics is translated into cell wall degradation and cell death by inappropriate or excess murein hydrolase activity has been under study for decades (see Bayles, 2000). One current hypothesis is that the hydrolases are normally constrained in their access to the PG substrates and that antibiotic encourages oligomerization of certain proteins, forming channels in the cytoplasmic membrane that allow passage of the PG hydrolases to reach their substrate. In bacteriophage λ infections of *E. coli* there are such channel proteins, holins and antiholins (Young et al., 2000), that control the timing of access of bacteriophage-encoded murein hydrolases to the PG. These may serve as a precedent for the action of related holin-antiholin systems in organisms such as *S. aureus* (Bayles, 2000).

Side chain modifications in penicillins

The natural side chain in the initial β-lactam antibiotic natural product after biosynthetic cyclization (chapter 13) is L-aminoadipoyl (Fig. 3.13). This is then

A

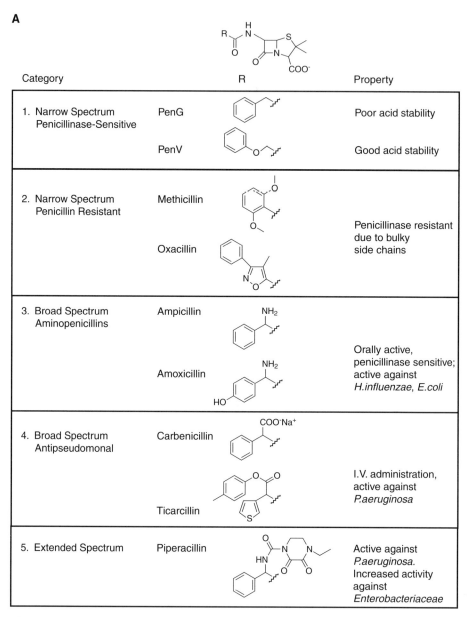

Figure 3.18 Different generations of (A) penicillins and (B) cephalosporins. (Adapted from Scholar and Pratt [2000], with permission.)

epimerized to the D-form and the ring-expanding dioxygenase generates cephalosporins with an olefin in the six ring and the same D-adipoyl side chain, followed by hydroxylation and acetylation at C_3 to yield cephalosporin C (O'Sullivan and Ball, 1983). As medicinal chemists tried to broaden the spectrum of antibacterial activity of the original β-lactams and to gain potency and combat developing resistance (discussed in chapter 8), they made many side chain variants by semisynthetic modifications, using the deacylated 6-aminopenicillanic acid or 7-aminocephem for reacylation with a variety of different kinds of side chains, screening for gain or optimization of the desired activity.

B

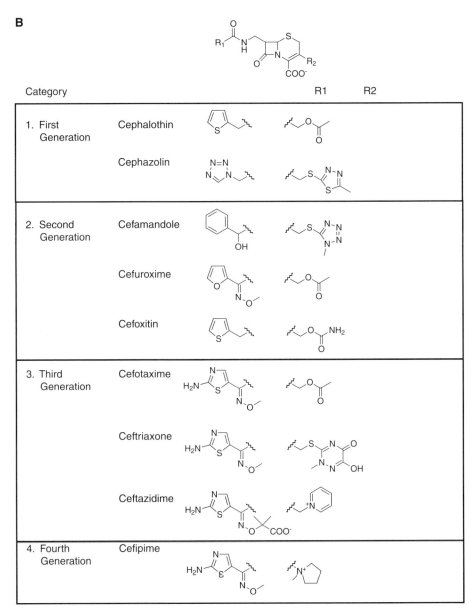

Figure 3.18 *Continued.*

This has led to multiple waves of semisynthetic β-lactams over the 50 years of their clinical use. Scholar and Pratt (2000) note five categories of penicillins (**Fig. 3.18A**) based on narrow- versus broad-spectrum activities and whether there is antipseudomonal activity. The early synthetic side chains, phenylacetyl in penicillin G and phenoxyacetyl in penicillin V, gave narrow-spectrum drugs, active for example against streptococci and neisseria, and were β-lactamase sensitive. Replacement of the unsubstituted aryl groups with the 2,6-dimethoxy substituents in methicillin, the napthyl moiety in nafcillin, and the phenyl-oxazolyl group in oxacillin created misalignment in β-lactamase active sites and consequent resistance to hydrolysis. For example, with the β-lactamase from S.

aureus the K_m values for hydrolysis for penicillin G and penicillin V were in the range of 2 to 4 μM, while the dimethoxy groups in methicillin raised the K_m value by 10^4 to 28,000 μM (Novick, 1962), making methicillin useful against staphylococcal infections. A broader spectrum of activity resulted when the phenylacetyl side chain was converted to the phenylglycyl chain by introduction of an amino group (ampicillin) or by the *p*-OH-phenylglycyl of amoxicillin, generating orally active penicillins with good bioavailability. These aminopenicillins are active against such gram-negative bacteria as *E. coli* and *Haemophilus influenzae*. To obtain antipseudomonal activity, requiring increased penetration through the restrictive porins of the pseudomonal outer membranes, further side chain modifications led to the development of such drugs as ticarcillin, a carboxyl ester derivative of a thiazolyl side chain, which is active by intramuscular and intravenous routes for hospital uses. Finally, for *P. aeruginosa* bacteremias in nosocomial (in-hospital) settings, the ureido derivative of ampicillin with a piperazino group, piperacillin, is an extended-spectrum intravenous penicillin.

Side chain modifications in cephalosporins: multiple generations

Cephalosporins are the most widely prescribed and largest-selling class of the β-lactam antibiotics. Side chain modifications have led to differential penetration through the porins in cell envelope structures and provide varied antibacterial and pharmacokinetic properties (see Scholar and Pratt, 2000). **Figure 3.18B** lists examples of first- to fourth-generation cephalosporins. Narrow-spectrum ("first-generation") examples include intravenous and oral drugs, with cephalothin a prototype. The narrow-spectrum drugs have the best activity against gram-positive pathogens, except methicillin-resistant *S. aureus* (MRSA), and are active against some gram-negative organisms, such as *E. coli* and klebsiella strains. The expanded-spectrum ("second-generation") cephalosporins, represented by intravenous drugs cefoxitin and cefamandole and oral drugs such as cefaclor and loracarbacef, are somewhat less effective against gram-positive but have a broader spectrum against gram-negative pathogens including *Bacteroides fragilis* and *H. influenzae*. The increased gram-negative activity stems from a combination of better penetration, increased affinity for binding to PBP targets, and lowered catalytic efficiency toward hydrolysis by β-lactamases. The side chains in both narrow- and expanded-spectrum cephalosporins built on the experience with penicillins, including thiazolyl and phenylglycyl side chains. The side chains in expanded- and broad-spectrum ("second-" and "third-generation") cephalosporins typically provide a couple of logs of resistance to β-lactamases. Also varied is the 3′ substituent on the hydroxyl of the six ring. In the broad-spectrum cephalosporins, gram-negative activity has been optimized and extended to cover *P. aeruginosa*, while retaining sufficient activity against gram-positive bacteria (e.g., methicillin-sensitive *S. aureus*), except for ceftazidime (Scholar and Pratt, 2000), such that they are useful for surgical prophylaxis. The "fourth-generation" cephalosporin molecule, cefepime, approved for use in the United States, has properties akin to the broad-spectrum cephems, but gains increased resistance to many β-lactamases. The favored acyl side chains on the β-lactam in the third and fourth generation of cephalosporins are aminothiazole oximes, some of which have charged carboxylates (e.g., ceftazidime, cefixime), which allow good penetration through the porins of gram-negative outer membranes while retaining high affinities against PBP targets. The 3′ substituents differ more widely, some with positively charged amines, which also affect intrinsic antibacterial activity and pharmacokinetics and distribution. For example, many of them penetrate well into the cerebrospinal fluid when meninges are inflamed (Scholar and Pratt, 2000) and are effective for treating meningitis.

Overall, the semisynthetic manipulation of cephalosporin side chains shows the ability for optimization against different subsets of pathogens, accounting for the dominant role in many infections where β-lactam antibiotics are prescribed. The cephalosporins also have excellent safety profiles, leading to broad use in hospitals in both preoperative and postoperative contexts. On the other hand, the success of cephalosporins may in the end have selected for bacteria with resistance determinants (see chapter 17).

Carbapenems and monobactams

Two carbapenems, imipenem and meropenem (Fig. 3.14), are approved for clinical use in the United States, with a third, ertapenem (MK-0826), in clinical development with the intent of once-daily dosage (see Fuchs et al., 2001). Imipenem and meropenem are water soluble, have low oral bioavailability, and are utilized in hospital settings against antibiotic-resistant infectious organisms, where they show broad-spectrum activity (see Table 4-9 in Scholar and Pratt, 2000). They tend to be resistant to most serine-based β-lactamases but are sensitive to hydrolysis by metallo-β-lactamases, as examined in chapter 8. Although imipenem is resistant to bacterial enzyme β-lactam ring-mediated hydrolysis, in vertebrates dehydropeptidase I in renal epithelial cells hydrolyzes the lactam. Cilastatin, a dehydropeptide mimic that inhibits the renal hydrolase, is thus given with the carbapenem. Meropenem with a C-methyl substituent is not susceptible to the renal enzyme. Ertapenem has a prolonged half-life compared to the earlier carbapenems, probably due to serum protein binding, and is proposed for once-a-day dosing. Both carbapenems have useful antipseudomonal activity (Livermore and Woodford, 2000).

One monobactam antibiotic, aztreonam (Fig. 3.14), is in human clinical use. The acyl side chain is the same as in ceftazidine, while the lactam has an N-sulfonate substituent on the other side. The spectrum of antibacterial activity (Scholar and Pratt, 2000) is such that it is useful only against gram-negative pathogens, with good activity against *P. aeruginosa*. It appears to target PBP3 at low concentrations and has low susceptibility to the lactamases of the gram-negative target pathogens.

The clavam scaffold is found in clavulanate (Fig. 3.13) (see also chapter 13). Clavulanate on its own is a poor substrate for PBP and so is not considered an antibiotic. Its utility derives from its "suicide substrate" properties with β-lactamases, discussed further in chapter 8.

Glycopeptide antibiotics act by complexing the un-cross-linked peptide strands and blocking transpeptidation

Two glycopeptide antibiotics in the vancomycin family have been approved for human clinical use, vancomycin itself (**Fig. 3.19**) and, outside of the United States, teicoplanin.

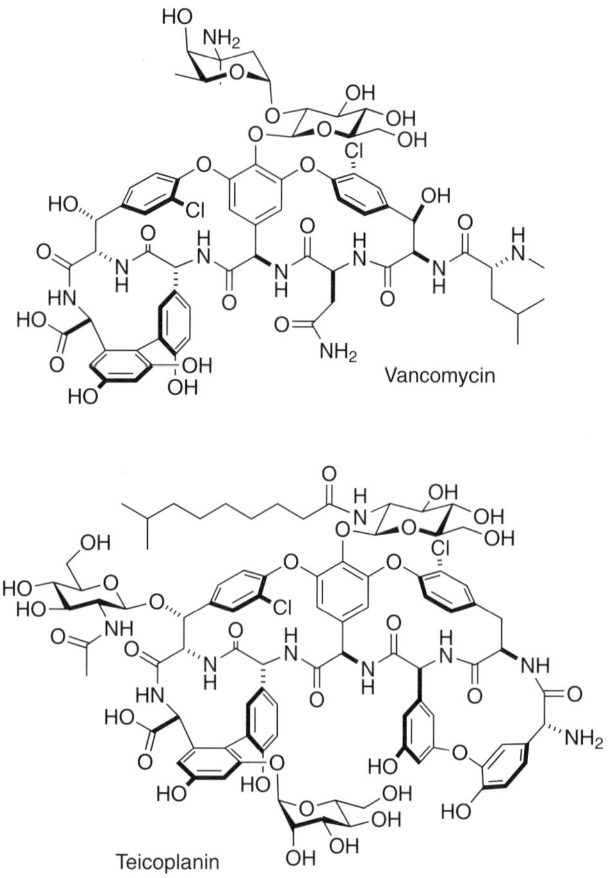

Figure 3.19 Structures of the glycopeptide antibiotics vancomycin and teicoplanin.

Figure 3.20 Sequestration of PG-D-Ala-D-Ala termini by vancomycin. (A) Five hydrogen bonds between the antibiotic and PG terminus; (B) space-filling model of the antibiotic and PG terminus.

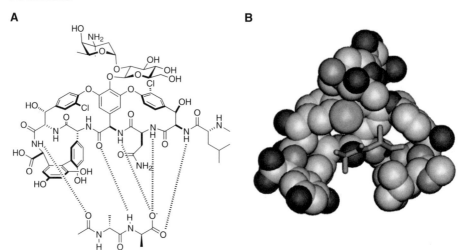

Teicoplanin differs in three ways from vancomycin: (i) the glycosylation number and placement is distinct; (ii) teicoplanin has a long-chain fatty acid substituent in amide linkage to the GlcNAc sugar attached to $PheGly_4$; and (iii) the cross-linked heptapeptide scaffold is different at residues 1 and 3, allowing four side chain cross-links (1-3, 2-4, 4-6, 5-7) in contrast to the three in vancomycin (see Hubbard and Walsh, 2002; Williams and Bardsley, 1999; and references therein). As noted in chapter 2, vancomycin and teicoplanin cannot penetrate the pores of the gram-negative outer membranes so are restricted to treating infections of life-threatening gram-positive pathogens such as staphylococcal, streptococcal, and enterococcal infections.

Both these antibiotics act not by inhibiting the transglycosylases or transpeptidases per se, but rather by complexation of the substrate PG units that have

Figure 3.21 PG termini interacting with vancomycin and teicoplanin: (A) un-cross-linked strands on preexisting PG; (B) the lipid II substrate before polymerization into PG.

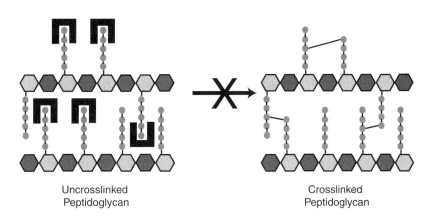

A

Uncrosslinked
Peptidoglycan

Crosslinked
Peptidoglycan

B

Lipid II

$O-PO_2$
O
PO_2
O

$O-PO_2$
O
PO_2
O

$O-PO_2$
O
PO_2
O

C55   C55   C55

Inner Membrane

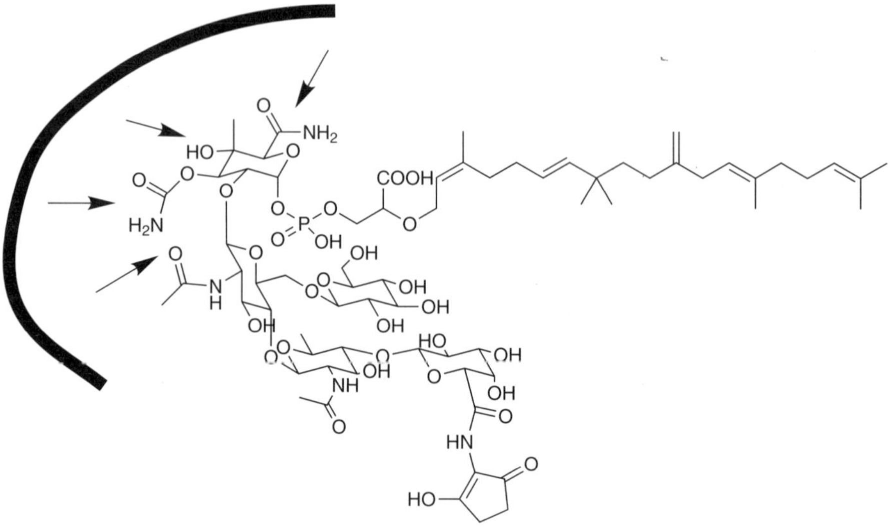

Figure 3.22 Model for moenomycin interaction with target transglycosylases. (From Kurz et al. [1998], with permission.)

the pentapeptidyl tails terminating in D-Ala$_4$-D-Ala$_5$. This substrate sequestration effectively shuts down transpeptidation by making the N-acyl-D-Ala-D-Ala acceptor unavailable to the transpeptidases (Fig. 3.20). In this sense the sequestration of substrate is analogous to the sequestration proposed for lipid II by ramoplanin (also a lipoglycopeptide antibiotic) (Lo et al., 2000). The complex has been characterized first by NMR and then by X-ray (see Williams and Bardsley, 1999) to involve molecular recognition of a not yet cross-linked N-acyl-D-Ala-D-Ala terminus of a PG-pentapeptidyl strand by the underside of the rigid, cup-shaped vancomycin via a series of five hydrogen bonds (see Walsh et al., 1996b; Williams and Bardsley, 1999). The space-filling model shows the optimized tightness of fit of antibiotic for its target. There are two kinds of PG units that have the intact pentapeptide strand, the lipid II molecules at the periplasmic face of the membrane, and also strands as yet un-cross-linked in polymerized PG (Fig. 3.21). The steric blockade of the transpeptidation can also have effects on transglycosylases, especially in the bifunctional, high-molecular-weight PBPs. Different members of the vancomycin glycopeptide antibiotic family have different tendencies to dimerize, and this may enable an enhanced avidity for complexation with PG termini (Williams, 1996). We will return to these mechanisms in chapter 10 with a discussion of the molecular mechanisms of glycopeptide antibiotic resistance in one type of opportunistic human pathogens, vancomycin-resistant enterococci (VRE). Given that vancomycins and penicillins work on two different aspects of the PG cross-linking, one might expect to, and does, observe synergy of antibacterial effects in combination.

Moenomycin as an inhibitor of the transglycosylase activity of PBP1B

In contrast to the many β-lactam antibiotics that inhibit the transpeptidase activity of the bifunctional transglycosylase/transpeptidase activities of the high-molecular-weight PBPs, there are very few natural product antibiotics that target the transglycosylase active site. Moenomycin A (Kurz et al., 1998) is one such compound (**Fig. 3.22**), used as a growth promoter in animal feed (Ritter and Wong, 2001).

Moenomycin has a 25-carbon lipid alcohol, moecinol, linked via a phosphoglycerate to a pentasaccharide tail in phosphodiester linkage. NMR analysis has provided a model for the three-dimensional structure with the proposal that the E and F rings of the carbohydrate moiety interact, as a substrate analog, with the target transglycosylase to shut down addition of the disaccharyl pentapeptide units in PG layer growth. The moecinol tail is probably a membrane anchor that preconcentrates the antibiotic at the external side of the cytoplasmic membrane where PBP1 enzyme molecules are located. Libraries of constituent disaccharides have been made, but so far without retention of useful activity (see Ritter and Wong, 2001, for review).

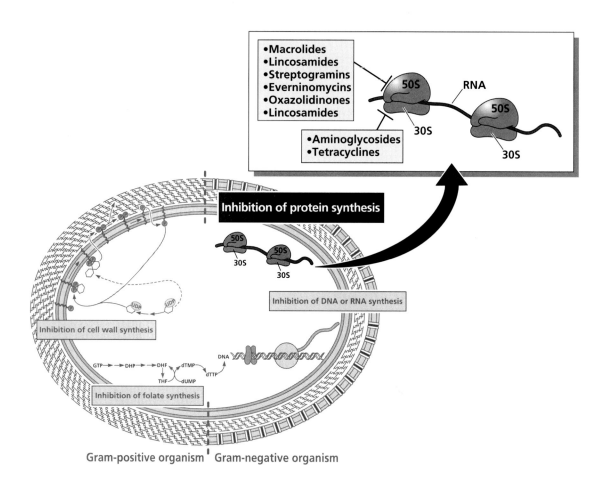

Antibiotics that block bacterial protein biosynthesis.

chapter *4*

Antibiotics That Block Bacterial Protein Biosynthesis

This chapter deals with the various classes of antibiotics that exert their bacteriostatic or bactericidal action by blockade of one or more of the protein biosynthetic steps that occur on the 30S and 50S subunits of the bacterial ribosome. The figure on the facing page shows a blowup of the relevant portions of Fig. 2.2, emphasizing that some antibiotics block processes at the 50S ribosome and others act at the 30S ribosome.

Bacterial ribosome structure and the peptidyltransferase cycle

Given the centrality of protein biosynthesis to cellular function and the large number of steps involved, from activation of the 20 proteinogenic amino acid monomers by the aminoacyl-tRNA synthetases, to the many steps in chain initiation, chain elongation, and chain termination of the growing polypeptides on the ribosome, it is natural that many natural product antibiotics target one or more steps in protein biosynthesis. Before analyzing the sites and mechanism of action of ribosome-inhibiting antibiotics, a short summary on the ribosome is presented.

In bacteria the ribosome is a two-subunit nucleoprotein particle, about two-thirds RNA and one-third protein, of molecular weight 2.5 to 2.6 MDa. The small subunit, 30S, contains about 20 proteins and a 16S ribosomal rRNA of about 1,500 ribonucleotides. Typically the large, 50S subunit has about 30 proteins, a 23S rRNA of about 2,900 ribonucleotides, and a 5S rRNA (122 nucleotides). The two large rRNAs, with about 4,500 nucleotides, are both scaffold and catalyst for peptide bond formation. The X-ray structure of the 70S ribosome from *Thermus thermophilus* has been reported at a resolution of 5.5 Å, sufficient to reveal the architecture of both the 30S and 50S subunits and their interactions (Yusupov et al., 2001) (**Color Plate 4.1**). **Color Plate 4.1A** shows the 30S subunit on the left, the 50S on the right, and an aminoacyl-tRNA in the interface. A 90° rotation in **Color Plate 4.1B** shows the view from the back of

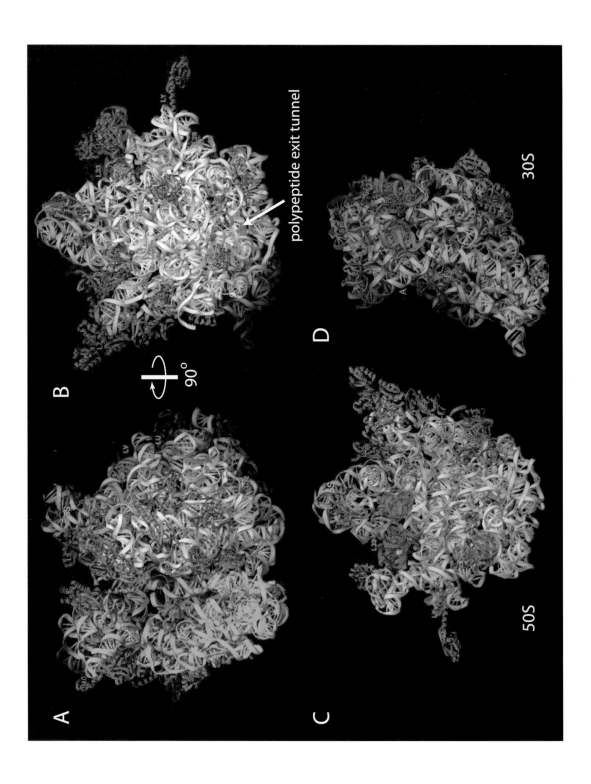

the 50S subunit with the exit tunnel for the nascent polypeptide chain indicated. **Color Plate 4.1C** gives an interface view of the 50S subunit with three tRNAs, occupying the P, A, and E sites (see below), and **Color Plate 4.1D** shows the corresponding interface view of the 30S subunit.

The X-ray structure of the 70S ribosome complements recent structures of the 30S subunit from the same organism (Wimberly et al., 2000), refined to 3 Å resolution, and the structure of the 50S subunit from *Haloarcula marismortui* (Nissen et al., 2000). The ensemble of structures has opened a new chapter in the study of ribosomes as protein-synthesizing machines and the mechanisms of blockade by antibiotics.

In addition to the 16S and 23S rRNA molecules that are crucial structural, recognition, and catalytic elements of the ribosome, two other RNA molecules, mRNA and tRNA, are required for protein synthesis. The mRNA provides the instructional template, and its path through the ribosome has recently been visualized by X-ray analysis (see reviews in Culver, 2001, and Yusupova et al., 2001). mRNA threads through two tunnels in the 30S subunit, with only a short stretch protruding through to the interface between the 30S and 50S subunits (**Color Plate 4.2A**). That stretch of mRNA contains the six nucleotides that comprise the aminoacyl (A) and peptidyl (P) codons (**Color Plate 4.2B**), nucleotides +6 to +1. The exit site codon (E), at -1 to -3 bases, is in the upstream tunnel just in front of the -5 to -12 region, the Shine-Dalgarno sequence, that base pairs with the anti-Shine-Dalgarno sequence at the 3′ end of the 16S rRNA to form the double helix that sets the register for mRNA translation. The tRNA molecules transfer the amino acids to the ribosome and provide the anticodon trinucleotides for Watson Crick base pairing at the A and P sites at the 30S-mRNA interaction site.

The aminoacylated end of the P and A tRNAs reach away from the 30S subunit into the 50S subunit at domain V of the 23S rRNA. The peptidyl chain is translocated onto the aminoacyl-tRNA in the A site by the peptidyltransferase activity in each peptide-chain-elongation cycle of the ribosome. The peptidyltransferase activity derives from the catalytic ribozyme activity of this portion of the 23S rRNA with no obvious assistance from proteins (see Nissen et al., 2000) (**Fig. 4.1**).

In each catalytic cycle of elongation, the 30S subunit functions as a decoding unit to select the proper aminoacyl-tRNA with its anticodon that will fit the A-site codon. Once the correct aminoacyl-tRNA is docked in the A site, the aminoacyl moiety tethered 75 Å away at the CCA end of that tRNA is oriented into a productive conformation to attack the adjacent peptidyl chain, itself oriented at the CCA end of its tRNA, elongating the growing peptidyl chain as it is translocated onto the attacking aminoacyl group. At this juncture this is an

Color Plate 4.1 Interaction of 30S and 50S subunits and location of tRNAs in the A site, P site, and E site. (A) The *T. thermophilus* ribosome 30S subunit is shown on the left, the 50S subunit is at right. (B) 90° rotation from (A) shows the back of the 50S subunit and the location of the exit tunnel for the nascent polypeptide chain. (C) View of the 50S subunit from the 50S/30S subunit interface with tRNAs in P, A, and E sites. (D) View of the 30S subunit interface. (From Yusupov et al. [2001] with permission.)

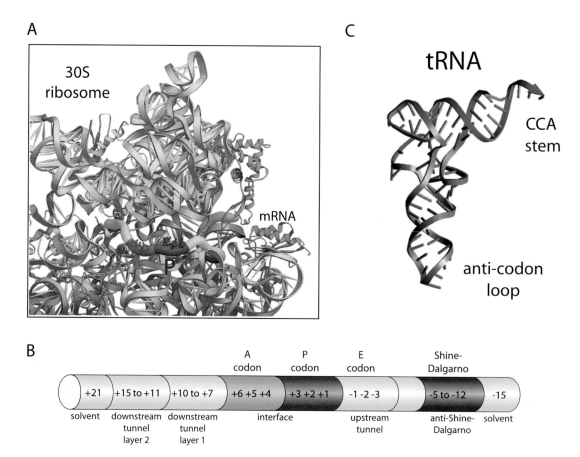

A

30S
ribosome

mRNA

C

tRNA

CCA
stem

anti-codon
loop

B

			A codon	P codon	E codon	Shine- Dalgarno	
+21	+15 to +11	+10 to +7	+6 +5 +4	+3 +2 +1	-1 -2 -3	-5 to -12	-15
solvent	downstream tunnel layer 2	downstream tunnel layer 1	interface		upstream tunnel	anti-Shine- Dalgarno	solvent

Color Plate 4.2 (A) Threading of the mRNA into the 30S subunit decoding region; (B) placement of the A, P, and E codons of the mRNA in the decoding site; (C) architecture of a tRNA highlighting the anti-codon loop that recognizes the codons on mRNA and the CCA tail where the amino acid is covalently tethered and activated. (From Culver [2001] with permission.)

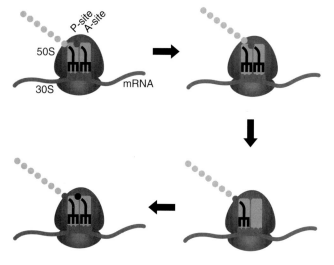

50S

P-site
A-site

30S

mRNA

Figure 4.1 Schematic of peptide bond formation at the ribosome.

empty, deacylated tRNA in the P site (**Fig. 4.1**) and the peptidyl group is tethered to a tRNA still docked in the A site. For the next round of elongation, the deacylated tRNA moves to the E site, the peptidyl-tRNA relocates to the P site, and the A site becomes open for the next aminoacyl-tRNA to be brought in and decoded by the 30S-mRNA complex. The orchestration of the movement of mRNA, to present a new triplet codon at the A site in the interface between 30S and 50S to allow decoding, and of the three tRNAs, to shuttle between the E, P, and A sites, is not yet understood.

The peptidyltransferase center in the 50S subunit has been defined in domain V of the 23S rRNA by cocrystallization of a transition-state analog, a peptidyl puromycin phophonamidate (**Color Plate 4.3**) that mimics the tetrahedral geometry of the intermediate in peptidyltransferase RNA catalysis. This allows definition of P-site and A-site rRNA nucleotides in relation to the bound analog and has suggested mechanisms for functions of individual RNA bases in the peptide bond-forming steps (Nissen et al., 2000). It has also facilitated definition of the polypeptide exit tunnel, about 100 Å long, that allows passage of the growing polypeptide chain through the 50S subunit to the outside (**Color Plate 4.4**).

It is clear that the low observed error rates in protein synthesis, about one mistake in 10^4 elongation cycles, requires proofreading and editing for maintenance of this high fidelity during amino acid incorporation at the ribosome (see Rodnina and Wintermeyer, 2001, for review). Evidence has accrued over the years for a multistep discrimination to distinguish between the cognate aminoacyl-tRNA in a sea of noncognate aminoacyl-tRNAs. The aminoacyl-tRNAs are brought to the ribosome in complex with a chaperone protein, EF-Tu, which is a latent GTPase. After initial binding to the ribosome, the aminoacyl-tRNA can either dissociate or proceed to base pair in the anticodon-codon helix interaction, leading to reorientation and a longer-lived complex (**Fig. 4.2**). At this point, the GTPase activity of EF-Tu is activated, presumably by conformational change, and GTP cleavage to bound GDP and P_i occurs, followed by product P_i release. The GDP stays bound, promoting a specific conformation of EF-Tu.GDP. When peptide bond formation occurs over in the peptidyltransferase center of the 50S subunit, the now deacylated tRNA is released from the A site by the GDP form of EF-Tu. It is presumed that local structures of rRNA in the 30S and 50S subunits are relaying signals that decoding information has occurred and that the aminoacyl end of the aminacyl-tRNA should orient productively for peptide bond formation.

Antibiotics could interrupt the timing and specificity of any of these steps, and such disruptions are likely to slow down growth and/or be lethal to the bacteria. **Figure 4.3** shows examples of major classes of antibiotics targeted to the 30S subunit (spectinomycin, the aminoglycosides kanamycin and streptomycin, tetracycline) or to the 50S subunit (clindamycin, chloramphenicol, linezolid, and macrolides such as erythromycin, clarithromycin, azithromycin, and tylosin). Structures of antibiotics bound to rRNA target sites in the 30S and 50S subunits have appeared in the past two years (e.g., Carter et al., 2000; Schlunzen et al., 2001). For example, cocrystallization of the three antibiotics paromomycin, spectinomycin, and streptomycin with the target 30S subunits indicated alteration of delicate balances between rRNA conformational states, causing disruption

A

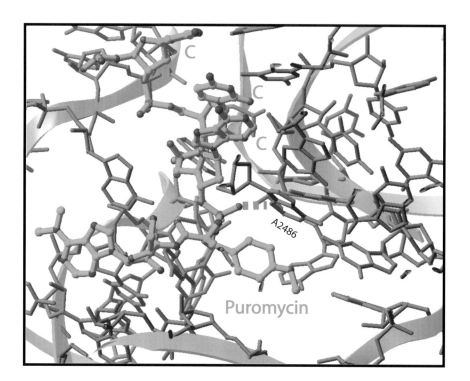

Color Plate 4.3 The peptidyl transferase center on the 50S ribosomal subunit. (A) Docking of the CCdAp-puromycin complex at the peptidyl transferase center of the 50S subunit; (B) two-dimensional projection of the interaction of CCdAp-puromycin with A_{2486} and analogous geometry of the tetrahedral intermediate during peptide bond formation at the same site on the ribosome.

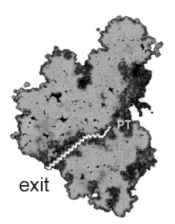

Color Plate 4.4 The polypeptide exit tunnel through the 50S ribosome.

of translocation (spectinomycin), decoding (paromomycin), and translational accuracy (streptomycin) (Carter et al., 2000). This work is likely to be a harbinger of many studies to come that pinpoint the action of antibiotics on one or more of the constituent steps in ribosome function.

The erythromycin class of macrolide antibiotics

Erythromycin is a 14-membered macrocyclic lactone produced by the streptomycete *Saccharopolyspora erythraea*. The aglycone arises from a modular poly-

Figure 4.2 Steps in binding, codon recognition, GTPase activation, proofreading, and peptidyl transfer in peptide bond formation. (Modified from Rodnina and Wintermeyer [2001].)

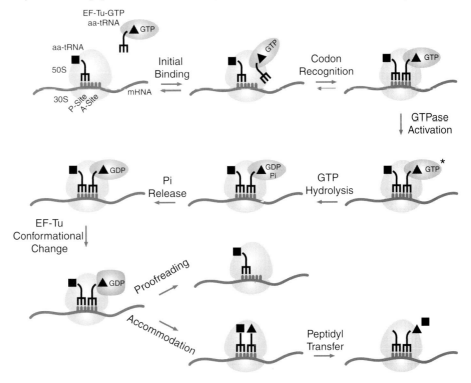

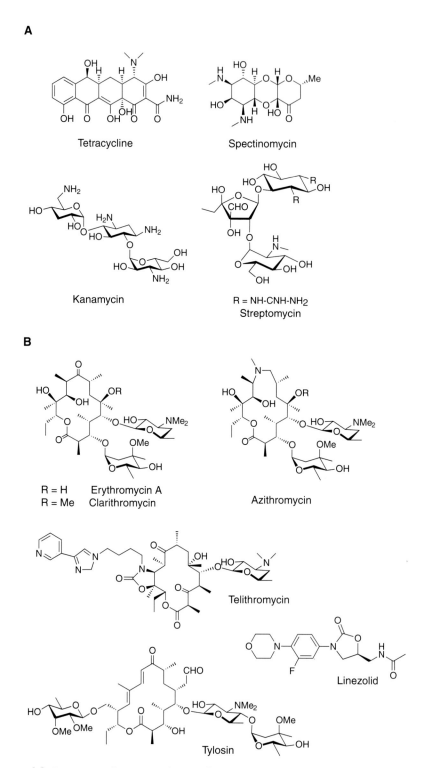

Figure 4.3 Structures of some antibiotics that act at (A) the 30S subunit or (B) the 50S subunit of bacterial ribosomes.

ketide synthase assembly line, as will be examined in chapter 12, and is then bis oxygenated and bis glycosylated to produce the active antibiotic; 15-membered semisynthetic (azithromycin) and 16-membered naturally occurring macrolides such as tylosin are also active (Fig. 4.3). The architecture of the macrolactone and the interactions of the sugars are key determinants of binding and specificity for interaction with the 23S rRNA in the six-nucleotide region 2058-2062. Erythromycin binding blocks polypeptide translation with the net effect of release of peptidyl-tRNA intermediates prematurely, by blocking the approach to the elongating peptide's exit tunnel (Ban et al., 2000; Schlunzen et al., 2001). The drug also blocks assembly of 50S subunits, presumably through this interaction with 23S rRNA. The 50% inhibitory concentartion (IC_{50}) for translation inhibition in *Staphylococcus aureus* cells is about 0.2 μg/ml (Goldman et al., 1990) and the K_d for stoichiometric binding to the 23S rRNA component of the 50S subunit is about 1 nM. Erythromycin has proven safe and effective in adults and children and has been used in both inpatient and outpatient settings.

Expanded-spectrum macrolides such as azithromycin and clarithromycin (Fig. 4.3) fill an important therapeutic niche for treatment of respiratory infections (Scholar and Pratt, 2000). They are semisynthetic molecules—clarithromycin with a methoxy at C_6 and azithromycin with an expanded, 15-membered macrolide and an inserted nitrogen—that have an altered macrolide conformation. Azithromycin and clarithromycin have IC_{50} values about equivalent to that of erythromycin (see Champness, 2000, for review), cause less gastrointestinal tract irritation, are more stable to the acid pH of the stomach, have better tissue penetration, and have longer half-lives, allowing once- or twice-daily dosing. In the narrow- and expanded-spectrum macrolides the cladinose sugar is required for antibiotic activity.

Broad-spectrum macrolides, with the 3-OH oxidized to a ketone, removing the site of attachment of the cladinose sugar, known as ketolides (e.g., telithromycin) (Bronson and Barrett, 2001a), are in late stages of clinical development, and telithromycin has recently been approved in the United States. Such ketolides show about a 1-log improvement in IC_{50} values (0.02 to 0.04 μg/ml) (Capobianco et al., 2000; Douthwaite et al., 2000) and do not induce rRNA methylation resistance gene expression (see chapter 10). The successive generations of macrolides have been optimized for altered properties including acid stability in the stomach and activity against macrolide-resistant pathogens (chapters 9 and 10). All three generations of macrolides must take advantage of architectural differences in the 23S RNA of bacterial ribosomes versus their eukaryotic counterparts to provide selectivity for killing of the bacteria. The recent X-ray analysis of macrolide antibiotics bound to bacterial ribosomes (see below) gives some insight into this selectivity. Members of this class of drugs have also been heavily investigated as targets for diversity generation by combinatorial biosynthesis, as will be discussed in chapter 15.

Tylosin, a 16-membered macrolide with a macrolactone two carbons larger than that of erythromycin and distinct sugars, targets the 23S rRNA at essentially the same site and is used in veterinary medicine. Kinetic analysis of both tylosin and erythromycin binding to the ribosome suggest an initial collisonal complex followed by a slow isomerization step, resulting in tightened binding and slow dissociation. Return from the isomerized RI* complex can be very slow. For tylosin as inhibitor I, the ribosome·I* complex accumulates over the collisional RI by 600/1.

$$\text{Ribosome} + I \leftrightarrow \text{Ribosome·I} \leftrightarrow \text{Ribosome·I*}$$

For the ribosome-erythromycin* complex the ratio is 10/1, indicating longer-lived inhibition for the tylosin complex (Dinos and Kalpaxis, 2000). In direct assays of peptidyltransferase activity, erythromycin does not block activity while tylosin does. Footprinting analysis had indicated that erythromycin binds adjacent to the peptidyltransferase center of the 50S and blocks passage of the nascent peptidyl chain into the exit tunnel through the 50S subunit. This has now been directly validated by X-ray analysis of macrolides bound to the 23S rRNA in the 50S subunit of the bacterium *Deinococcus radiodurans* (Schlunzen et al., 2001).

Erythromycin and the expanded-spectrum 14-membered macrolide antibiotics clarithromycin and roxithromycin all bind at the entrance to the polypeptide export tunnel (**Color Plate 4.5A**), allowing about a six- to eight-oligopeptidyl-tRNA buildup before elongation is blocked and prematurely terminated. The narrow- and expanded-spectrum macrolides have three structural elements—macrolactone, desosamine, and cladinose sugars—and this ensemble makes up to seven hydrogen bonds with 23S rRNA. No ribosomal proteins are in molecular contact with the macrolide antibiotics. The 2′-OH of the desosamine makes hydrogen bonds to N_1 and N_6 of A_{2058} in 23S RNA (**Color Plate 4.5B**), explaining the key requirement for A_{2058} for susceptibility to macrolides (Vester and Douthwaite, 2001). In eukaryotes A_{2058} is changed to G_{2058}, explaining at least part of the target selectivity of the erythromycin class of drugs to bacterial ribosomes (Schlunzen et al., 2001). The 6-OH, 11-OH, and 12-OH substituents on the macrolactone may also make hydrogen bond contacts to 23S RNA for orientation of the antibiotic. The cladinose ring makes no crucial interactions and is replaced in the broad-spectrum ketolides with retention and even gain of activity.

Although the macrolides do not directly block the peptide bond-forming step at the peptidyltransferase center of the 50S subunits, it has been known that they are competitive with lincosamide antibiotics that are direct peptidyltransferase inhibitors. Indeed, a single mutation at A_{2058}, to any of the other three bases (G, C, or U), induces a tripartite resistance to macrolides, lincosamides, and streptogramin B family members (MLS_B resistance), suggesting physical overlap (see Vester and Douthwaite, 2001, for review). Schlunzen et al. (2001) have provided direct validation with the cocrystal structure of the lincosamide antibiotic clindamycin (**Color Plate 4.5C and 4.5D**), in which the 2′- and 3′-OH groups of the sugar moiety of the antibiotic form hydrogen bonds to the same exocyclic N_6 amino group of A_{2058}. An overlay of clindamycin binding and erythromycin binding shows partial physical overlap (Color Plate 4.5C). Clindamycin has separately been known to interact with both the A site and the P site of the peptidyltransferase center; thus a model building of the 3′ ends of the A- and P-tRNAs produces the composite in Color Plate 4.5C, showing the placement of clindamycin and erythromycin relative to the two tRNAs which position the peptidyl donor and aminoacyl acceptor in peptide bond formation that is the core reaction of the ribosome. Finally, the antibiotic chloramphenicol, now in restricted usage due to toxicity concerns, has also been cocrystallized

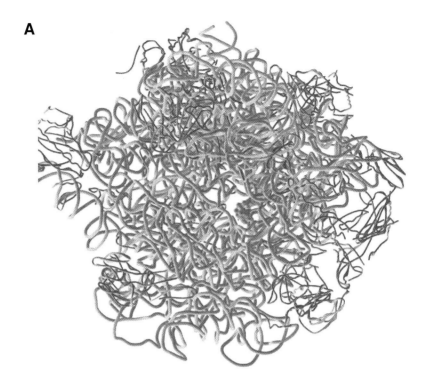

Color Plate 4.5 Mode of action of macrolide antibiotics: (A) binding of macrolides at the 50S polypeptide exit tunnel; (B) interaction with the 23S RNA bases; (C) overlap with the binding sites for clindamycin and chloramphenicol as well as the A-site and P-site tRNAs; (D) inventory of the molecules that are overlapped in panel C. In direct assays of peptidyl transferase activity, erythromycin does not block activity. (From Nissen et al. [2000] with permission.)

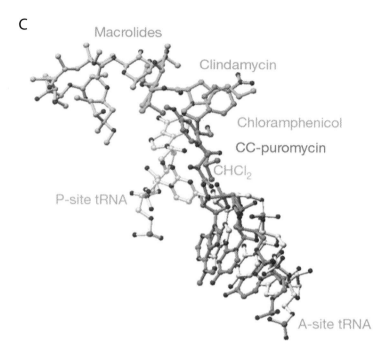

C

Macrolides

Clindamycin

Chloramphenicol

CC-puromycin

CHCl₂

P-site tRNA

A-site tRNA

D

Macrolides

Clindamycin

Chloramphenicol

Puromycin

A C C C

Color Plate 4.5 (*continued*)

with the *D. radiodurans* 50S subunit by this same research team (Schlunzen et al., 2001). It is known that chloramphenicol blocks aminoacyl-tRNA interaction with the A site of the peptidyltransferase center, and that is indeed where chloramphenicol is bound.

The location of five antibiotics in the cavity of the peptidyltransferase center of the bacterial 50S subunit of the ribosome will certainly enable new efforts in rational design of antibacterials targeted at protein synthesis.

Synergistic nonribosomal peptide combinations: Synercid

A large variety of streptomycetes and actinoplanes (Champness, 2000) make a pair of antibiotics of the virginiamycin (also called pristinamycin and streptogramin) family, termed group A and group B (Barriere et al., 1998) or, alternatively, group I and II, that work synergistically to block polypeptide translation by the 50S subunit of bacterial ribosomes at 23S rRNA sites partially overlapping those targeted by the macrolides. We will use the term pristinamycins for the therapeutic pair recently approved as Synercid (Livermore, 2000) (**Fig. 4.4**) and the alternate generic term virginiamycins in chapter 11 when discussing regulation of the timing of antibiotic synthesis. The group I pristinamycins are nonribosomal cyclic peptidolactones with the side chain alcohol of an *N*-aryl-Thr$_1$ connected to the carbonyl of PheGly$_6$. The group II pristinamycins are polyketide/polypeptide hybrids with an oxazole-pro (derived from a ser-pro dipeptide precursor) moiety embedded in a polyketide lactone backbone (chapter

Figure 4.4 Structures of the pristinamycin I (quinuprustin) and pristinamycin IIA (dalfopristin) components of the peptide antibiotic Synercid.

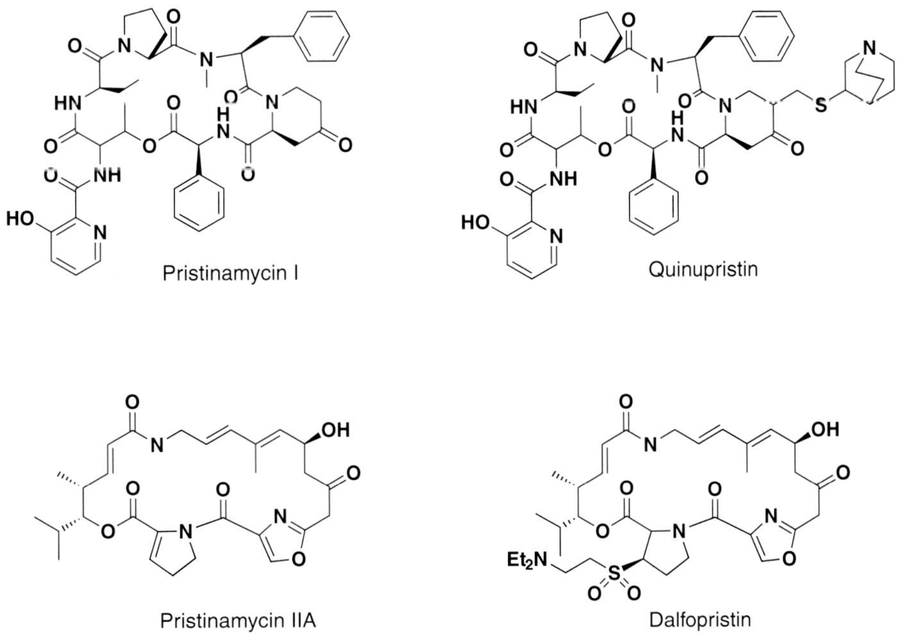

13). The particular pristinamycins I and II of the Synercid combination are semisynthetic versions, with a thioether substitution on the 4-oxopipecolyl residue of the quinupristin and a diethylaminoethylsulfone substituent on the prolyl ring of the dalfopristin component (Fig. 4.4). The modifications improve water solubility and have allowed clinical approval for the significant indication of treatment of vancomycin-resistant enterococcal (VRE) infections.

Tetracyclines and glycylcyclines

The tetracyclines have been known since 1948 with the discovery of chlortetracycline and then tetracycline from *Streptomyces aureofaciens* and then oxytetracycline from *S. rimosus* (**Fig. 4.5**). More-recent members of the class include the 6-deoxy-5-hydroxytetracycline (doxycycline), introduced in 1967, and minocycline, introduced in 1972 (Chopra and Roberts, 2001). The lack of new versions of tetracycline in the past 30 years reflects a declining role as front-line therapy in many human infections, but the ongoing clinical development of tigilcycline, a glycylcycline that inhibits efflux, indicates continued interest in this polyketide antibiotic class. The 19-carbon four-ring cyclic skeleton is derived from a starter molecule and eight molecules of malonyl CoA (see chapter 12) by iterative action of a polyketide synthase (Rawlings, 1999). Tetracyclines are largely bacteriostatic, working at the 30S ribosomal subunit to block binding of the incoming aminoacyl-tRNAs to the A site. Selectivity against bacterial versus eukaryotic ribosomes is due to both structural differences in RNA of the ribosomal subunits and selective concentration in susceptible bacterial cells (Chopra and Roberts, 2001). The determination of the structure of the 30S ribosomal subunit from *T. thermophilus* (Carter et al., 2000; Pioletti et al., 2001) with bound drug has revealed a major binding site and a lower-affinity binding site for tetracycline (**Color Plate 4.6A**).

The major site has only RNA, not protein, interacting with tetracycline, near the acceptor (A) site for aminoacyl-tRNA binding in a groove 20 Å wide and

Figure 4.5 Structures of tetracycline, chlortetracycline, oxytetracycline, doxycycline, a glycylcycline (DMG-MINO), and tigilcycline.

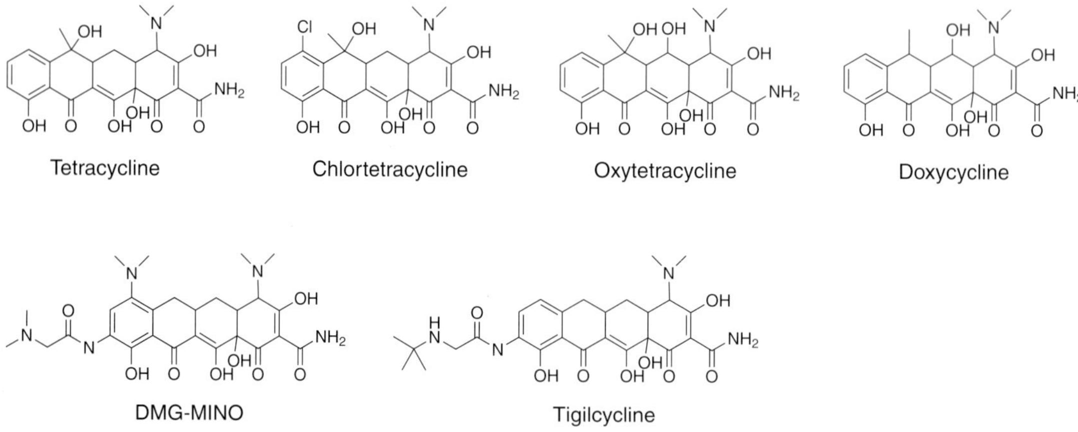

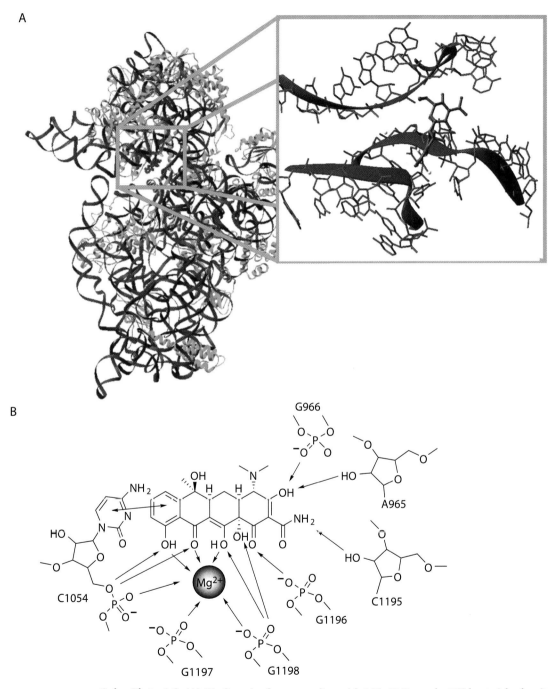

Color Plate 4.6 (A) Binding site for tetracycline with 16S rRNA on the 30S bacterial subunit of the ribosome; (B) interactions of tetracycline with helix 34 of 16S RNA. (From Schlunzen et al. [2001] with permission.)

7 Å deep. As shown in **Color Plate 4.6B**, the oxygens of internucleotide phosphodiester links in 16S rRNA helix 34 form electrostatic interactions, directly or through a Mg ion to the bottom edge of tetracycline. The bound structure suggests that while tetracycline will not block initial binding of aminoacyl-tRNA and the hydrolysis of GTP by the initiation factor EF-Tu that attends the tRNA delivery, the subsequent rotation of aminoacyl-tRNA into the A site would be blocked by tetracycline. The aminoacyl-tRNA would then be prematurely released, terminating that cycle without peptide bond formation.

Because of gradual development of resistant bacteria through the decades of use of tetracyclines and their derivatives (mechanism discussed in chapter 9), their use in first-line therapy has declined. However, programs to attack the resistance mechanisms are ongoing. For example, substitution of tetracycline at the 9-position with glycine amide functionality produces a compound, DMG-DMDOT (Color Plate 4.6B), with activity against tetracycline-resistant *Escherichia coli* and *S. aureus* as well as against methicillin-resistant *S. aureus* (MRSA) (see Chopra and Roberts, 2001, for reviews; Chu et al., 1996).

In addition to the tetracycline efflux mechanisms to be discussed in chapter 9, a second class of resistance is exemplified by the TetO and TetM proteins, which have been termed ribosomal protection proteins. It is now known that TetO and TetM are structural mimics of the elongation factor EF-G, a GTPase responsible for translocation of aminoacyl- and peptidyl-tRNAs from the A and P sites to the P and E sites in translocation cycles. An electron microscopic analysis (Spahn et al., 2001) of TetO binding shows overlap with the EF-G binding site but failure to induce the ribosome conformational changes that lead to translocation. Instead, the GTP hydrolysis by TetO is proposed to disturb helix 34 in 16S rRNA, leading to a lower-affinity conformation for tetracycline and its release. Thus GTPase action is used to pry tetracycline off the ribosome and relieve inhibition of protein biosynthesis.

Aminoglycoside antibiotics

Aminoglycosides have been widely used for decades, following the discovery of streptomycin in 1944 (see Piepersberg, 1997, for review), in many clinical settings for antibacterial infections due to their bactericidal action and their observed synergy with other antibiotics. It has been suggested that the alternate term aminocyclitols should be used to encompass the broad variation of structures in this antibiotic class (Piepersberg, 1997). They are hydrophilic sugars with multiple amino groups, protonated at physiological pH to function as polycations and target accessible regions of polyanionic 16S rRNA on the 30S ribosome, notably the A site for aminoacyl-tRNA binding (Carter et al., 2000). Several generations of aminoglycosides have been tested clinically, with tobramycin, gentamicin, and amikacin (**Fig. 4.6**) prominent family members in contemporary clinical use. The biosynthesis of the two major classes of aminoglycosides is taken up in chapter 14. The aminoglycosides show renal toxicity and ototoxicity, which is a limiting constraint. The ototoxicity is thought to be through aminoglycoside-iron chelates which reduce O_2 to oxygen radicals that destroy hair cells in the ear. Aminoglycosides are potent drugs against gram-negative bacteria but not

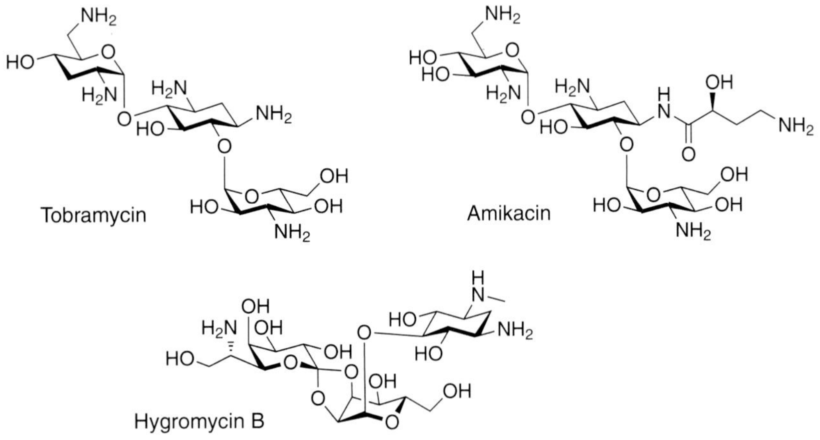

Figure 4.6 Aminoglycoside antibiotics: tobramycin, amikacin, and hygromycin B.

very effective against gram-positive organisms (Scholar and Pratt, 2000), although the combination of aminoglycosides and β-lactams is used to treat enterococcal infections. Synergy with lactam antibiotics is observed, and combinations of gentamicin, tobramycin, or amikacin with ticarcillin or piperacillin are effective against infections caused by *Pseudomonas aeruginosa*. There are several routes of enzymatic deactivation in resistant bacteria, as will be noted in chapter 8.

The structure of an aminocyclitol, hygromycin B, bound to the *T. thermophilus* ribosome 30S subunit has been solved by X-ray analysis (Carter et al., 2000) (**Color Plate 4.7A**) and a single binding site at the top of helix 44, near the A, P, and E sites for tRNA, has been observed. The contacts are to the RNA bases rather than backbone atoms, leading to high sequence specificity, in an extended array. Given the fact that hygromycin B has been reported to sequester tRNA at the A site of the ribosome, it is possible that drug binding blocks a required conformational transition during the peptide bond-forming translocation process. Streptomycin binding at the 16S subunit has been similarly characterized by X-ray analysis (**Color Plate 4.7B**) (Carter et al., 2000), giving powerful insights into how the aminocyclitols bring the translocation steps of protein biosynthesis in the ribosome to a halt.

Linezolid: a synthetic oxazolidinone antibiotic

The only totally synthetic antibiotic in clinical use that blocks protein synthesis at the ribosome is linezolid (Fig. 4.3), approved by the U.S. Food and Drug Administration in 2000. The core pharmacophore of linezolid is the oxazolidinone ring, and it has been described as the first structurally novel antibiotic to be introduced in three decades (Tally and DeBruin, 2000). It has been reported that linezolid-resistant mutants (Kloss et al., 1999) map to the 23S rRNA sites near the peptidyltransferase center, consistent with recent kinetic studies showing that oxazolidinones are competitive inhibitors of both A-site and P-site sub-

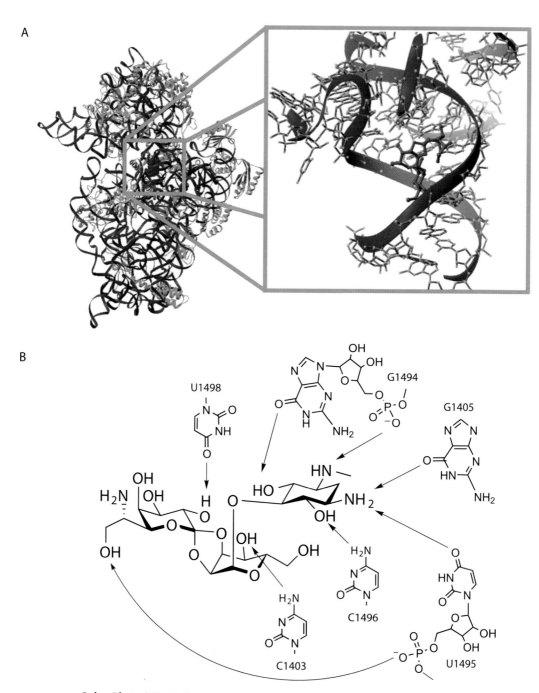

Color Plate 4.7 Binding site for (A) the aminoglycoside hygromycin B and (B) streptomycin with the 16S rRNA of the 30S ribosomal subunit.

strates (Patel et al., 2001). The mechanism of action has been proposed to be occupancy of the P site in the peptidyltransferase center of the ribosome, blocking the first peptide bond-forming step in protein synthesis (Patel et al., 2001). Linezolid is most active against gram-positive bacteria including VRE and has high oral bioavailability. Its therapeutic niche will be clarified as time from approval lengthens and clinical experience accumulates.

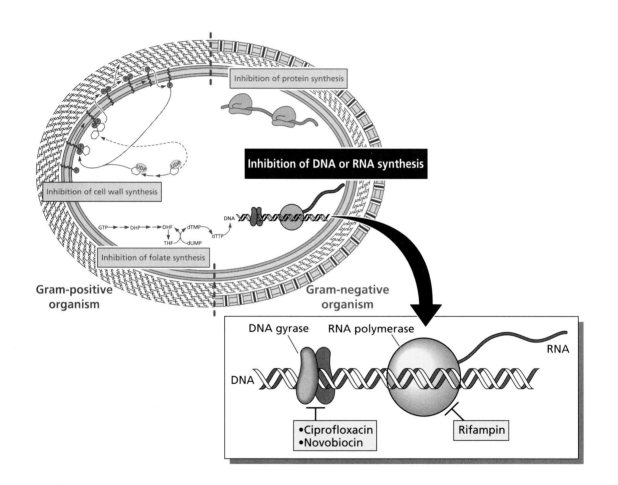

Antibiotics that block DNA and RNA replication.

chapter 5

Antibiotics That Block DNA Replication and Repair: the Quinolones

The third major functional grouping of antibiotics are those that block DNA replication and repair. The figure on the facing page highlights the relevant subsection of Fig. 2.2 and the inhibition of DNA and RNA synthesis by the quinolone and rifamycin classes of antibacterial drugs. The rifamycin class of peptide/polyketide antibiotics are taken up in the next chapter.

DNA gyrase as a target of quinolones and coumarins

Inhibition of DNA replication and repair enzymes would seem a logical target for antibacterial action by natural products elaborated by microbes to kill their neighbors. One such class of molecules, the coumarins, represented by such streptomycete metabolites as novobiocin and coumermycin (**Fig. 5.1A**), has been studied for many years and served to pinpoint enzymes called DNA type II topoisomerases, specifically DNA gyrase (**Table 5.1**), as the killing target (Maxwell, 1997). But it is a synthetic class of molecules, the fluoroquinolones, represented by levofloxacin and ciprofloxacin (**Fig. 5.1B**), that have become very widely used because of their activity against both gram-negative and gram-positive bacteria in urinary tract infections, osteomyelitis, community-acquired pneumonia, and gastroenteritis (Greenwood, 2000; Scholar and Pratt, 2000). The newest generation of quinolones in particular, such as gatifloxacin (**Fig. 5.1C**), have increased potency against gram-positive pathogens (Bronson and Barrett, 2001a). Ciprofloxacin has gained much recent notoriety as an FDA-approved drug for killing *Bacillus anthracis* in anthrax infections.

The DNA topoisomerases change the linking number in supercoiled DNA by making transient cuts in the DNA substrate and then passing the DNA to be relaxed topologically through the transient break, either one strand at a time (type I) or both strands at the same time (type II) (Table 5.1) (see Maxwell, 1997, and Wang, 1996, for reviews). Topoisomerases are essential for cell viability in both prokaryotic cells and eukaryotic cells; the quinolone inhibitors of the

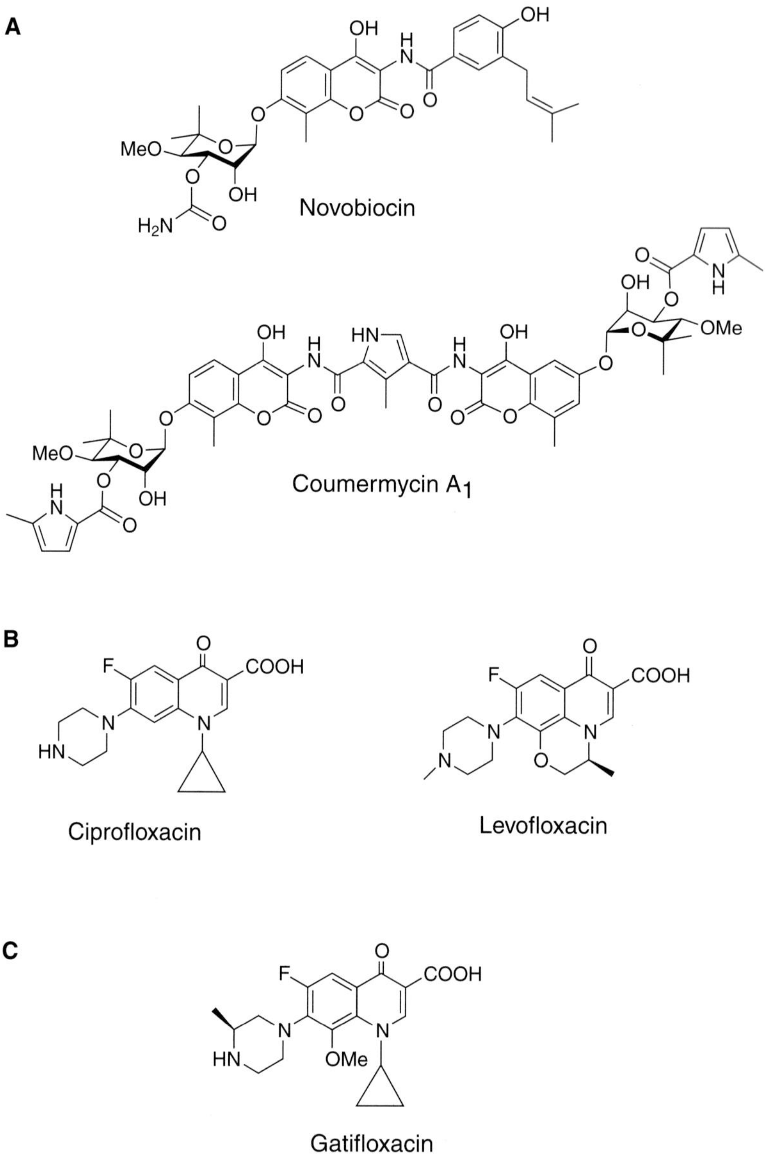

Figure 5.1 Antibiotics that inhibit DNA gyrase and topoisomerase IV: (A) aminocoumarin antibiotics; (B) quinolones (ciprofloxacin and levofloxacin); and (C) new quinolones (gatifloxacin).

type II topoisomerases in bacterial cells are potent antibacterials with enough selectivity to be useful, while inhibitors of the human topoisomerases include camptothecin and etoposide, which are used in cancer chemotherapy to kill rapidly growing tumor cells.

DNA gyrase is thought to be important for controlling DNA topology in DNA replication, recombination, and transcription, while topoisomerase (topo) IV is also implicated in DNA replication and decatenation of linked daughter chromosomes at the end of bacterial DNA replication (Pan and Fisher, 1997).

Table 5.1 Characteristics of *Escherichia coli* topoisomerases

Enzyme	Type	Gene(s)	Major enzyme function
Topoisomerase I	I	topA	Relaxes negative supercoils
Topoisomerase II (DNA gyrase)	II	gyrA gyrB	Introduces negative supercoils; relaxes positive supercoils
Topoisomerase III	I	topB	Decatenates replication intermediates and interlinked DNA dimers
Topoisomerase IV	II	parC parE	Decatenates DNA; removes positive and negative supercoils

Some quinolones have been reported to have selectivity for topo II (DNA gyrase) over topo IV while other quinolones show the reverse behavior. In turn, topo IV has been suggested to be the primary target in pathogenic *Staphylococcus aureus* strains, while in *Streptococcus pneumoniae* strains, the primary target varies between topo II and topo IV (Ng et al., 1996). Takei et al. (2001) recently evaluated 15 quinolones against *S. aureus* MS5935 and subdivided the drugs into three classes. One group (norfloxacin, ciprofloxacin, levofloxacin, and others) seemed to target topo IV preferentially while another class (sparfloxacin, nadifloxacin) was more selective for DNA gyrase (topo II). A third set of quinolones (gatifloxacin, moxifloxacin, and others) targeted topo II and topo IV equally in parent and mutant *S. aureus* strains.

The catalytic cycle of DNA gyrase

The bacterial DNA gyrase found in all bacterial cells is an A_2B_2 heterotetrameric enzyme, encoded by the *gyrA* and *gyrB* subunits. The homologous topo IV isomerase encoded by the *parC* and *parE* genes follows the same mechanism. DNA gyrase introduces negative DNA supercoils in a double-stranded circular DNA substrate. Cozzarelli (1980) noted the requirements for this topological insertion as first a twisting of DNA to produce a conformer with a positive node (**Fig. 5.2**), double-strand cleavage of the back segment, passage of the double-strand through the break, then double-strand resealing on the front side.

The type II catalytic cycle is mechanistically remarkable, and the architecture of the topoisomerases appropriately complex, as revealed by the X-ray structure of a large fragment of the yeast topo II (Berger et al., 1996) (**Fig. 5.3**). After

Figure 5.2 Model for supercoil formation by bacterial DNA gyrase. (From Cozzarelli [1980].)

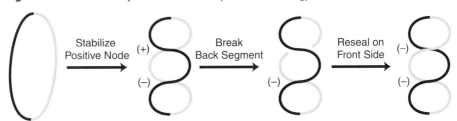

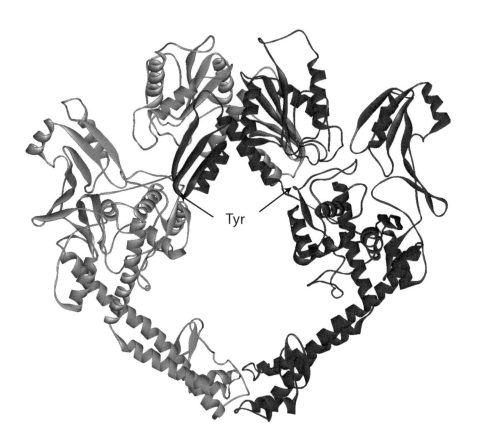

Figure 5.3 X-ray structure of the dimeric 92-kDa fragment of yeast topoisomerase II. (From Berger et al. [1996].)

double-stranded DNA is bound in an initial enzyme-substrate (ES) complex, the nucleophilic phenolic hydroxyl of Tyr_{122} (*Escherichia coli* numbering) on one of the two GyrA subunits attacks an internucleotide phosphodiester bond on one of the DNA strands, cleaving that strand to yield the free 3'-OH end, and captures the 5' end as a covalent DNA-phosphotyrosyl covalent intermediate (**Fig. 5.4A**). Meanwhile, the equivalent Tyr in the second GyrA subunit attacks the internucleotide phosphodiester bond on the other DNA strand four nucleotides downstream to complete the double-strand cut and make the second DNA-5'-P-tyrosyl enzyme intermediate on the complementary strand. This completes the DNA cleavage step and yields two free 3' DNA ends, still base paired elsewhere in the double helix, and two covalently tethered 5'-GyrA DNA ends. The double-strand gap has a four-base overhang, but it is likely that there is local unwinding and widening of the gap, perhaps driven by a conformational change in the enzyme-cut DNA covalent intermediate to widen the gap such that the enzyme can now accommodate passage of the 20-Å-wide double helix (**Fig. 5.4B**) through the gap to effect topological relaxation.

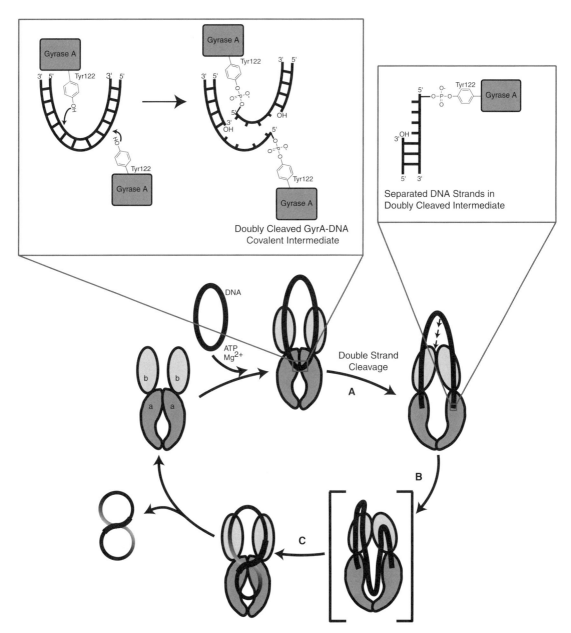

Figure 5.4 Schematic of DNA gyrase mechanism: (A) double-strand DNA cleavage and double covalent enzyme formation; (B) double-strand passage to lower linking number; and (C) religation of doubly cut DNA.

There is a DNA gate region in the yeast topo II enzyme that has corroborated the indicated model for double-strand passage. Clearly there must be dramatic changes in the conformation of both enzyme and passaging DNA at several stages in the catalytic cycle. At this point the enzyme has to autorepair the double-strand breaks, religating the cut DNA. This can be achieved isoenergetically by having each of the 3′-OH ends of the DNA strands attack the 5′-P-

Tyr$_{122}$ enzyme on each GyrA subunit, generate the pentacovalent phosphorane adduct, and then expel the Tyr$_{122}$-phenolate leaving group to religate each strand. This is the enzyme-product (E·P) complex, and the relaxed, intact double-stranded DNA can dissociate or undergo another catalytic cycle of topological linker number reduction: double-strand cuts, DNA passage through the gap in the covalent enzyme-substrate intermediate, followed by double-strand ligation. DNA gyrase is distinct from topo IV and other type II topoisomerases in being able to drive the equilibrium in the other direction, not to relaxation but to supercoiling, by using ATP cleavage to ADP and P$_i$ as the thermodynamic driving force (Maxwell, 1997).

Figure 5.5 Possible mechanism for quinolone base stacking to stabilize the covalent enzyme intermediate with double-strand DNA cuts.

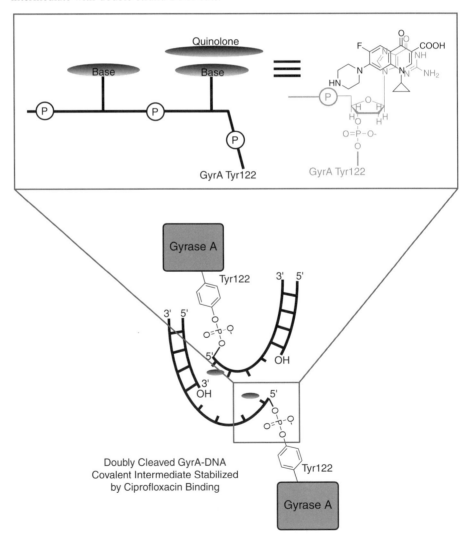

Mechanism of action of quinolone antibacterials

Thousands of fluoroquinolones have been synthesized around the core planar heterocyclic nucleus that gives the family its name (Wolfson and Hooper, 1989). Extensive analysis has indicated that quinolones affect the double-strand cleavage/double-strand religation equilibrium in gyrase and topo IV catalytic cycles, such that the cleaved complex accumulates. The DNA-5'-P-Tyr$_{122}$ covalent intermediates on each GyrA subunit are prevented from reversible religation in the presence of the fluoroquinolones. There has been speculation about whether quinolones speed up the double-cleavage step of bound DNA or selectively slow the double-religation step, without definitive evidence for either interpretation. The mechanism by which quinolones induce the accumulation of the doubly cut covalent DNA-enzyme intermediate is likewise still mysterious. There are hot spots on both the GyrA and GyrB subunits that induce quinolone resistance, suggesting interaction of both enzyme subunits with bound drug, and it is also likely that the quinolone interacts with the cleaved DNA. Speculation on both base-stacking of the planar fluoroquinolone heterocycle and Mg^{2+}-mediated complexation to one or more of the DNA phosphate groups has been advanced, along with the idea that the quinolone ring intercalates at the 3' end of the cut DNA in the space vacated by the displaced 5' portion of the cut DNA (**Fig. 5.5**). X-ray analysis of a quinolone-enzyme-cleaved DNA intermediate may be the only way to resolve this ambiguity and spur quinolone drug design to a new level.

As the quinolone-covalent gyrase-doubly cut DNA intermediate accumulates, the killing action is thought to be from the downstream effect this block has on the progression of DNA replication forks which are halted by this (Maxwell, 1997). It may be that DNA repair machinery is recruited, attempts to come to the rescue, and fails as the recalcitrant quinolone-stabilized gyrase-DNA intermediate persists. This may be the signal that turns on the signaling processes that lead to the rapid killing of bacteria induced by the quinolones.

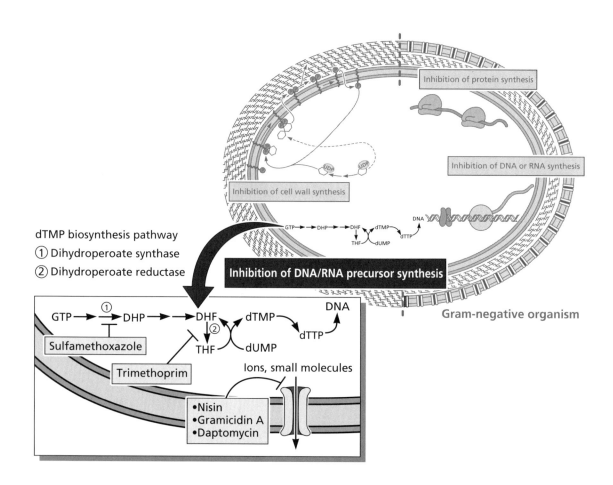

dTMP biosynthesis pathway
① Dihydroperoate synthase
② Dihydroperoate reductase

Inhibition of protein synthesis

Inhibition of DNA or RNA synthesis

Inhibition of cell wall synthesis

Inhibition of DNA/RNA precursor synthesis

Gram-negative organism

GTP → ① → DHP → DHF → ② → dTMP → dTTP → DNA

Sulfamethoxazole

Trimethoprim

THF — dUMP

Ions, small molecules

•Nisin
•Gramicidin A
•Daptomycin

Other validated targets for antibacterial drugs.

chapter 6

Other Targets of Antibacterial Drugs

The chapter opening figure is the fourth such diagram, are in each of chapters 3 through 6, that highlights the major grouping of antibiotics. This includes drugs that block precursor biosynthesis for nucleic acids as well as antibiotics that act to disrupt one or more aspects of bacterial membrane function.

Folic acid metabolism: the target for sulfamethoxazole-trimethoprim

The class of synthetic chemicals in longest use as effective antibacterials are the sulfa drugs, first tested in the 1930s as bacteria-killing molecules. The current generation of sulfa drug is sulfamethoxazole, used in combination with trimethoprim (**Fig. 6.1A**) for the treatment of patients with urinary tract infections and also for AIDS patients with *Pneumocystis carinii* infections (Scholar and Pratt, 2000). This drug pair also validates that combination chemotherapy can be an effective strategy in curing bacterial infections. Each of the drug molecules blocks a step in folic acid metabolism. Sulfamethoxazole blocks the enzyme dihydropteroate synthase in the biosynthetic pathway to folate, while trimethoprim inhibits dihydrofolate reductase (DHFR), a key enzyme providing the pyridime thymidylate for DNA biosynthesis (**Fig. 6.1B**). Thus, the rationale for the combination is synergistic blockade of two different steps in the biochemistry of this essential coenzyme. Bacteria have to make the folate skeleton de novo, while eukaryotes can scavenge folate from dietary sources and transport it into cells. The dihydropteroate synthase target is totally absent from humans while the DHFR has enough structural differences that selective inhibition can be achieved.

Dihydropteroate is assembled enzymatically from the 7,8-dihydropterin pyrophosphate precursor, itself elaborated from the common nucleotide GTP and cosubstrate *p*-aminobenzoate (PABA). The chemical transformation is unusual, the construction of a CH_2-NH amine bond by displacement of an alcoholate oxygen. In this case the oxygen had been converted into a low-energy-leaving

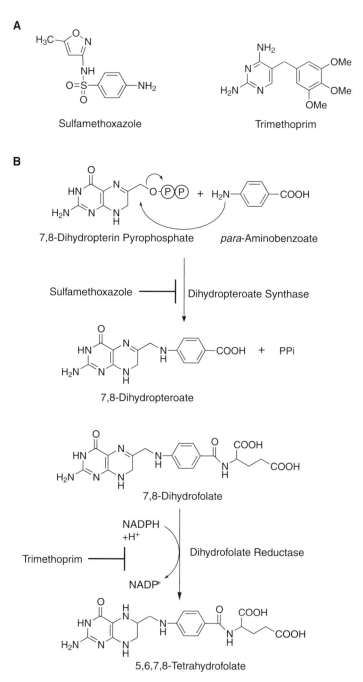

Figure 6.1 (A) The sulfamethoxazole-trimethoprim combination; (B) the reactions catalyzed by the two target enzymes, dihydropteroate synthase and dihydrofolate reductase.

group by its prior derivatization as a pyrophosphate moiety. The product dihydropteroate is subsequently glutamylated enzymatically to complete the enzymatic construction of the folate skeleton (**Fig. 6.2**). When sulfonamide-containing aryl amines were observed to be antibacterial, the mechanism was eventually traced to their mimicry of PABA in this enzymatic reaction. Sulfanilamide (**Fig. 6.3**), for example, is a very simple PABA mimic, while sulfamethoxazole has the heterocycle on the sulfonamide nitrogen. These are competitive inhibitors of PABA in the dihydropteroate synthase active site and can even serve as alternate substrates. When that flux occurs, the pterin has been dragged off to a metabolic dead end since those adducts are not substrates for the pteroyl glutamyltransferases. An X-ray structure of the *Escherichia coli* enzyme complexed with dihydropterin pyrophosphate and sulfanilamide has been determined (Achari et al., 1997), validating the mechanism of inhibition.

Trimethoprim blocks the enzymatic recycling of the folate coenzymes from 7,8-dihydrofolate (DHF) to 5,6,7,8-tetrahydrofolate (THF) oxidation state by DHFR. DHFR is part of a three-enzyme metabolic cycle (**Fig. 6.4**), which converts the CH_2OH group of the amino acid serine into the C_5-CH_3 methyl group of 2'-dUMP (= dTMP) (thymidylate) by the sequential action of serine transhydroxymethylase, thymidylate synthase, and DHFR (Walsh, 1979). Since dTMP is the source of one of the four nucleotides, dTTP, required for DNA replication, the cell growth comes to a halt when its availability is interrupted. The thymidylate synthase reaction is at the center of this cycle, using 5,10-CH_2-THF as cosubstrate with dUMP, to reductively install the transferring CH_2 as the C_5-methyl (CH_3) group, at the expense of oxidation of the THF skeleton to DHF. The cycle cannot run again until DHF is reduced to THF because only in that tetrahydro oxidation state can the N_5 nitrogen attack and capture the $CH_2=O$ released from serine.

DHFR is essential to all cells. Its selective inhibition by trimethoprim in bacteria yields an antibacterial drug, cycloguanil's action on the enzyme in malarial parasites gives an antimalarial agent, and methotrexate's action in human cells leads to its wide use as a drug in cancer chemotherapy regimens. The K_i for bacterial DHFRs for inhibition of DHF reduction by trimethoprim is about 5 to 15 nM, very potent indeed, while the 50% inhibitory concentration for human DHFR is about 300,000 nM (Scholar and Pratt, 2000), a selectivity for bacterial over vertebrate DHFRs of 60,000-fold. X-ray structures of both types

Figure 6.2 The bacterial biosynthetic pathway from GTP to pteroyl-polyglutamate (folate).

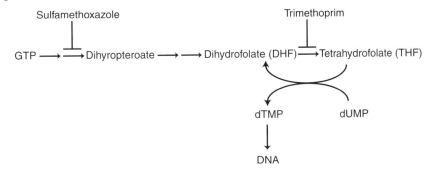

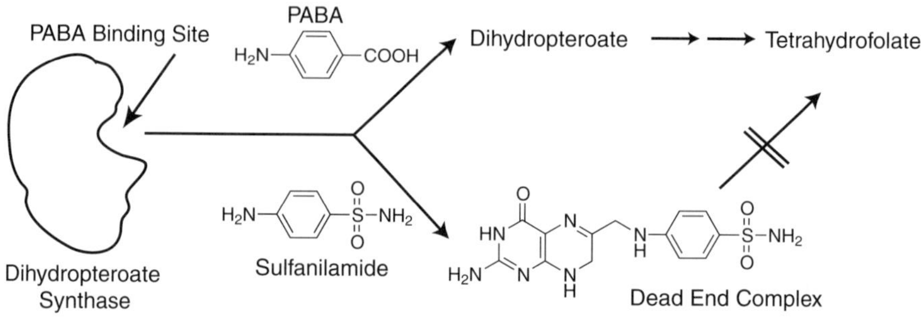

Figure 6.3 Sulfa drugs as competitive inhibitors and alternate substrates for dihydropteroate synthase.

of DHFR enzymes are available to aid in continued efforts to maximize selectivity.

Evaluation of the merits of a dihydropteroate synthase inhibitor and a DHFR inhibitor used in combination suggested that while sulfonamides shut off de novo synthesis of folate, folate pool levels would take several generations to decline, making for a slow killing mechanism. Addition of trimethoprim traps the folate coenzyme molecules in the useless DHF form after each cycle of dUMP synthesis, leading to a rapid depletion of the THF form of the coenzyme. For sensitive bacteria in acute urinary tract infections, trimethoprim can display up to 100-fold synergy with sulfa drugs (Scholar and Pratt, 2000, Table 7-5). The

Figure 6.4 Three-enzyme folate cycle involved in conversion of dUMP to dTMP for DNA biosynthesis.

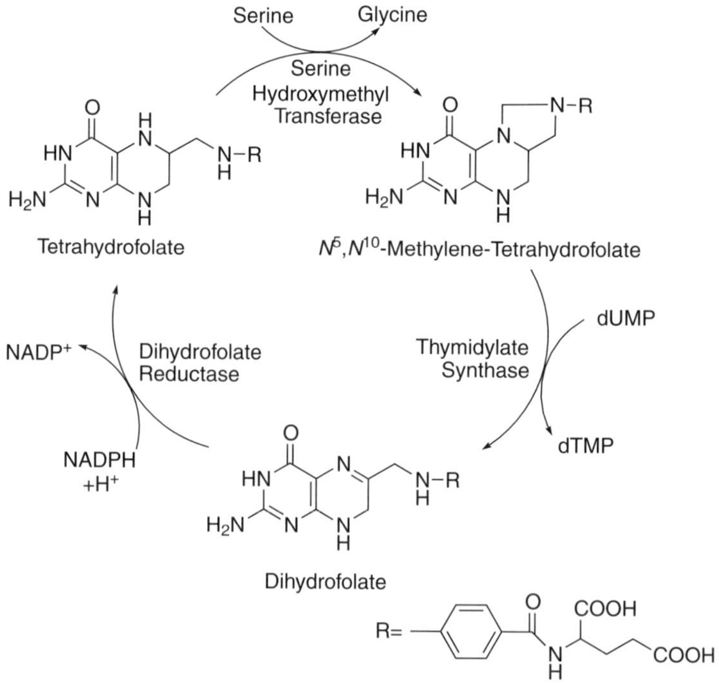

choice of a fixed combination of sulfamethoxazole and trimethoprim (see Scholar and Pratt, 2000) also matched their in vivo half-lives of 9 to 12 hours, so that levels of both drugs would be effective throughout the dosing period. Resistance has developed to both sulfonamides and trimethoprim (chapter 17) after years of clinical use, arguing for the need for structurally novel replacements for drugs for these target enzymes.

Peptide antibiotics

Bacteria, fungi, plants, higher eukaryotes, and even humans make antimicrobial peptides, including magainins from frogs and defensins from humans (Hancock and Chapple, 1999). In previous chapters we have noted the nonribosomally derived peptides that give rise to β-lactam antibiotics, glycopeptide antibiotics of the vancomycin class, the lipoglycopeptides ramoplanin and teicoplanin, and the quinupristin-dalfopristin combination Synercid. These, as we shall note further in chapter 13, incorporate unusual amino acid constituents, are highly modified against protease breakdown, and are often conformationally constrained into a restrictive architecture that underlies specific biologic recognition and function. Analogously, the ribosomally produced peptide microcin B17 has 14 of its 43 backbone peptide bonds modified into eight five-membered ring heterocycles before it reveals its DNA gyrase activity (chapters 14 and 15).

Some bacterial nonribosomal peptides, including bacitracin, gramicidin S, and polymyxin B (**Fig. 6.5**), while cyclized to restrict conformation and preorganize (gramicidin S is a cyclic β-sheet), probably act nonspecifically as membrane-inserting cationic hydrophobic peptides. Bacitracin also has the specific property of inhibiting the recycling of the C_{55} undecaprenol pyrophosphate in bacterial membranes by cation-dependent complexation with the lipid rather than the enzyme. These membrane-seeking properties bring toxic liabilities and all three of these peptides are too toxic, by virtue of membrane disruption in vertebrate cells, to be used systemically. They do have a well-defined niche in topical antibiotic formulations (Anonymous, 1999; Anonymous, 2001). Synthetic cyclic peptides of six to eight residues with alternating D- and L-centers have been reported to stack into β-tubules, insert into bacterial membranes, and increase permeability as antibacterial agents (Fernandez-Lopez et al., 2001).

Polymyxin has a net charge of +5 and goes to both outer membranes and inner membranes of gram-negative bacteria. There are mutations in genes involved in outer membrane lipopolysaccharide metabolism that increase resistance to polymyxin, by incorporation of 4-aminoarabinose moieties on the anionic lipid A to reduce its net charge and electrostatic attraction to polymyxin (Baltz, 1997). A proposed mechanism of action for cationic peptides with gram-negative bacterial membranes is shown in Fig. 6.5. It is possible that all lipopeptide antibiotics have some component of membrane penetration and membrane disruption to their bioactivity. For example, the lipopeptidolactone daptomycin (**Fig. 6.6**), in complex with Ca^{2+} ions, may exert part of its antibacterial activity through such membrane-seeking, surface-active behavior. Another part of the action of daptomycin in particular may be the blockade of biosynthesis of the lipoteichoic acid component of the outer membranes of

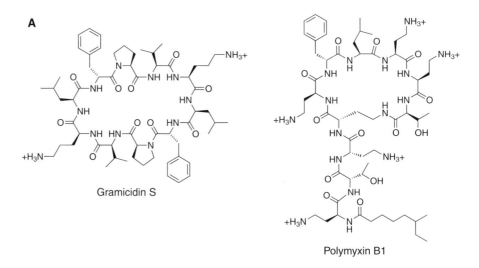

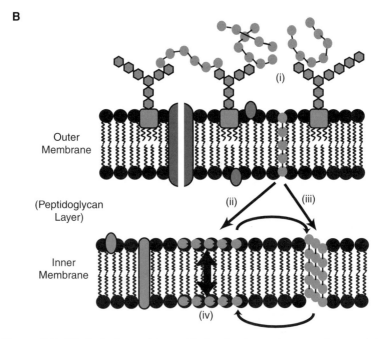

Figure 6.5 (A) Cationic peptide antibiotics that insert into membranes. (B) Schematic for membrane insertion and disruption in gram-negative bacteria (adapted from Hancock and Chapple [1999], with permission). (i) The unfolded cationic peptides associate with the negative charge on the membrane or bind to the cationic binding sites on lipopolysaccharide, to cross the outer membrane. (ii) They then bind to the negative charge on the cytoplasmic membrane surface and the folded, amphipathic peptide inserts into the membrane interface, (iii) aggregating into micelle-like complexes or (iv) flip-flopping across the membrane. Some peptides can then dissociate from the membrane into the cytoplasm.

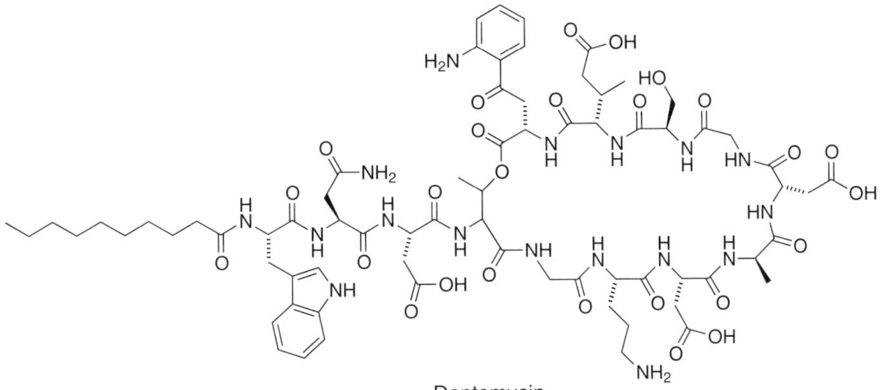

Figure 6.6 Structure of the lipodepsipeptide antibiotic daptomycin.

gram-positive bacteria (Baltz, 1997). Daptomycin is in phase 3 clinical development for the treatment of serious gram-positive infections (Tally and DeBruin, 2000).

In addition to the peptide antibiotics produced by microbes, there are about 500 known peptides produced by multicellular organisms (see Zasloff, 2002, for review) to serve as broad-spectrum antimicrobial agents. These tend to be linear peptides that arise by proteolytic processing of protein precursors and can function as membrane-seeking, amphipathic peptides by presenting hydrophobic and positively charged patches of side chains to insert into microbial membranes at micromolar concentrations. Resistance development may be slow because of the membrane insertion mechanism, while some selectivity may arise because the outer membranes of bacteria have more anionic molecular constituents than do animal cell membranes. Epithelial tissues and cells therein may release a "cocktail" mixture of such peptides that can be important constituents of innate immunity mechanisms. It remains to be seen whether the cationic linear peptides of the magainin and defensin families will be safe enough and efficacious enough to warrant development beyond topical administration (in which systemic toxicity is mitigated by the route of delivery).

A second set of peptides with antibiotic activity are produced by gram-positive bacteria and are classified as lantibiotics because they all contain the unusual double-headed thioether-containing amino acid lanthionine (**Fig. 6.7A**) or its β-methyl lanthionine congener. These are ribosomally produced peptides that are posttranslationally modified to introduce the thioether cross bridges (**Fig. 6.7B**), then cleaved to remove an N-terminal signal sequence (see Hansen, 1997, for reviews; Jack et al., 1995) (see chapter 14 for lantibiotic biosynthesis).

Type A lantibiotics are cationic peptides with an elongated, amphiphilic, corkscrew geometry that insert into membranes and act as depolarizing agents, like the nonribosomal peptides noted above. By contrast, type B lantibiotics are compact, globular peptides (see **Fig. 6.8** for the structure of mersacidin). Both mersacidin and nisin Z (Breukink et al., 1999) have been reported to complex lipid II (chapter 3), although the details of that interaction have not been characterized. Similarly, the 19 residue actigardin blocks cell wall biosynthesis, possibly at the lipid I/II stages.

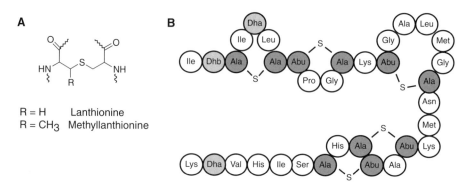

Figure 6.7 (A) Lanthionine and methy lanthionine: key constituents of lantibiotic peptides; (B) five thioether cross-links in the lantibiotic nisin.

A set of proline-rich antibacterial peptides, originally isolated from insects, are thought to be taken up by peptide transporter import pumps into bacterial cytoplasm and interact with their ultimate targets inside bacterial cells. One such peptide is pyrrhocoricin (Kragol et al., 2001), a 20-residue linear peptide, glycosylated on the single threonine by insect producers. The sugar is not required for antibacterial activity and the 20-residue peptide has been shown to bind to the 70-kDa bacterial heat shock chaperone protein DnaK of *E. coli* and block its ATPase activity. This interrupts the folding and chaperone activity of DnaK. Kragol et al. (2001) propose that pyrrhocoricin and the related proline-rich pep-

Figure 6.8 (A) Mersacidin's primary and three-dimensional structure (from Schneider et al. [2000]) and (B) target molecule lipid II.

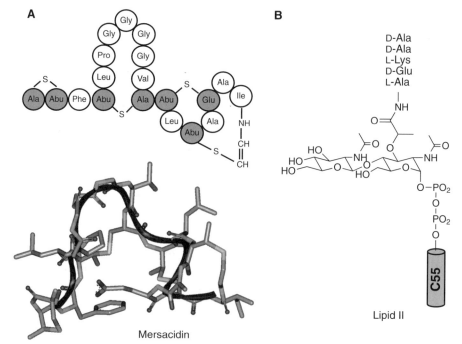

tides drosocin and apidaecin kill bacteria by also blocking the opening and closing of the helical lid of the DnaK binding pocket, required for folding of proteins in that chaperone binding pocket. They argue for the design of strain-specific antibacterial peptides and peptidomimetics based on different DnaK sequences in target pathogens.

Rifamycins in tuberculosis

Rifampin (also known as rifampicin) is a semisynthetic version of rifamycin B (**Fig. 6.9**), a natural product of the ansamycin antibiotic class, isolated originally from an actinomycete known as *Streptomyces mediterranei* and later reclassified as *Nocardia mediterraniae* (Lancini, 1983). The ansa designation means "handle," referring to the aliphatic chain running between the nonadjacent connecting centers on the substituted naphthalene backbone. Rifampin is used clinically only as part of combination regimens for killing the slow-growing pathogen *Mycobacterium tuberculosis*. The drug is an RNA polymerase inhibitor, the only one in clinical use for blocking bacterial transcription. Bacterial RNA polymerase has a core tetramer of $\alpha\beta\beta'\gamma$ subunits and a dissociable σ subunit that directs the core polymerase to transcribe particular classes of genes. Different σ factors can be expressed in bacteria under different growth conditions as one mechanism for targeting the core polymerase to transcribe distinct subsets of genes. Rifampin binds to the β subunit of the RNA polymerase enzyme at an allosteric site, not at the active site (Campbell et al., 2001), as defined by resistant mutations in clinical isolates of *M. tuberculosis* and *M. leprae* (Spratt, 1994; Toney et al., 1998). Recently the X-ray structure of the *Thermus aquaticus* (*Taq*) core RNA polymerase, the 400-kDa $\alpha_2,\beta\beta'\omega$ complex, with bound rifamycin was determined (Campbell et al., 2001) (**Fig. 6.10**) and validated that rifamycin directly blocks the elongating RNA chain by binding in the DNA/RNA tunnel of the β subunit, about 12 Å away from the polymerization site for incoming ribonucleoside triphosphates. Rifamycin is bound by hydrophobic side chain interactions to the residues of the β subunit and by hydrogen bonds to the key −OH groups at positions 1, 2, 9, and 10 of the antibiotic. The structure shows how blockade of RNA elongation by rifamycin binding selectively blocks elongation at the di or trinucleotide stage. Clinical isolates of rifamycin-resistant *M. tuberculosis* have mutations in the β subunit residues that recognize rifamycin, with about three-quarters of the resistance arising from mutations in side chains of residues 406

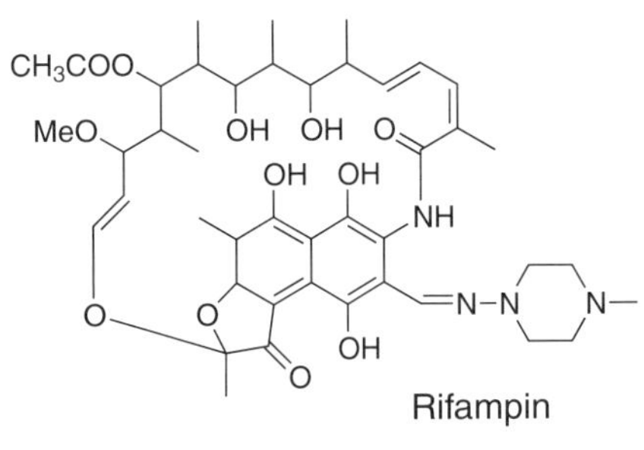

Figure 6.9 Structure of the antituberculosis drug rifampin from the rifamycin family.

CH₃COO

MeO

OH   OH   O

OH   OH

NH

O

O

OH

=N−N   N−

O

Rifampin

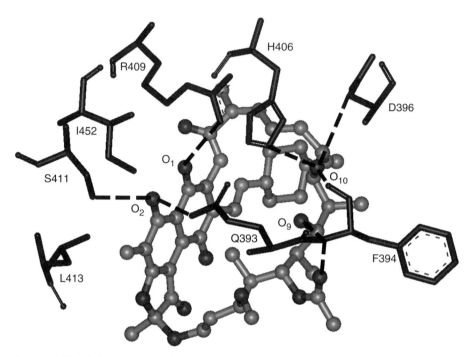

Figure 6.10 Binding site for rifamycin on its target protein, the β subunit of RNA polymerase. (From Campbell et al. [2001].)

and 411 (Spratt, 1994). Resistance development is relatively rapid if rifampin is used as a single agent (Heep et al., 2000), explaining one of the reasons combination therapy is used for tuberculosis (see chapter 11 of Scholar and Pratt, 2000). The 50% inhibitory concentration against mycobacterial RNA polymerase is in the range of 0.005 to 0.1 μg/ml and eukaryotic RNA polymerases are at least 100-fold less sensitive.

Antibiotic Resistance

S ECTION III EXAMINES RESISTANCE TO THE ANTIBACTERIAL DRUGS that have been discussed in section II. Chapter 7 introduces the topic of resistance in antibiotic-producing microbes that must have developed self-protection mechanisms to avoid self-destruction during antibiotic production. The three main intrinsic mechanisms in antibiotic producers are (i) inactivation of the antibiotic, (ii) efflux of the antibiotic, and (iii) modification of the susceptible molecular target. These mechanisms presage the resistances that are acquired as susceptible bacterial pathogens become resistant. Chapter 8 takes up inactivation of antibiotics in the context of both β-lactam hydrolysis and aminoglycoside covalent modification. Chapter 9 details the families of efflux pumps found in pathogens. Chapter 10 describes protein modifications in penicillin-binding proteins that underlie the methicillin-resistant *Staphylococcus aureus* (MRSA) phenotype, 23S rRNA methylation prevalent in erythromycin resistance, and reprogramming of peptidoglycan intermediates in vancomycin resistance.

Bacteria	Case mortality	% of isolates resistant to:	
		Methicillin	Vancomycin
Coagulase-negative Staphylococcus	21%	80%	—
Staphylococcus aureus	25%	30%	—
Enterococcus faecalis	25%	—	20%

Incidence and severity of methicillin- and vancomycin-resistant infections. —, not determined.

chapter 7

Natural and Producer Immunity versus Acquired Resistance

During the five to six decades that antibiotics have been in ever-widening therapeutic use, the development of antibiotic resistance has followed. The historical observations are that whenever a new antibiotic, broader-spectrum forms of an existing antibiotic, or a new class of antibiotics is introduced into widespread use in people, clinically significant resistance appears. It may be a matter of months (penicillin resistance was detected as early as 1945) or it could take years: vancomycin resistance took almost 30 years (1987) after clinical introduction (1954). The long delay was probably due to limited use of vancomycin in the first 25 years, but as it advanced to the front of the therapeutic line, resistance emerged. Also, as we shall note in chapter 10, while clinically significant resistance to β-lactams can occur through the action of one gene product, the hydrolytic β-lactamase, the vancomycin-resistant enterococcus (VRE) phenotype requires a five-gene resistance cassette to have been assembled. The outbreaks of resistance can be geographically scattered and to all major antibiotic classes. **Figure 7.1** shows a map of outbreaks in the United States over the 11-year period from 1983 to 1994 of pathogens resistant to both penicillins and cephalosporins, to the fluoroquinolone ciprofloxacin, to the macrolide erythromycin, and to the glycopeptide vancomycin. Similar patterns have continued since 1994, as noted in chapter 17.

Antibiotic-resistant bacteria are selected for in hospital settings much more rapidly than in the outside community. In hospitals there is intensive and essentially constant exposure of bacteria to antibiotics. In these microenvironments there is selective pressure for antibiotic-resistant bacteria to maintain those determinants, survive, and even dominate the bacterial populations. In a large population of bacteria, say 10^8, exposed to a drug there is a competition between death of all the bacteria and the development of rare mutations that confer resistance. Given the short replication time for bacterial division (as short as 20 to 30 minutes) and a typical frequency of one error per 10^7 bases as their DNA polymerases copy DNA, then the 100 million bacteria will contain about 10 mutants in the population. If these mutations are randomly dispersed in the

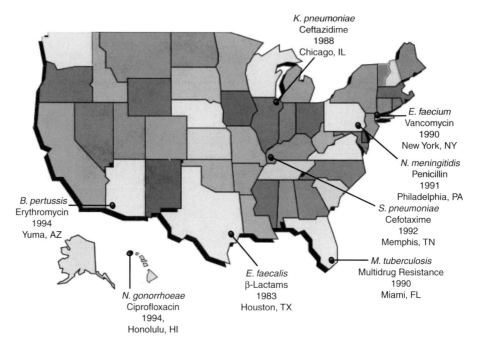

K. pneumoniae
Ceftazidime
1988
Chicago, IL

E. faecium
Vancomycin
1990
New York, NY

N. meningitidis
Penicillin
1991
Philadelphia, PA

B. pertussis
Erythromycin
1994
Yuma, AZ

S. pneumoniae
Cefotaxime
1992
Memphis, TN

M. tuberculosis
Multidrug Resistance
1990
Miami, FL

E. faecalis
β-Lactams
1983
Houston, TX

N. gonorrhoeae
Ciprofloxacin
1994,
Honolulu, HI

Figure 7.1 Recent outbreaks of antibiotic-resistant bacteria in the United States over the 11-year period 1983–1994.

genome of a bacterium the size of *Escherichia coli*, with 3,000 genes, then 0.3% (10/3,000) of the genes will have one mutation. If one of these gene mutations is in a target for an antibiotic and the mutation confers some degree of resistance that renders that bacterium less sensitive, then it will have a selective survival advantage. As its sensitive neighbors die, it will persist and have space to grow and dominate the culture and may disseminate effectively.

In addition to the independent evolution of point mutations to create resistant genes, such genes can be collected on transposable DNA elements (transposons), which are mobile genetic elements that can transpose between DNA sequence elements on both larger mobile elements (plasmids) and on bacterial chromosomes (conjugative transposons) (see Whittle et al., 2001). Thus the genes responsible for the VanA phenotype of vancomycin resistance are typically on a transposon embedded in a plasmid in VRE cells. Analogously, the TEM-1 β-lactamase is often carried by the transposon TN3 (Amyes, 2001). Plasmid-sized DNA elements can integrate into specific attachment sites on chromosomes to create antibiotic resistance islands, as found in *Salmonella enterica* serovar Typhimurium DT104 (chapter 17) and methicillin-resistant *Staphylococcus aureus* (MRSA) (this chapter). This allows multiple resistance genes to be maintained together. All these routes ensure rapid spread and stable maintenance of collections of antibiotic resistance genes through bacterial populations. Jain et al. (1999) have suggested that extensive horizontal gene transfer is a continuing process among bacteria.

The resistant strain will continue to be selected for by the continuing presence of antibiotic in the microenvironment, e.g., in a hospital ward. **Figure 7.2**

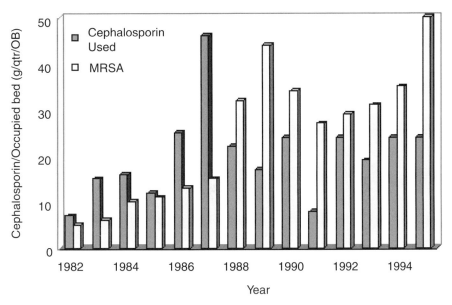

Figure 7.2 Time course for development of resistance to cephalosporins by MRSA.

shows a clear temporal relationship over a 12-year period between the use of cephalosporins and the emergence of MRSA (Hiramatsu et al., 2001). The effects can also occur in a compressed period of time. For example, patients admitted for surgery are given antibiotics prophylactically and then for a few days post-surgery to reduce the probability of infectious complications. A study of nasal culture history in such a patient population indicated (**Fig. 7.3**) that on pread-mission, a given aliquot size contained 10^5 *S. aureus* bacteria, essentially all sen-sitive to methicillin (MSSA) (Schentag et al., 1998). Following surgery and medication with cefazolin (a cephalosporin), 90% of the patients were sent home at 2 days postsurgery, without infectious complications. The nasal bacterial count was down 100-fold to 10^3 and was a mixture of sensitive, borderline-resistant, and resistant staphylococci. For those patients who remained in the hospital and

Figure 7.3 Progression of bacterial populations in surgical patients from MSSA to MRSA to VRE in a three-week time frame. (From Schentag et al. [1998], with permission.)

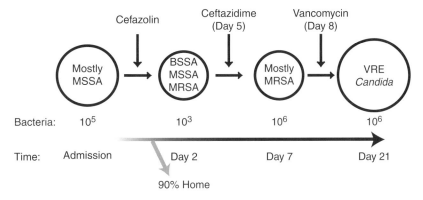

were switched on day 5 to a second cephalosporin (ceftazidime), when assayed on day 7, the bacterial count was up 1,000-fold to 10^6 and was mostly MRSA. These patients were then switched to a 2-week course of vancomycin, and for those still in the hospital on day 21, the nasal cultures revealed 10^6 VRE as well as some *Candida*. Because of the short division time of bacteria, the selection for drug-resistant, life-threatening pathogens can be remarkably rapid.

By the above argument, bacterial resistance to antibiotics is not a matter of if but only a matter of when. This logic argues there will be a constant need for cycles of new antibiotic discovery and development. As soon as an antibiotic is introduced for widespread clinical use, the selection of resistant organisms will start and a finite therapeutic lifetime will occur before resistance of pathogens becomes sufficiently widespread to lessen that drug's efficacy. Then one needs the next generation (e.g., we are at fourth-generation cephalosporins and third-generation erythromycins) or whole new classes of antibiotics. This is further emphasized by the list of bacteria in **Table 7.1** that are resistant to different classes of antibiotics used clinically. A recent review of methods to assess antimicrobial resistance is provided by Cockerill (1999).

Many antibiotics that have been developed into approved antibacterial drugs have MICs or sometimes 50% inhibitory concentrations, often in Petri plate assays, in the range of 1 μg/ml. For antibiotics with molecular weights $\leq$500

Table 7.1 Bacterial resistance to various classes of clinically used antibiotics

Antibiotic	Structural class	Target	Mutant/ plasmid	Efflux	Porin	Inact.	Target alteration
Ampicillin	Penicillin	E	+/+	✓	✓	✓	✓
Ceftriaxone	Cefalosporin	E	+/+	✓	✓	✓	✓
Imipenem	Carbapenem	E	+/+	✓	✓	✓	✓
Fosfomycin	Phosphonic acid	E	+/+		✓	✓	
Gentamicin	Aminoglycoside	R	+/+	✓		✓	✓
Chloramphenicol	Phenylpropanoid	R	+/+	✓		✓	✓
Tetracycline	Polyketide (II)	R	+/+	✓		?	✓
Erythromycin	Macrolide	R	+/+	✓		✓	✓
Clindamycin	Lincosamide	R	+/+			✓	✓
Synercid	Streptogramin	R	+/+	✓		✓	✓
Telithromycin	Ketolide	R	+/+	✓		✓	✓
Ciprofloxacin	Fluoroquinolone	D	+/+	✓			✓
Vancomycin	Glycopeptide	E	+/+				✓
Sulfisoxazole	Sulfonamide	M	+/+				
Trimethoprim	—	M	+/+				
Rifampin	Ansamycin	P	+/+			✓	✓
Fusidic acid	Steroid	T	+/+	✓			✓
Linezolid	Oxazolidinone	R	+/−				✓
Novobiocin	Coumarin	D	+/+				✓
Isoniazid	—	M	+/−				
Pyrazinamide	—	M	+/−				
Nitrofurantoin	Nitrofuran	M	+/−			(✓)	
Polymyxin	Peptide	E	+/−	✓			✓
Capreomycin	Peptide	R	+/−			✓	✓
Mupirocin	Pseudomonic acid	T	−/+				✓

Inact., inactivation; D, replication; E, envelope; M, metabolism; P, RNA polymerase; R, ribosome; T, translation; —, nonstandard structural class.

Adapted from a poster on Mechanisms of Antibiotic Action and Resistance, C. Walsh, J. Trauger, P. Courvalin, J. Davies (2001), *Trends in Microbiology, The Lancet Infectious Disease, Current Opinion in Microbiology, Trends in Molecular Medicine*.

g/mol, this would be in the ~2 μM concentration range. For example, 50% inhibitory concentrations of oxazolidinones for susceptible organisms are in the 1-μg/ml range, while tetracycline MIC around 0.1 μg/ml may be typical. Vancomycin MICs are often in the range of 0.1 to 0.5 μg/ml; MICs of quinolones such as ciprofloxacin are reported in the range of 0.05 to 0.5 μg/ml for sensitive organisms. Macrolides of the erythromycin family may have MIC in the 0.01- to 1-μg/ml range. The potencies have translated into useful dosing ranges for treatment of infections in humans. As bacteria develop antibiotic resistance determinants and mechanisms, when MIC reach or exceed 8 μg/ml the organisms may be classified as moderately resistant. Organisms for which MICs are above 32 μg/ml are generally viewed as clinically resistant to the antibiotic.

How do antibiotic producers escape their own destruction?

Many observers have noted that antibiotic producers could be vulnerable to their own chemical weapons of destruction and must have worked out strategies for their own protection and immunity. This has led to the general concept that antibiotic resistance genes and mechanisms must have coevolved with antibiotic biosynthetic capability for a just-in-time self-protection scheme. In the next section of this chapter we shall examine some examples that give insights into the variety of autoprotection mechanisms in play in antibiotic-producing bacteria and the timing that switches on the protection as antibiotic production is geared up.

As a general rule, though, natural product antibiotics are made by enzymatic machinery within the bacterial cell and the mature antibiotics are secreted molecules. The armamentarium of almost every antibiotic producer examined includes one or more transmembrane protein pumps presumably dedicated to pumping out the antibiotics as they are made and before they accumulate to harmful concentrations within a producing cell (**Fig. 7.4A**). When clusters of

Figure 7.4 Schematics of antibiotic efflux protein pumps: (A) general scheme; (B) function for lantibiotic efflux pumps.

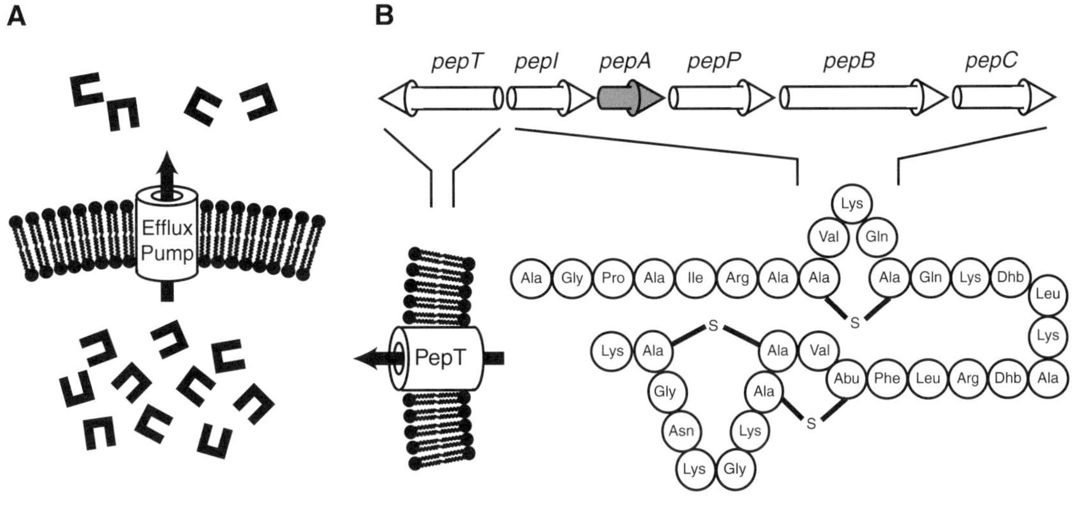

antibiotic genes have been sequenced, one typically finds genes encoding such antibiotic export pumps within the transcriptional clusters, ensuring the coordinate production of the export pumps as antibiotics roll off the enzymatic assembly lines (chapters 12 and 13). In the Pep lantibiotic cluster, *pepA* encodes the precursor to the antibiotic peptide and *pepT* encodes the pump. It may be that many of the later stages of antibiotic assembly, e.g., the protein complex making the lantibiotic proteins (Brotz and Sahl, 2000) (**Fig. 7.4B**), are physically coupled at the membrane to the pumps such that antibiotic synthesis and vectorial efflux from the bacterial cytoplasm are kinetically coupled.

The existence of genes in antibiotic producers that provide intrinsic resistance or autoimmunity also provides a potential reservoir for those genes to be acquired, through a variety of gene transfer mechanisms, by the bacteria that are the intended targets of the antibiotics. Given the resistance gene reservoirs, various transposon and other mobile genetic elements as transfer vehicles, and the selective pressure for bacteria to survive in an antibiotic-rich microenvironment once they have acquired the resistance genes, it is to be expected that the pilfering of such genes would be a common route to acquired resistance. We shall see this exemplified particularly clearly when comparing the autoprotection strategy in the glycopeptide antibiotic producers and the mechanism by which pathogenic enterococci become VRE.

Self-protection in macrolide producers

Streptomycetes produce most of the polyketide-based macrolide antibiotics, including erythromycin, the related 14-membered ring macrolide oleandomycin, and the 16-membered ring homolog tylosin (**Fig. 7.5**; also see Table 11.1). Oleandomycin differs from erythromycin in enzymatic modification of the C_8-CH_3 locus into an epoxide. Three strategies for self-resistance have been described in

Figure 7.5 Structures of the macrolide antibiotics erythromycin A, oleandomycin, and tylosin.

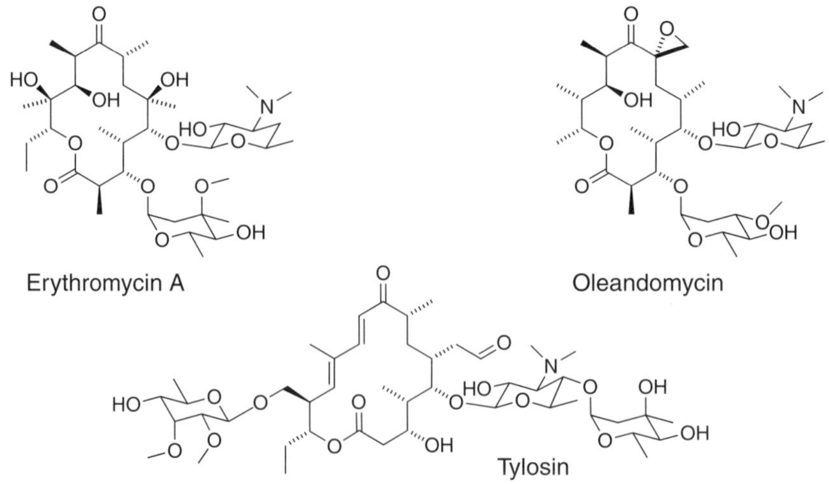

Erythromycin A

Oleandomycin

Tylosin

macrolide producers and presage acquired resistance mechanisms in human pathogens. The first is modification, by tandem action of the Erm methyltransferase, of the exocyclic amino group of one adenine residue, A_{2058}, in 23S RNA for mono- or dimethylation. This N-methylation interferes with erythromycin binding to that high-affinity site on the 50S ribosome (**Fig. 7.6**; also see chapter 4). This resistance mechanism is found in erythromycin and tylosin producers (Fierro et al., 1987; Quiros et al., 1998) but not in oleandomycin producers. The second mechanism is the expression of macrolide-exporting transport proteins, powered by ATP hydrolysis and known as ATP-binding cassette (ABC)-type proteins. Confirmation of export pump function comes from overexpression of these ABC proteins and increased resistance to erythromycin, discussed further in chapter 9.

The third self-resistance mechanism, deciphered by Salas and colleagues (Quiros et al., 1998) in the oleandomycin-producing *Streptomyces antibioticus*, involves enzymatic modification at the end of the biosynthetic pathway to keep the macrolide in an inactive form while it is still intracellular. The complementary piece of this elegant self-protection scheme is that once the macrolide is secreted it runs into an extracellular enzyme that converts it into its active form. The transient protecting group is a glucosyl group, encoded by a glucosyltransferase, *oleI*, within the oleandomycin gene cluster. **Figure 7.7** shows that the OleI glucosyltransferase uses UDP-glucose and regiospecifically glucosylates the C_2-OH of the desosamine sugar attached to C_5 of the macrolactone. The resulting macrolide, now with a desosaminyl-2,1-glucose disaccharide at C_5, is inactive as an antibiotic, because the newly introduced glucosyl moiety blocks binding to the 50S ribosome subunit. This causes no harm to the producing *S. antibioticus* cell, even if it accumulates to otherwise toxic levels before being pumped out by the ABC-type pump, the OleB protein.

On the other hand, this tri-sugar-containing macrolide, even when shipped out, is also not toxic to any of the neighboring bacteria. To reactivate the antibiotic properties of this latent glucosyl-oleandomycin, *S. antibioticus* also secretes a glycosidase, the product of the *oleR* gene (Quiros et al., 1998), that now re-

Figure 7.6 Enzymatic mono- and dimethylation of A_{2058} in 23S rRNA in macrolide resistance. SAM, *S*-adenosylmethionine; SAH, *S*-adenosylhomocysteine.

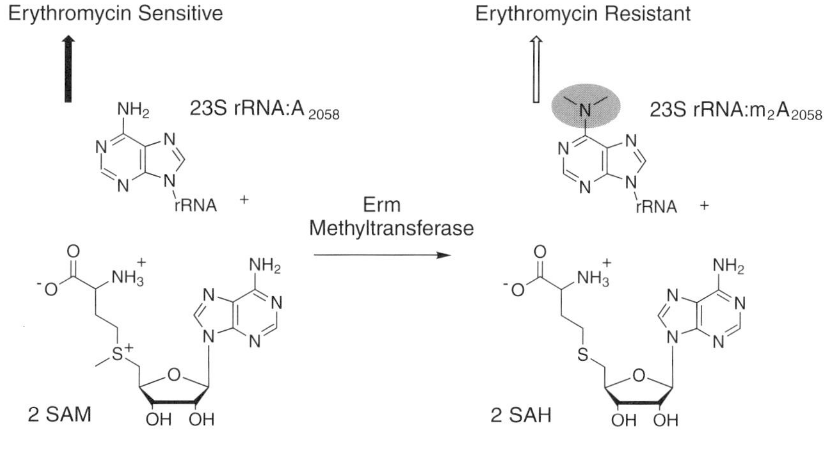

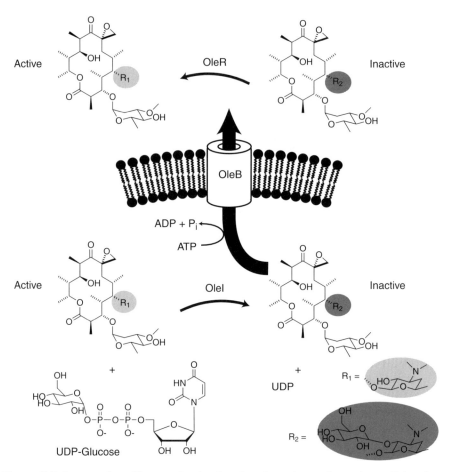

Figure 7.7 Strategy for self-protection by the oleandomycin producer: intracellular gluco-sylation to an inactive precursor of oleandomycin by OleI, export by the OleB pump, and extracellular reactivation by the glycosidase OleR.

moves the glucose hydrolytically and produces the form of oleandomycin capable of binding to the 50S ribosome (Fig. 7.7). This decoy mechanism does not seem to be followed by the erythromycin-producing *Saccharopolyspora erythraea*, although the EryBI enzyme is homologous to OleR, suggesting that at one time such a glycosylation (inside)/deglycosylation (outside) strategy may have been in play for some phase of the evolution of erythromycin producers, perhaps before export pumps became optimized or the rRNA methylase strategy, found in *S. erythraea* but not *S. antibioticus*, evolved. One last feature of note in *S. antibioticus* self-protection is the observation that the OleB transport/efflux pump will pump out the glucosyl-oleandomycin. It has yet to be determined if OleB has a lessened affinity for oleandomycin itself, once deglycosylated in the extracellular milieu by OleR. A lower affinity for reuptake of oleandomycin would bias the net flux of the pumping system to send glucosyl-oleandomycin out of the cell.

It remains to be seen how general is the cloaking of intracellular antibiotics by glycosylation or other covalent modification. There is a hint that off-pathway intermediates in the bahlimycin glycopeptide antibiotic biosynthetic pathway are glycosylated in what may be a protective surveillance function (Bischoff et al., 2001). As will be discussed in chapter 14, there is cognate logic in streptomycin producers where intracellular streptomycin is inactive because of phosophorylation which is enzymatically removed after export.

Self-protection in aminocoumarin producers

In the biosynthesis of the gyrase-targeted aminocoumarin antibiotics (chapter 5), it is likely that the coumarin ring is generated relatively early in the biosynthetic pathway (see chapter 14), and several of the intermediates on the way to novobiocin could therefore be potential inhibitors of the target enzyme, DNA gyrase. The producing streptomycetes have been tested for DNA gyrase susceptibility and intrinsic resistance has been observed. These determinants map to the GyrB subunit and are likely to be mutations in the extended ATP binding site which desensitize the site to novobiocin binding (Tsai et al., 1997). This is a case of modification of the target by mutation to retain essential catalytic activity while decreasing binding affinity for the inhibitor. It presages the molecular bases of resistance of pathogens by GyrB mutations after exposure to coumarin antibiotics (Maxwell, 1997).

Protection during antibiotic production in vancomycin family producers

The vancomycin group of antibiotics are made by streptomycetes and by actinoplanes. The gene clusters for a vancomycin analog, chloroeremomycin (van Wageningen et al., 1998) (**Fig. 7.8**), and for the variant heptapeptide scaffold of teicoplanin (Sosio et al., 2000) and A47934 (Pootoolal et al., 2002), a nonglycosylated version of teicoplanin from *Streptomyces toyocaensis*, have been sequenced. The details of biosynthetic logic will be covered in chapter 13 and the mechanisms of acquired resistance in VRE in chapter 10, where we note that the VRE phenotypes arise from a reprogramming of the enzymes that make the D-Ala-D-Ala terminus of the peptidoglycan pentapeptide precursor to the D-Ala-D-lactate terminus. This reduces affinity to vancomycin by 1,000-fold (Bugg et al., 1991) and creates the autoimmunity.

This dipeptide to depsipeptide transition is effected by three enzymes encoded by *vanH, vanA,* and *vanX* (see Walsh et al., 1996b). VanH, VanA, and VanX equivalents are found in tandem both in the S. *toyocaensis* producer of A47934 (Marshall et al., 1998) and in the teicoplanin producer, near the teicoplanin biosynthetic cluster (Sosio et al., 2000). The physiology of *S. toyocaensis* has been examined. Cultures are sensitive to A47934 during logarithmic growth when the antibiotic is not being made. During that phase of the life cycle the peptidoglycan chains have D-Ala-D-Ala produced by a normal D-Ala-D-Ala ligase. When the organism enters stationary phase and turns on the genes for antibiotic production it also presumably turns on *vanH, vanA,* and *vanX* to make D-Ala-D-lactate, by the A protein, known as ddlM in this organism (Marshall et al.,

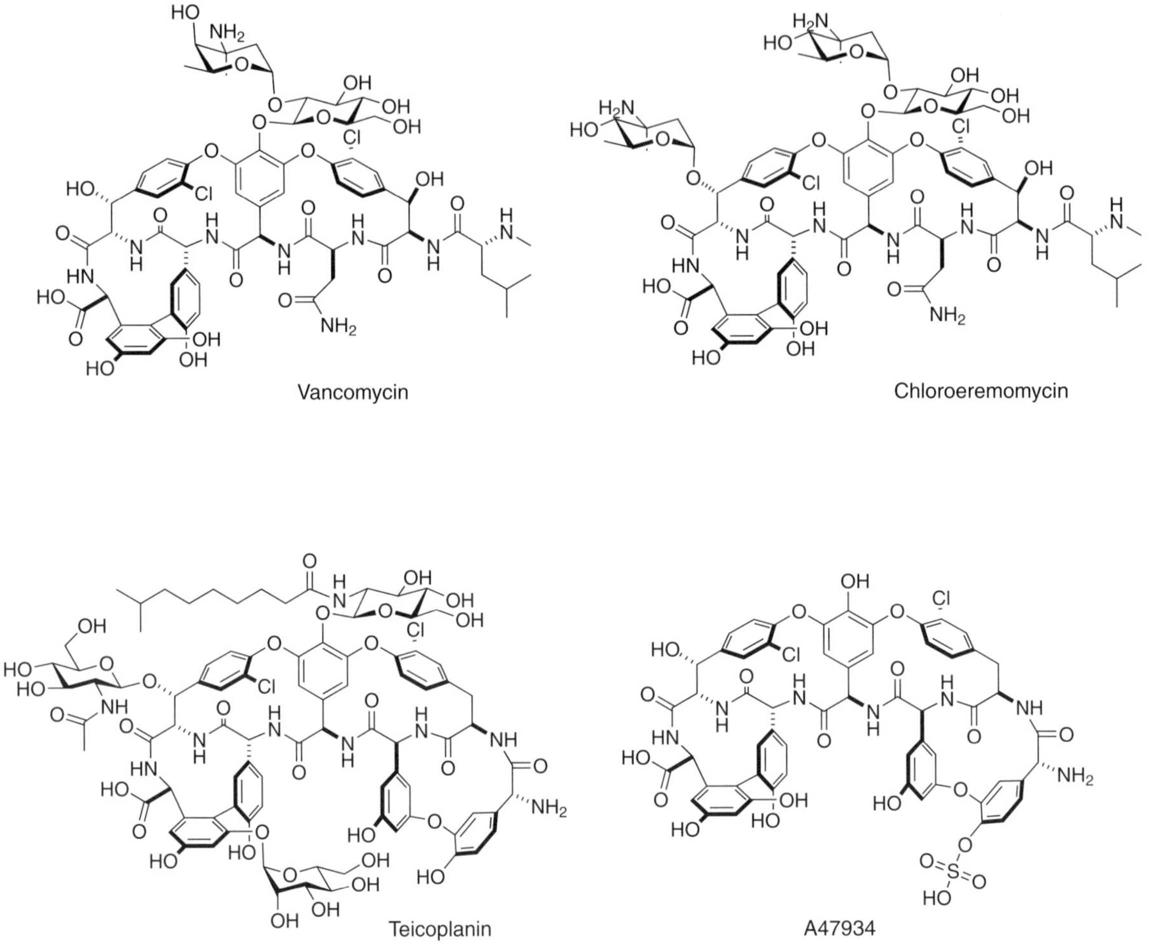

Figure 7.8 Glycopeptide antibiotics.

1997), reprogramming the peptidoglycan layer to insensitivity to the antibiotic which is now being made (**Fig. 7.9**). So the switch occurs in a temporally co-ordinated manner.

Protective strategy in mitomycin producers

Streptomyces lavendulae produces the quinone-containing mitomycin C, which is an antitumor antibiotic by virtue of DNA covalent cross-linking at CpG se-quences in both DNA strands after bioreduction (**Fig. 7.10A**) of the benzoqui-none portion of the drug by electrons possibly from the respiratory chain of the bacteria. The producing streptomycetes contain a resistance gene, *mcrA*, that encodes a flavoprotein with a flavin adenine dinucleotide cofactor that partici-pates in redox-mediated protection. Mitomycin C is a prodrug in its oxidized form at the completion of its biogenesis. It has to undergo one or two electron

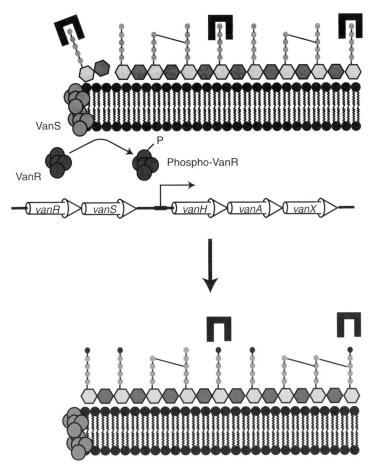

Figure 7.9 Regulation of the *vanH, vanA,* and *vanX* genes allows cell wall restructuring to glycopeptide antibiotic insensitivity at the time of antibiotic biosynthesis.

reductions and then it can rearrange by loss of methanol to a quinone methide which now can covalently capture DNA. It is proposed that the redox-active flavin adenine dinucleotide coenzyme of the McrA immunity protein reoxidizes the reduced form of mitomycin in competition with, and thereby blocking the rearrangement to uncover, the DNA-reactive functional group (**Fig. 7.10B**). This is the first example reported of a redox-mediated self-protection mechanism in an antibiotic producer (Sheldon et al., 1997) and emphasizes the amazing biochemical and physiological diversity that antibiotic producers will employ to provide self-immunity to their own chemical weapons.

Natural and acquired resistance in pathogenic bacteria

The examples in the four previous sections typify the kinds of acquired resistance mechanisms that have presumably been accumulated, some from the reservoir

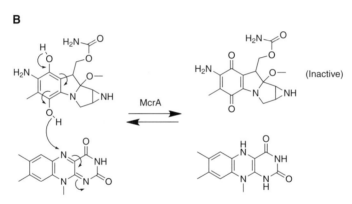

Figure 7.10 Mitomycin: (A) DNA cross-linking by bioreductive alkylation; (B) enzymatic reoxidation of dihydro mitomycin by McrA for self-protection.

of these genes in producer organisms and some from evolution of housekeeping enzymes to new specificities, by soil bacteria in the hundreds of millions of years that they have coevolved with antibiotic-producing neighbors.

The complete genomes of two major human bacterial pathogens, *Pseudomonas aeruginosa* and MRSA, reveal different strategies (Kuroda et al., 2001; Stover et al., 2000) for self-protection.

P. aeruginosa strains can be key culprits in life-threatening bacteremias in burn patients, causative agents in urinary tract infections in patients with urinary catheters, and causative agents in pneumonias in patients on respirators and in chronic lung infections of cystic fibrosis patients. But these pseudomonads are generally much less virulent than *S. aureus* and are often termed opportunistic pathogens because they establish dangerous infections largely in immunocompromised hosts. Two attributes in the first analysis of *P. aeruginosa* PA01's 5,570 open reading frames occasioned note (Stover et al., 2000). First were the large number of two-component regulatory systems—55 sensor kinases, 89 response regulator transcription factors, and 14 sensor/response regulator fusion proteins—allowing for flexibility in response to environmental inputs and integration of many extracellular inputs that may make *P. aeruginosa* a successful pathogen (Rodrigue et al., 2000). Second were the large number of outer membrane porins: 19 members of the OprD family, 34 genes of the TonB family, and 18 in the OprM gene family. Pseudomonads are intrinsically resistant to many or most antibiotics because they keep a low net intracellular concentration. The porin capacity is one index, and a correlated one is the efflux pumps (described in detail in chapter 9), with 10 of the Mex subfamily and 20 of the Bmr subfamily. These pumps can confer protection against foreign compounds, ensuring that the efflux/influx ratio is far on the side of efflux.

The highly virulent MRSA and VRSA (vancomycin-resistant *S. aureus*) strains of *S. aureus* are more virulent human pathogens in disease and have been termed professional pathogens in contrast to the opportunistic ones noted in the preceding paragraph. The genomes of the N315 MRSA strain and the Mu50 VRSA strain (Kuroda et al., 2001) reveal 3 or 4 large gene clusters in pathogenicity islands and 26 to 28 gene clusters on mobile genetic elements. Both types of clusters reflect mechanisms for *S. aureus* to pick up genes from elsewhere and bring them on board for virulence and pathogenicity functions. All told, transposons and insertion sequences make up 7% of these *S. aureus* genomes, while they are almost totally absent from another gram-positive bacterium, *Bacillus subtilis*. Almost 70 novel open reading frames implicated in virulence were found by Kuroda et al. (2001). In terms of specific gene pickups that lead to antibiotic resistance, **Table 7.2** (based on data of Kuroda et al., 2001) notes nine genes that confer antibiotic resistance in the MRSA and VRSA strains, including both *blaZ* and *mecA* for β-lactam resistance (chapters 8 and 10), *ermA* for erythromycin resistance (chapter 10), *ant4′*, *ant9′*, and *aacA-aphD* for aminoglycoside modification (chapter 8), and *tetM* and *qacA* for drug efflux pumps (chapter 9). A pathogenicity island termed SSC$_{mec}$ contains the *bleO, blaZ, mecA, ermA*, and *ant4′* genes and is obviously a genetic determinant that contributes to the prowess of MRSA strains as professional pathogens (Hiramatsu et al., 2001).

Susceptibility of bacteria to antimicrobial drugs has classically been tested with phenotypic assays that evaluate the ability of an antibiotic to inhibit bacterial growth under some specified set of growth conditions. Various formats can be used, including disk diffusion, agar dilution, and broth dilution assays.

Table 7.2 Antibiotic resistance genes found in MRSA

Protein	Gene	Antibiotic resistance
Bleomycin resistance protein	*bleO*	Bleomycin
PBP2′	*mecA*	β-Lactams
β-Lactamase	*blaZ*	β-Lactams
rRNA methylase	*ermA*	Erythromycin, pristinamycins
O-NucleotidylTransferases	*ant 4′, ant 9′*	Aminoglycosides
Acetylase-phosphotransferase	*aacA-aphD*	Aminoglycosides
TetM efflux protein	*tetM*	Tetracyclines
QacA	*qacA*	Antiseptics

For example, disks impregnated with a colorless cephalosporin substrate, nitrocefem, can be used to test for β-lactamase-producing bacteria. Ring opening of the lactam ring of nitrocefem leads to elimination of an electron-rich nitroaromatic substituent that is yellow, so the assay scores development of color. More recently, methods that directly evaluate antibiotic resistance genotype rather than phenotype susceptibility have come into common use (reviewed by Cockerill, 1999), especially when prevalent mutations causing resistance are known and can be readily screened for genetically. For example, the presence of the *mecA* gene in staphylococcal clinical isolates is readily detected by PCR of a region of *mecA*, followed by gel electrophoresis analysis. The presence of the *mecA* gene is readily detected on ethidium bromide staining of the gel (Cockerill, 1999). Analogously, the acquisition of genes of the TEM β-lactamase family, conferring clinical resistance to ceftazidime, cefotaxime, and aztreonam (see chapters 3 and 8) in *Klebsiella pneumoniae* and *E. coli* isolates, is readily detected by PCR and restriction fragment length polymorphism analysis (Cockerill, 1999). Rifampin resistance in *Mycobacterium tuberculosis* is detected by PCR analysis of mutations in the *rpoB* gene encoding the β subunit of RNA polymerase while fluoroquinolone resistance is detected by PCR analysis and DNA sequencing of fragments of the *gyrA* gene encoding the GyrA subunit of DNA gyrase, accounting for effectively all clinical quinolone resistance (Cockerill, 1999).

In summary, the three methods of self-protection in macrolide antibiotic producers noted in **Fig. 7.11** set the stage for the understanding of the three major strategies for bacterial resistance to antibiotics that we will explore in chapters 8 to 10. The first is exemplified by temporary inactivation of the intracellular form of the antibiotic in oleandomycin producers. The cognate in resistant pathogens can be characterized as enzymatic destruction of the antibiotic, as is the case for β-lactam hydrolysis, aminoglycoside modification, and fosfo-

Figure 7.11 Analogy between producer self-protection and bacterial resistance.

Method of Producer Self-Protection	Temporary Intracellular Inactivation of Antibiotic	Efflux of Produced Antibiotic	Modification of Target in Producer
Example of Macrolide Producer Self-Protection	Glycosylation of Oleandomycin 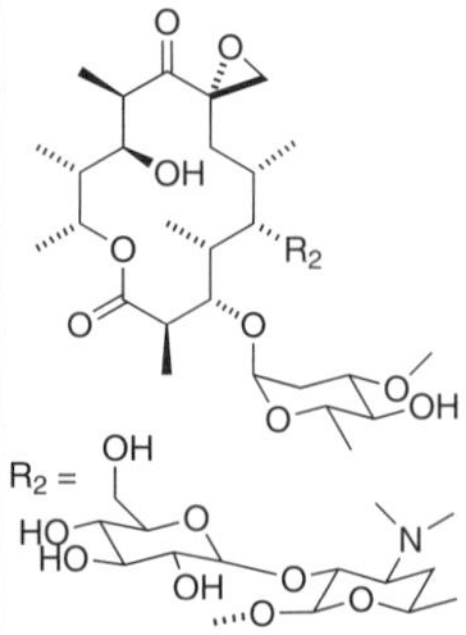	Export of Oleandomycin by OleB 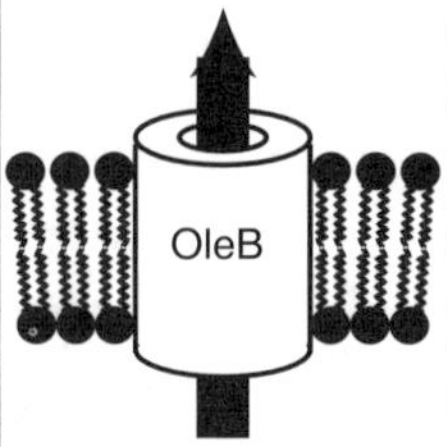	Dimethylation of Adenine in 23S rRNA 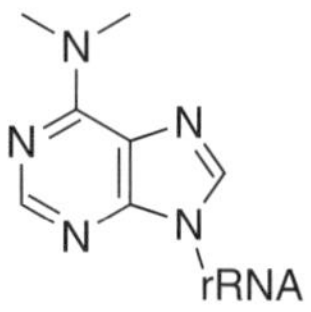 / 23S rRNA:m$_2$A2085
Analogous Mode of Clinically Observed Bacterial Resistance	Inactivation of Antibiotic	Efflux of Antibiotic	Modification of Target

mycin capture by glutathione (chapter 8). The efflux of intracellular antibiotics practiced by producers, and shown by the action of the OleB pump, presages a general strategy to lower the ambient concentration of antibiotics in the cells of the pathogens. This can be a combination of lowered rates of influx, operating mostly in gram-negative bacteria through the outer membrane permeability barrier, coupled to accelerated rates of efflux. The efflux pump proteins can have narrow specificity, e.g., TetB protein for tetracycline, or have broad selectivity, as with the multidrug efflux pump proteins (chapter 9). The third mechanism is for the pathogen to alter the target protein such that it still retains its physiologic function but now has a lower affinity for antibiotic binding (chapter 10). In some erythromycin producers this strategy is enacted by A_{2058} N,N-dimethylation in 23S rRNA to make a resistant 50S ribosome subunit. The alteration of the target in pathogens can be mutations in or replacement of the wild-type protein, as in penicillin-binding proteins, or an alteration in a substrate for a key enzyme, as in the D-Ala-D-lactate reprogramming.

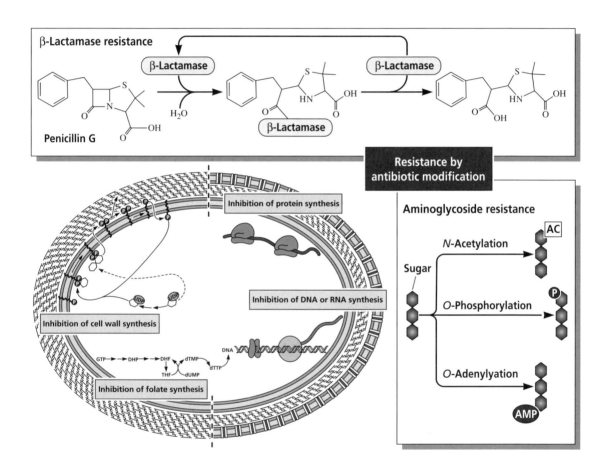

Modification of antibiotics by resistant bacteria.

chapter 8

Enzymatic Destruction or Modification of the Antibiotic by Resistant Bacteria

This chapter is the first of three (chapters 8 to 10) that deal with the three major mechanisms of antibiotic resistance. The chapter opening figure highlights a section of Fig. 2.2 that summarizes resistance by antibiotic modification.

Enzymatic inactivation of antibiotics occurs with several of the natural product antibiotic classes but has not yet been observed as a major route of resistance development for the classes of synthetic antibacterials: the sulfamethoxazole-trimethoprim combination, the fluoroquinolones, or the oxazolidinones. This may reflect the time of exposure of the bacteria to natural products, putatively hundreds of millions of years, versus the 70 years or less for the man-made antibiotics. This criterion might suggest that novel antibiotics made from libraries of synthetic chemicals not found in nature might also be slow to be inactivated by this mechanism. Of course, the other two inactivation routes, discussed in chapters 9 and 10, can still be in effect.

The most widespread mode of clinical resistance development to β-lactam antibiotics is the expression of β-lactamases that hydrolyze the antibiotic (Bush and Mobashery, 1998). An estimate of $30 billion in annual economic loss to the U.S. population from disease caused by lactamase-producing resistant bacteria has been suggested (Palumbi, 2001).

Destruction of β-lactam antibiotics by β-lactamases

Subfamilies of β-lactamases: active-site serine hydrolases

β-Lactamases hydrolyze the four-membered β-lactam ring in both penicillin and cephalosporin classes of antibiotics as well as the carbapenem series (**Fig. 8.1**). They thereby destroy the antibacterial activity by deactivating the chemical warhead in the molecule, the strained β-lactam that is the chemically reactive acylating group for modifying the active-site serine side chains in the penicillin-binding proteins (PBPs) (the transpeptidases and carboxypeptidases in peptidoglycan [PG] cross-linking; see chapter 3). β-Lactamase activity was detected

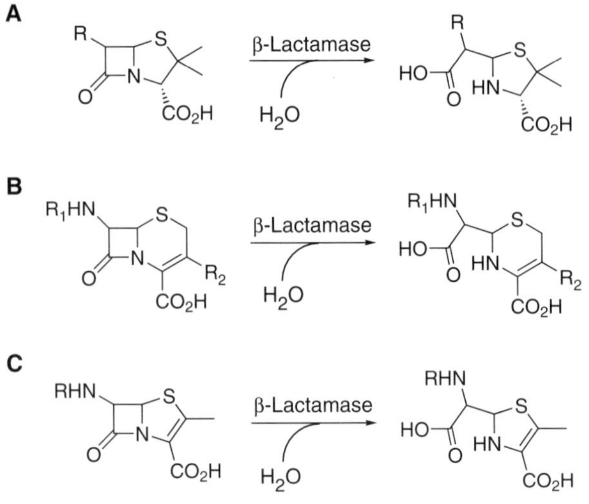

Figure 8.1 Hydrolytic ring opening and deactivation of (A) penicillins, (B) cephalosporins, and (C) carbapenems by β-lactamases.

a few years before clinical use of penicillins in humans, indicating its presence in soil bacteria that combat the natural product penicillins, and by now more than 190 β-lactamases have been described (Bush and Mobashery, 1998; Thomson and Moland, 2000) and categorized into class A, B, C, and D lactamases (Bush and Mobashery, 1998). The A, C, and D classes are active-site serine enzymes, with architectural and mechanistic similarities to the PBPs (Knox, 1995; Knox et al., 1996) (**Fig. 8.2**), suggesting evolution from PBPs.

In the A, C, and D classes of β-lactamases the same type of penicilloyl-O-Ser enzyme covalent intermediates are formed as in the catalytic cycle of PBPs that attack and open the β-lactam ring and become self-acylated (chapter 3). There is no such covalent penicilloyl enzyme intermediate in the catalytic cycle of the zinc-dependent, class B β-lactamases (**Fig. 8.3**), which has consequences for the failure of class B lactamases to be inhibited by certain drugs, as discussed below.

It has been argued that PBPs may have evolved into β-lactamases several times independently, to generate the different orientations of the active-site residues in the class A, C, and D lactamases (see Massova and Mobashery, 1998, and references therein). The difference in outcome, turnover for lactamases and suicide for the PBP transpeptidases, arises from the different lifetimes of the acyl-O-Ser enzymes. In the penicloyl-PBP acyl enzyme of the transpeptidases, water is excluded from the active site and hydrolysis is exceedingly slow (with a half-time for deacylation of about 90 min, compared to 4 ms for the N-acyl-D-Ala-D-Ala acyl enzyme from the normal substrate) (Fisher et al., 1980), and correspondingly the penicilloyl enzyme lifetime is long, the transpeptidase activity is inactivated, and PG cross-linking is halted (see Knox et al., 1996, for review). By contrast, the lactamase activity involves hydrolysis, not capture of the acyl-O-Ser enzyme by an amine; water has free access to the penicilloyl-O-Ser enzyme active site; and the deacylation rate is fast (**Fig. 8.4**), 2,600 s^{-1} for the TEM-1 β-lactamase. The net difference in deacylation rates of the same penicilloyl-O-Ser enzyme intermediate in the lactamase versus PBP is 2.7×10^7. The β-lactamase-producing gram-negative bacteria secrete this surveillance en-

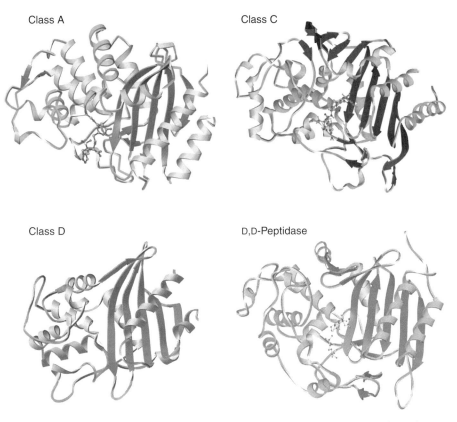

Class A   Class C

Class D   D,D-Peptidase

Figure 8.2 Structures of class A, C, and D β-lactamases and homology to the fold of a D,D-peptidase (PBP). (Figure provided courtesy of J. Knox.)

Figure 8.3 Hydrolysis of the β-lactam ring of penicillins by class A, C, and D lactamases involves covalent penicilloyl enzyme intermediates, while the class B zinc-dependent lactamases carry out direct attack by water

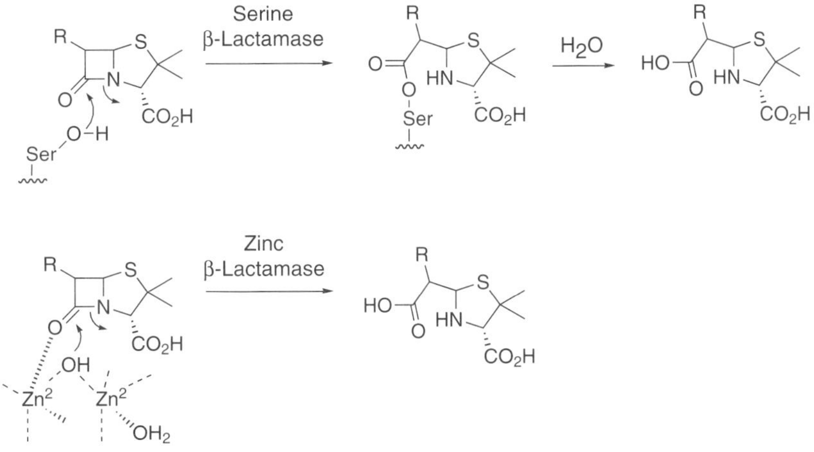

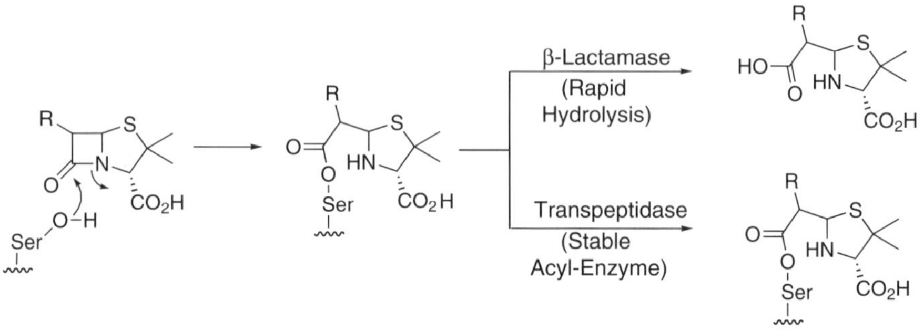

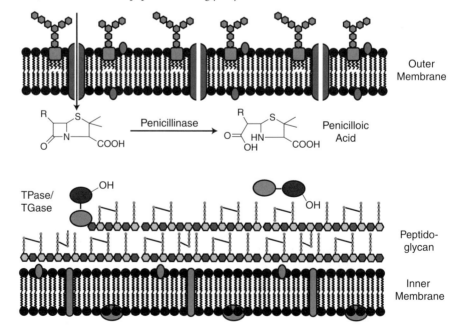

Figure 8.4 Different half-lives for the acyl-*O*-Ser enzyme intermediates control the outcomes with penicilloyl-PBPs versus penicilloyl-β-lactamases.

zyme into the periplasmic space so that β-lactam antibiotics have to run the gauntlet of these hydrolytic enzymes to reach their targets at the surface of the cytoplasmic membrane (**Fig. 8.5**), making it difficult for any intact β-lactam to reach its target PBP.

The TEM-1 (Datta and Kontomichalou, 1965) and related TEM-2 lactamases, prevalent in gram-negative bacteria such as *Escherichia coli* and *Klebsiella pneumoniae*, are encoded on transposable elements and move rapidly through these populations (Amyes, 2001; Wiedemann et al., 1989). Extended-spectrum cephalosporins such as ceftazidime and cefotaxime (structures in **Fig. 8.6**; also see chapter 3) were developed to combat resistance provided by TEM-1 and

Figure 8.5 β-Lactamases in bacterial periplasms hydrolyze penicillins and cephalosporins before they reach their target PBPs at the outer face of the cytoplasmic membrane. TPase/TGase, bifunctional transpeptidase/transglycosylase.

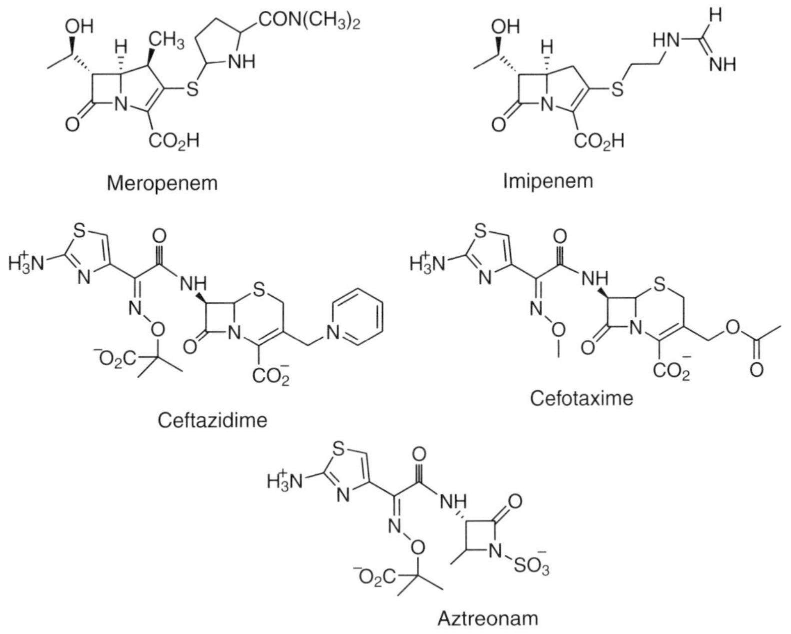

Figure 8.6 Structural modifications in the acyl side chains of β-lactam antibiotics to build in slow processing by β-lactamases. X-ray analysis of extended-spectrum β-lactam antibiotics with β-lactamase cocrystals shows that the bulky side chain provides a severe steric block to proper positioning of water in the deacylation step and accounts for the very low k_{cat}s for enzymatic hydrolysis.

related β-lactamases. In turn, subsequent widespread cephalosporin use is thought to have selected for sequential mutants in the TEM lactamases, producing hydrolytic enzymes that have improved affinity for these lactam scaffolds and consequent extended-spectrum lactam resistance (see chapter 17). Many variants of TEM lactamases have been isolated and sequenced (e.g., Goussard and Courvalin, 1999). For recent progress on determination of X-ray structures of lactams and lactam-derived acyl enzyme intermediates in the active site of lactamases, see Beadle et al. (2002).

Metallo-β-lactamases: zinc-hydrolases

The class B lactamases are zinc enzymes, containing a binuclear zinc cluster in the active site (Toney et al., 1998; Wang et al., 1999). Unlike the class A, C, and D lactamases, which do lactam ring opening via covalent acyl enzyme intermediates, noted above, the class B lactamases use zinc to activate a water molecule and catalyze its direct addition to the β-lactam ring (Fig. 8.3). The metallo-β-lactamases of type B are thought to be the major subclass of hydrolases that destroy the carbapenem antibiotics such as imipenem (thienamycin) and meropenem (Fig. 8.6). The widespread use of carbapenems in Japan (Kurokawa et al., 1999) has probably been instrumental in selecting for the IMP-1 version of the zinc-β-lactamase first seen in *Serratia marcescens* and *Pseudomonas aeruginosa*. The carbapenemases have been described as a clinical problem in waiting for pseudomonal infections (Livermore and Woodford, 2000) but the more acute carbapenem resistance problems in *P. aeruginosa* are efflux mechanisms, as noted in chapter 9. Many bacteria that produce the type D metallohydrolases also produce a type A, C, or D lactamase (Rasmussen and Bush, 1997); for example, a clinical isolate of *S. marcescens* carries a type A and a type B *bla* gene on a plasmid (Yano et al., 1999).

Strategies to neutralize β-lactamases

Two approaches have been taken in the decades since lactam-resistant clinical isolates began to diminish the efficacy of penicillins and cephalosporins as antibiotics. The first has been to develop semisynthetic β-lactams which were slower substrates for attack by the hydrolytic lactamases. The second approach has been to screen for inhibitors and inactivators of lactamase activity and then combine these molecules with a β-lactam. Both approaches have had their successes (Knowles, 1985).

Slow substrates for the β-lactamases

The search for semisynthetic lactams that would retain antibiotic potency but have increased efficacy against lactamase producers turned up several molecules that made it into clinical therapeutics. Essentially this is a strategy to find substituents on the β-lactam chemical warhead that block β-lactamase binding and/or catalysis but do not interfere with PBP binding and acylation. The monocyclic monobactams fall in this category, aztreonam being an example (Fig. 8.6). Also in this category are the carbapenems, with sulfur in the five ring replaced by carbon (Fig. 8.6); this is the strategy in meropenem and the thienamycin component of imipenem. Much of the effort to find lactams that would not be hydrolytic substrates for lactamases focused on the cephalosporin 4/6 bicyclic scaffold with alteration of the acyl side chain, leading to such drugs as ceftazidime and cefotaxime (Fig. 8.6) that extended the spectrum of antibiotic activity to treat many β-lactamase-producing pathogens (also see chapter 3). The rationale was that the bulky acyl side chains on the 7-amino group of the lactam scaffold permitted formation of the acyl-PBP intermediates but blocked the processing by the lactamases.

The carbapenem thienamycin is a slow substrate for lactamase hydrolysis for a different reason. The initial acyl enzyme intermediate (**Fig. 8.7**) can undergo a double-bond isomerization in the five-membered ring from a Δ^2 to a Δ^1 olefin, an eneamine to an imine, and the latter form of the acyl enzyme is slower to hydrolyze by 50,000-fold (see Massova and Mobashery, 1998). The stereochemistry of the hydroxyethyl side chain, 1R instead of the usual 1S in penicillins, is also an important determinant for blocking water attack in the deacylation of the acyl enzyme. Slow hydrolysis means a long lifetime for the acyl enzyme, so the catalytic destructive power of the lactamase is slowed by orders of magnitude while it is tied up in this covalent adduct. A variant of thienamycin, meropenem (see Mitscher et al., 1999) (Fig. 8.6), has a methyl substituent on the five ring to provide steric hindrance to binding to β-lactamases.

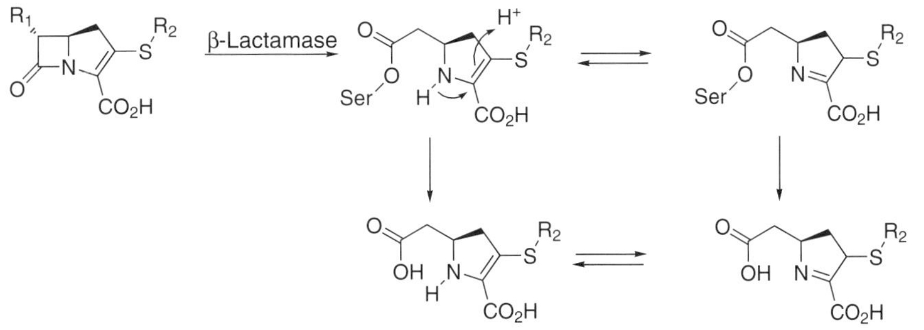

Figure 8.7 Isomerization in the ring-opened acyl enzyme form of the carbapenem thienamycin during destruction by β-lactamase slows net hydrolysis.

Mechanism-based inactivators of β-lactamases

The second approach, screening for mechanism-based inactivators of the β-lactamases, builds philosophically on the pattern seen with the carbapenem-derived acyl enzyme. It relies on a rearrangement of the initial acyl-O-lactamase covalent enzyme into an alternate covalent acyl enzyme form that is much slower to hydrolyze. Two types of mechanism-based inactivators, or suicide substrates, for β-lactamases have become clinically successful (Maiti et al., 1998). The first is the natural product clavulanate, an enol ether–β-lactam from *Streptomyces clavuligerus*, and the second class is represented by penicillin sulfone and a substituted congener tazobactam (**Fig. 8.8**). In both clavulanate and the penicillin sulfones, the structural alterations weaken the C-O bond or the C-S bond, respectively, such that the attack by the lactamase active-site serine-OH on the β-lactam carbonyl leads also to fragmentation of the 4/5 ring junction, as indicated in **Fig. 8.9**. Subsequent rearrangements can follow, with further fragmentation and accumulation of a rearranged acyl enzyme (Massova and Mobashery, 1998). The net effect in the clavulanate processing by class A β-lactamases is a conjugated acyl enzyme much less rapidly attacked by water for deacylation and a comparable deactivation of the subsequent ring-opened acyl enzyme derived from the penicillin sulfones. More-stable acyl enzyme forms of lactamase means this antibiotic-destroying catalyst is tied up in knots as long as the acyl enzyme persists. Neither clavulanate nor the sulfones are potent enough as β-lactam antibiotics to be used on their own so they are used in combinations (Fig. 8.8). For example, the combination of amoxicillin and clavulanate, known as Aug-

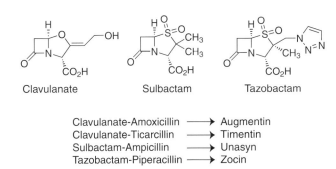

Clavulanate   Sulbactam   Tazobactam

Figure 8.8 Clavulanate, sulbactam, and tazobactam: mechanism-based inactivators of β-lactamases.

Clavulanate-Amoxicillin ⟶ Augmentin
Clavulanate-Ticarcillin ⟶ Timentin
Sulbactam-Ampicillin ⟶ Unasyn
Tazobactam-Piperacillin ⟶ Zocin

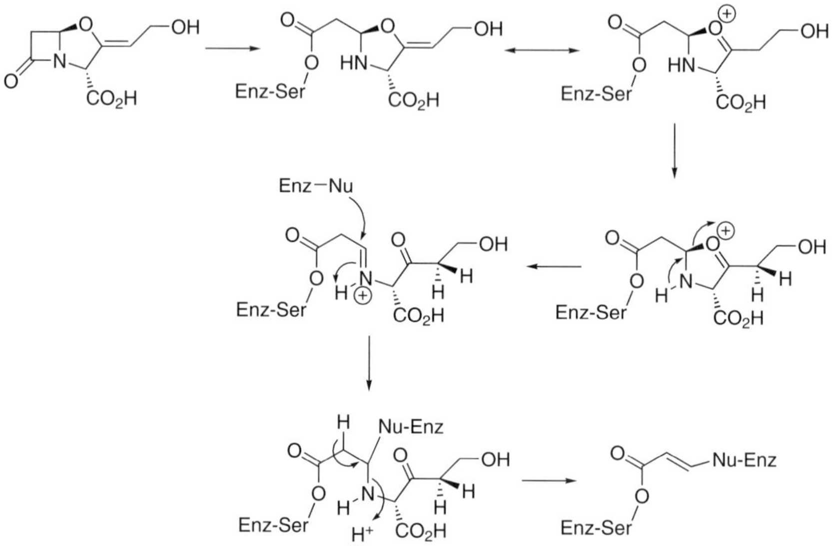

Figure 8.9 Rerouting of the acyl enzyme intermediate by clavulanate and penicillin sulfone to inactivate β-lactamases.

mentin, for the augmenting powers that clavulanate confers to amoxicillin, has been the most widely used form of penicillin in recent years. In the scheme of Fig. 8.5, clavulanate will inactivate enough penicillinase (β-lactamase) molecules to allow amoxicillin to survive in a β-lactamase-producer's periplasm to cross that space intact. Amoxicillin can thus run the gauntlet and reach its PBP targets at the cytoplasmic membrane (e.g., the transpeptidase [TPase] domain of a bi-functional TPase/transglycosylase high-molecular-weight PBP). The corresponding combination of sulbactam and ampicillin is known as Unasyn, and tazobactam and piperacillin are sold as Zosyn. (Fig. 8.8). While it is clear that these mechanism-based inhibitors will target only the serine-based lactamases and not the class D metallolactamases (Fig. 8.3), it is observed that the sulbactams and clavulanates are most active against class A lactamases and lack useful activity against the class C lactamases (Bronson and Barrett, 2001a), so there is room for further development of mechanism-based lactamase inhibitors.

A β-lactamase inhibitory protein (BLIP) has been isolated from *Streptomyces clavuligerus*, the clavulanate producer, where it may serve as an immunity protein to protect the antibiotic-producing organism. BLIP has picomolar to nanomolar K_i values for binding to several β-lactamases (e.g., 0.1 to 0.6 nM for TEM-1) (Rudgers et al., 2001), and the X-ray structure of the complex of BLIP and the TEM-1 β-lactamase has been solved (Strynadka et al., 1996), showing that residues 46-51 of BLIP make a type II' β-turn in the active-site region of the TEM lactamase, leading to insights into protein-based inhibitors and suggesting that β-turn peptidomimetics would be useful inhibitors (Rudgers et al., 2001). A second protein, BLIP-II, from *Streptomyces exfoliatus*, has also had its structure solved in complex with the TEM-1 β-lactamase, showing a distinct fold from BLIP and a second way to block the active site of TEM-1, as a competitive inhibitor of lactam binding with a remarkably potent 27 pM K_i (Lim et al.,

2001). The physiological function of BLIP-II appears to be in streptomycete sporulation, where it may inhibit one or more of the streptomycete PBPs to redirect PG biosynthesis toward spore formation.

Inhibitors of metallo-β-lactamases

The utility of carbapenems in the treatment of both gram-negative and gram-positive infections is becoming compromised by enzymatic hydrolysis and de-activation. While carbapenems as noted above are largely resistant to the class A chromosomal serine-based β-lactamases, they are rapidly hydrolyzed by the class B zinc-β-lactamases (Rasmussen and Bush, 1997), for example, in *Bacteroides fragilis* strains isolated from surgical patient infections. The X-ray structure of the CcrA metallo-β-lactamase from *B. fragilis* has been reported (Toney et al., 1998) and used for structure-based design of biphenyl tetrazole inhibitors that coordinate to the active-site zinc and thereby are specific for this metallo-lactamase class. A 50% inhibitory concentration of 0.4 μM for the most potent biphenyl tetrazole inhibitor was observed, and this was cocrystallized to confirm active-site binding and zinc ligation by one of the nitrogens of the tetrazole ring. These may be promising leads for molecules to add to carbapenems, much the way clavulanate or sulbactam is added to a β-lactam to get a combination that overcomes class B lactamase-mediated resistance. A series of tricyclic natural products with modest activities toward this subgroup of lactamases has also been described (Payne et al., 2002).

Regulation of β-lactamase gene expression and/or autolysis in the presence of penicillin

β-Lactamase genes can be embedded in bacterial chromosomes, such as the *ampC* gene in enteric bacteria or the *blaZ* gene in *Staphylococcus aureus*, or they can be carried on multiple-copy plasmids or transposons, as is the case for the TEM-1 *bla* gene in a variety of high-level penicillin-resistant gram-negative bacteria found in clinical isolates. *bla* genes are not usually constitutively expressed but get turned on when β-lactam antibiotics show up in the microenvironment. Recently the signaling systems for detecting external β-lactams have been sorted out for *E. coli*, *S. aureus*, and *Streptococcus pneumoniae* and reveal different paths of signal transduction that could be targets for reversing lactamase-mediated resistance.

E. coli

In *E. coli* the *ampG, ampD*, and *ampR* genes control expression of the *ampC*-encoding β-lactamase (Jacobs et al., 1997). The *ampG* gene encodes a trans-membrane protein thought to act as a permease that imports a cell wall peptidoglycan fragment released by disruption of cell wall–cross-linking enzy-matic machinery when a β-lactam begins to acylate PBPs and disrupt the orderly process of PG extension and remodeling. The molecule transported by AmpG is the disaccharyl tripeptide GlcNAc-anhydroMurNAc-L-Ala-D-γ-Glu-*meso*-DAP (**Fig. 8.10**), released by consecutive action of three enzymes. First is endopepti-

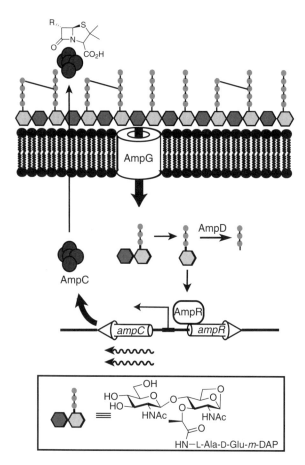

Figure 8.10 The anhydromuramyl tripeptide signaling pathway for induction of *ampC* expression in *E. coli*; transport into the cytoplasm by AmpG and ligation to AmpR to relieve transcriptional repression of *ampC*; and secretion of AmpC into the periplasm.

dase action to cleave the cross-links holding peptide strands together. Then comes action of lytic transglycosylases, catalyzing addition of the C_6-OH of a glucosyl group in a glycan strand to the 1-position, cleaving the inter sugar linkage and releasing the disaccharide as the 6,1-internal hemiacetal (the anhydroMurNAc). The tripeptide chain comes from shortening of the tetrapeptide or pentapeptide chain by action of L,D-carboxypeptidase, the third enzyme required to produce the signaling fragment. Now the GlcNAc-anhydroMurNAc tripeptide, a soluble small molecule, can diffuse to the outer domain of AmpG, bind, and be transported into the cytoplasm (**Fig. 8.10**), where it can dissociate from AmpG. The disaccharyl tripeptide released into the cytoplasm can now be recognized as a ligand for AmpR, the transcription factor, and convert it to an activated form that turns on the transcription of *ampC*, and β-lactamase expression begins. The AmpC lactamase is translated with an N-terminal signal sequence that targets it for transport to the cytoplasmic membrane and secretion into the periplasmic space, where it will start to destroy the β-lactam antibiotic hydrolytically (e.g., as in Fig. 8.5). The AmpD protein is also in the cytoplasm and is an amidase enzyme, cleaving the GlcNAc-anhydroMurNAc tripeptide. Thus it contributes at a basal level to the negative regulatory circuit, keeping the disaccharyl tripeptide concentration low and the *ampC* gene off (Jacobs et al., 1997). When the import of the signaling disaccharyl tripeptide is at higher levels due to antibiotic-induced disruption of PG assembly, presumably the amount in the cytoplasm overwhelms the AmpD capacity and escapes to bind to AmpR.

S. aureus

In *S. aureus* two routes to clinically relevant resistance have been observed. The first is due to expression of the chromosomally encoded BlaZ lactamase, a class A lactamase, discussed below, and the second is the expression, in methicillin-resistant *S. aureus* (MRSA), of a novel, penicillin-insensitive PBP2A, encoded by the *mecA* gene, as will be described in chapter 10. The expression of the BlaZ β-lactamase activity is inducible; expression is off in the absence of penicillins and cephalosporins in the microenvironment and turned on when they arrive at the outside of the cell. The sensing, transduction, and transcriptional activation functions are provided by two proteins encoded by the *blaR1* and *blaI* genes that are found just upstream of the *blaZ* gene (**Fig. 8.11**). All three genes are negatively regulated at rest by the BlaI protein, a 14-kDa protein that dimerizes and binds to promoter regions to repress transcription.

Figure 8.11 The *blaR1-blaI-blaZ* operon of *S. aureus* and the signal transduction pathway for expression of the BlaZ lactamase in *S. aureus*: tandem proteolysis of BlaR1 and BlaI for gene activation.

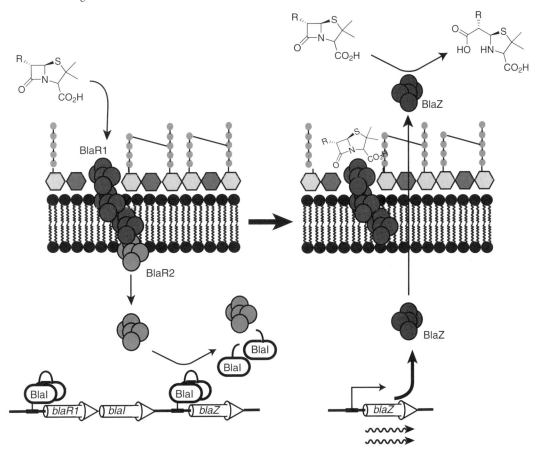

When a β-lactam antibiotic approaches the outer face of the cytoplasmic membrane in which a few copies of the transmembrane protein BlaR1 are embedded, the antibiotic is detected and the signal transduced. The exo domain of the 66-kDa BlaR1 is a PBP domain and initial signaling is through covalent acylation by the β-lactam, as for any PBP domain (Fig. 8.11). The formation of this penicilloyl enzyme covalent intermediate in the exo domain is sensed (perhaps by conformation change in this PBP domain) and occupancy transduced through the transmembrane domain and read out by the internal 30-kDa domain of BlaR1. The external PBP-type domain of BlaR is most related to class D β-lactamases (Massova and Mobashery, 1998), consistent with evolution of this binding/sensing domain from the class D lactamases (Ghuysen, 1991). This would be the reverse of the evolution of PBPs into lactamases, proposed in an earlier section of this chapter, suggesting protein evolution has gone both ways.

The intracytoplasmic 30-kDa domain of BalR1 has the hallmarks of the proenzyme form of a zinc-dependent protease. When a penicilloyl-O-Ser intermediate forms on the extracytoplasmic domain, the 30-kDa domain inside undergoes autocleavage between residues 293 and 294 to liberate the BlaR2 30-kDa cytoplasmic fragment. Precedents for autocleavage of the proenzyme forms of zinc proteases exist and may be mediated by a clustering effect in the penicilloyl BlaR1 exo domain (McKinney et al., 2001; Zhang et al., 2001). Remarkably, one proteolytic signal transduction event generates a second as BlaR1 induces proteolysis of the 14-kDa BlaI to an 11-kDa fragment that has apparently lost ability to dimerize and bind promoter DNA. The net repression of BlaZ and BlaR1 transcription is relieved, and transcriptional upregulation leads to BlaZ lactamase production, transport of BlaZ to the outside of the cell, β-lactam antibiotic hydrolysis, and lactam resistance.

The BlaR1-BlaI two-component system is logically analogous to the two-component sensor/response regulator systems used over and over again by bacteria for gene regulation in antibiotic production (CarR, CarI) and antibiotic resistance (VanS, VanR) (see chapter 15), but those use phosphoryl group transfer (from ATP to His-sensor to Asp-regulator) as the chemical information for state switching from "off" to "on." In the BlaR-BlaI two-component system the switch is proteolytic. Since proteolysis is biologically irreversible switching, while phosphoryl transfers are biologically reversible (by phosphatase action), the BlaR and BlaI proteins must be continually replenished, explaining their autogenous regulation. This system is not unique to *S. aureus* since a BlaR1 homolog has been detected in *B. fragilis* strains that also produce inducible β-lactamase.

Further, it turns out that the regulation of the *mecA* gene expression and the encoded PBP2A production that confers methicillin resistance in MRSA is regulated by entirely parallel logic, with a *mecR1* and *mecI* two-component system, again with gene clustering with *mecA* for coordinate regulation (**Fig. 8.12**). The exo domain of MecR1 is also a PBP, so covalent capture of a lactam as the lactamoyl-PBP acyl enzyme domain initiates transmembrane signaling with the same cascade of an in *cis* proteolysis of the cytoplasmic domain of MecR1 and then an in *trans* proteolysis to cleave the intact MecI and relieve repression of the *mecA* gene. The insertion of PBP2A, the *mecA* gene product, into the membrane allows PG cross-linking that is insensitive to methicillin and other β-lactam antibiotics. It may be that this two-component proteolysis logic will

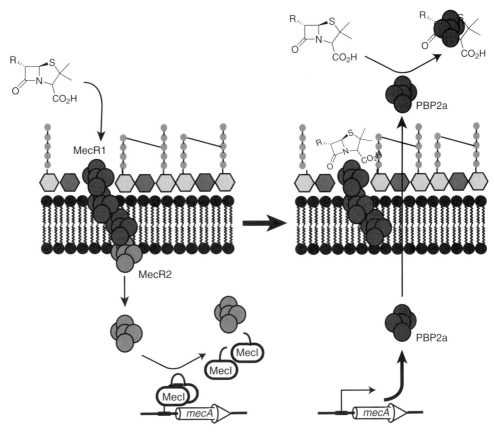

Figure 8.12 Signal transduction logic for regulated expression of the MecA PBP2A to confer methicillin resistance in MRSA.

be more general. In any event it raises the prospect that these signaling pathways for the two routes to inducible lactam resistance in *S. aureus* should be new targets for antibiotic screening and design.

S. pneumoniae

In *S. pneumoniae* external penicillin leads to an increase in autolytic peptidoglycan hydrolase activity and subsequent vulnerability to osmotic lysis and death. Genetic analysis (Novak et al., 2000) has indicated a signal transduction pathway logic distinct from those used by *E. coli* and *S. aureus*, described above.

As will be discussed elsewhere in this book (chapter 15), bacteria use two kinds of signaling systems to relay information from the external environment across the membrane to the cytoplasm for selective gene regulation. One is a two-component protein system, with a transmembrane signaling histidine protein kinase domain and a response regulator which acts as transcription factor. The second signaling system is dependent on the density of the bacterial culture and uses molecules secreted by one cell that diffuse into a neighbor, bind to a receptor/transcription factor, and activate downstream genes. These are known as quorum sensors and in gram-positive bacteria they tend to be small peptides. A two-component system (VncR-VncS) is required for cell killing by both vancomycin and penicillin (Novak et al., 2000), presumably triggering the upregulation of the gene for the major autolytic enzyme LytA, with VncS sensing derangement in the PG structure and dephosphorylating VncR to relieve repression of gene transcription. Just upstream of the *vncR* and *vncS* genes is an open reading frame encoding a 27-residue peptide, Pep[27], and a three-protein ATP-binding cassette-type ATPase pump to pump Pep[27] out to act as a quorum sensor and a death-inducing peptide on neighboring *S. pneumoniae* cells. The interaction of Pep[27] and antibiotics (e.g., as ligands for the transmembrane VncS?) to turn on the lytic cascade is not understood but may be a fruitful intersection for new antibiotic targeting in *S. pneumoniae*.

Aminoglycoside-modifying enzymes

The aminoglycoside (aminocyclitol) antibiotics do not have a reactive chemical warhead comparable to the β-lactam that is the core acylating unit embedded in all penicillins, cephalosporins, carbapenems, and monobactams. Instead we have noted that the aminoglycosides read specific regions of the 16S rRNA in the 30S ribosome subunit by a hydrogen bonding network (see chapter 4) through the various hydroxyl and amino substituents on the cyclitol rings to provide a high-affinity docking site for this class of antibiotics. The enzymatic destruction strategy for aminoglycoside-resistant bacteria is to covalently modify those specificity-conferring OH and NH_2 groups in the aminoglycosides and thereby interfere with recognition by the 16S rRNA. In some bacteria such as the gram-negative pathogenic *P. aeruginosa*, the outer membrane can also be a significant initial barrier to entry of aminoglycosides, both by decrease in the number of porin channels in the outer membrane and also by modifications to the lipopolysaccharide outer leaflet (Livermore, 2000; Poole, 2001).

Three kinds of enzymatic modifications of OH and NH_2 groups on aminoglycosides are common determinants of resistance and represent variants of normal electrophilic group transfer enzymes that participate in primary metabolism (see Kotra et al., 2000, and Wright, 1999, for review). ATP is one such reactant, used in both *O*-phosphoryl transfers, by attack of the γ-PO_3 group by an OH or NH_2 nucleophile, and *O*-adenylyl transfers, by attack of the aminoglycoside substrate nucleophile on the α-P of ATP to transfer the AMP moiety (**Fig. 8.13**). The second thermodynamically activated but kinetically stable cosubstrate in electrophilic group enzymatic transfers is acetyl-CoA and the NH_2 groups of the aminoglycosides attack the acetyl thioester moiety to transfer the acetyl group. All three reactions—phosphorylation, adenylation, and acetylation—are irreversible, driven by the -7 kcal/mol released and corresponding to a K_{eq} of 10^5 (Walsh, 1979) in favor of aminoglycoside modification.

It is likely that the antibiotic-inactivating enzymes will have evolved from adenyltransferases, phosphotransferases, and *N*-acetyltransferases that had been utilized for normal biosynthetic processes in the bacterial cells. For example, the determination of the X-ray structure of the APH(3')-IIIa phosphotransferase from enterococci revealed high similarity to eukaryotic serine/threonine protein kinases, consistent with an evolution from protein substrate −OH recognition for attack on the γ-PO_3 of ATP to recognition of the aminocyclitol framework

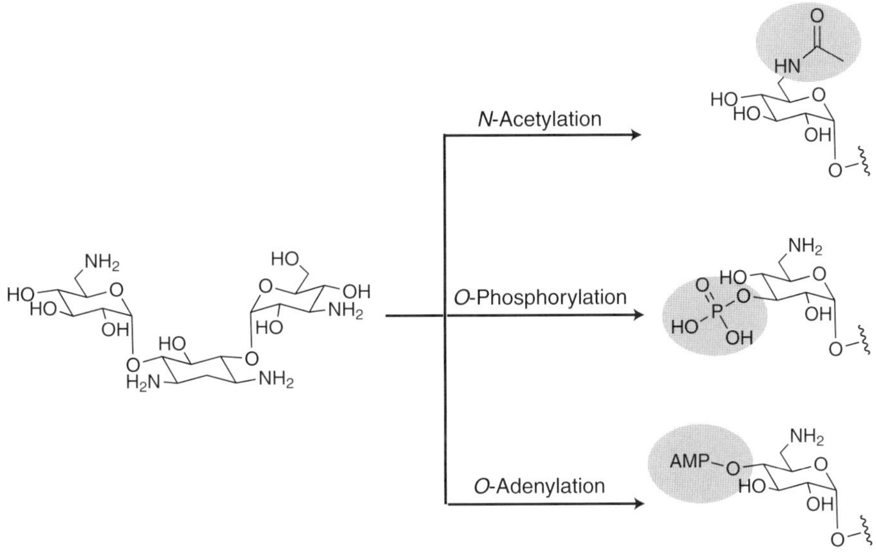

N-Acetylation

O-Phosphorylation

O-Adenylation

Figure 8.13 Three enzymatic routes to aminoglycoside deactivation: acetylation by acetyl-CoA, phosphorylation by ATP, and adenylation by ATP.

−OH (Hon et al., 1997) under selective pressure to survive. Given the multiplicity of OH and NH_2 groups in the successive generations of aminoglycosides to see clinical use, it is not surprising that modifying enzymes of distinct regiospecificity for acetylation, phosphorylation, and adenylation would arise. A typical pattern for covalent modification of a tricyclic aminoglycoside skeleton is shown in **Fig. 8.14**. Over 30 isoforms of these three kinds of enzymes have been described in aminoglycoside-resistant bacteria, including a fusion protein with two catalytic domains: an adenyltransferase and a phosphotransferase domain (Kotra et al., 2000). The *N*-acetyltransferases are classified according to their regioselectivity for acetylating—N_1, N_2', N_3—or N_6', with N_6' the most common subfamily of the aminoglycoside acetyltransferases, exhibiting broad specificity toward aminoglycoside scaffolds. The presence of the genes for the modifying enzymes on transmissible plasmids helps spread the resistance deter

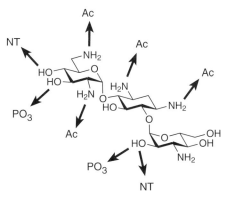

Figure 8.14 Patterns of regioselective enzymatic modification and deactivation of aminoglycoside antibiotics. NT, nucleotidyl transfer; PO_3, phosphoryl transfer; Ac, acetyl transfer.

minants and perhaps speed the evolution of catalytic activities toward newly introduced aminoglycosides.

Some strategies to subvert the enzymatic modifications have been reported by Mobashery and colleagues, studying one of the aminoglycoside O-phosphotransferases. For example, an aminoglycoside mimic once enzymatically phosphorylated rearranges to a reactive species that covalently modifies the O-phosphoryltransferase and takes it out of action (Roestamadji et al., 1995).

Analogous to the aminoglycoside-inactivating acetyltransferases is a family of virginiamycin/streptogramin-inactivating acetyltransferases, designated Vats (for virginiamycin acetyltransferases). We noted in chapter 4 that Synercid is a combination of a streptogramin A and streptogramin B component and that the Erm-mediated methylation of 23S rRNA leads to macrolide-lincosamide-streptogramin B (MLS_B) resistance, blocking binding of the streptogramin B component. The streptogramin A component can be removed by efflux (by mechanisms described in chapter 9) or by O-acetylation on the single free hydroxyl group (see Fig. 4.9 for dalfopristin structure). The X-ray structure of the VatD acetyltransferase from *Enterococcus faecium* (Sugantino and Roderick, 2002) has been solved, providing insight into the architecture of this drug-inactivating enzyme for the streptogramin A components.

Fosfomycin enzymatic deactivation

Fosfomycin is analogous to the β-lactam antibiotics in the sense that it also has a reactive chemical warhead, the three-ring epoxide, embedded in its simple chemical structure (**Fig. 8.15**). The epoxide is attacked by a reactive amino acid side chain, in this case the —SH of Cys rather than the —OH of Ser in the PBPs, in its target enzyme MurA at the start of peptidoglycan assembly (see chapter 3). The covalently derivatized active site of MurA leaves the enzyme unable to initiate the enolpyruvyl ether formation in UDP-GlcNAc conversion to UDP-MurNAc. Also analogous to destruction of the β-lactam ring by enzymatic capture of the reactive β-lactam by an alternate nucleophile, water in the case of the β-lactamases, the destruction of fosfomycin is catalyzed by enzymes that capture the epoxide with a soluble cosubstrate nucleophile, in this case the reactive thiolate anion of the tripeptide glutathione (γ-Glu-Cys-Gly). The fosfomycin glutathione S-transferase (FosA) is a manganese metalloenzyme (Bernat et al., 1997) (Fig. 8.15) that generates the ring-opened 2-OH thioether adduct in which the epoxide warhead has been deactivated as the glutathione thiol adds to C_1. Glutathione is the most abundant low-molecular-weight cellular thiol in most bacterial and eukaryotic cells, reaching levels of 1 to 10 mM. It is used for

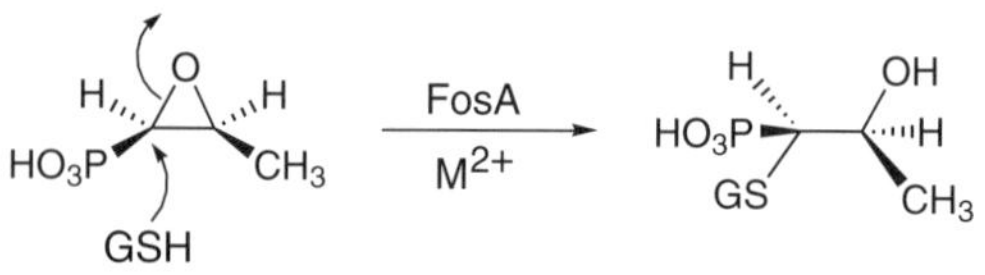

Figure 8.15 Enzymatic deactivation of fosfomycin by epoxide ring opening with glutathione.

protection and detoxification of reactive chemical groups, as in this example, by the high reactivity of its nucleophilic thiolate. The FosA enzyme has homology to both glyoxalase and metal-dependent catechol-cleaving dioxygenases (Bernat et al., 1997), consistent with an evolution from housekeeping enzymes of primary and secondary metabolism.

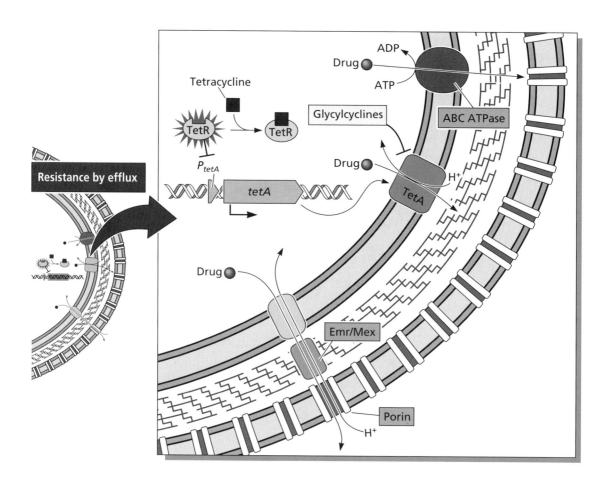

Resistance by action of H$^+$ and ATP-coupled efflux pumps in bacterial membranes.

chapter 9

Antibiotic Resistance by Efflux Pumps

The second major route by which drug resistance is manifested in bacteria is by the active export or efflux of antibiotics such that therapeutic concentrations are not attained in the bacterial cytoplasm. The chapter opening figure focuses on the portion of Fig. 2.2 that deals with resistance by active efflux of antibiotics.

The active efflux is mediated by transmembrane proteins, both in the cytoplasmic membranes and also in the outer membranes of gram-negative bacteria, with the transmembrane proteins acting as pumps that export the antibiotics, often against concentration gradients (**Table 9.1**). Active efflux can be clinically relevant for β-lactam antibiotics, macrolides, the pristinamycin peptides, fluoroquinolones, and most classically the tetracyclines. As we shall note below, some efflux pumps have relatively narrow specificity, e.g., the tetracycline pumps, while others have broad tolerance and confer multidrug resistance (Mdr) phenotypes. Bacteria have large numbers of efflux pumps, used physiologically for export of specific metabolites and to pump out foreign toxic substances. The integrated array of pumps with overlapping activities can lead to a remarkable capacity to pump out antibiotics either as a chromosomally encoded metabolic capacity, which makes *Pseudomonas aeruginosa* intrinsically antibiotic insensitive, or by acquisition of pump genes carried on plasmids and transposons.

Classes of membrane efflux pumps

From bioinformatic analysis four protein families of efflux pumps that can function in antibiotic resistance have been described (**Fig. 9.1**). The first three couple drug efflux to counterflow of protons, or sometimes to Na$^+$ ions, while the fourth family uses the hydrolysis of ATP to provide the energy for active transport of the antibiotic or other foreign compound out of the cell (Paulsen et al., 1996). The pumps driven by proton motive force (ΔpH) are categorized in the major facilitator subfamily (MFS), the small multidrug regulator (SMR) family,

Table 9.1 Summary of reported drug resistance profiles for multidrug-resistance-inducing efflux pumps (modified from Putman et al. [2000])

Drug	MFS 12-TMS cluster				MFS 14-TMS cluster		SMR	RND						ABC
	Blt	Bmr	EmrD	NorA	EmrB	VceB	EmrE	AcrB	AcrF	MexB	MexD	MexF	MexY	LmrA
Aminoglycosides		−					−	−		−	−	−	+	+
β-Lactams														
Carbapenems							−			+		−		−
Cephalosporins							−			+				+
Penicillins								+	+	+	−			+
Chloramphenicol		+	−	+	−	+	−	+		+	+	+		+
Glycopeptides							−	−	+					−
Lincosamides														+
Macrolides														
14-Membered		−		−	−	+	+	+	+	+	+	−	+	+
15-Membered										+	+			+
16-Membered														+
Novobiocin						−		+	+	+				
Quinolones														
Hydrophilic	+	+	−	+	−	−		+		+	+	+	+	+
Hydrophobic		+	−	+	+	+		+		+	+		+	+
Rifampin						+		+	+					
Sulfonamides										+				
Tetracyclines		−		−	−		+	+	+	+	+	+		+
Trimethoprim										+		+		−

From Putman et al. [2000], with permission.

Figure 9.1 Four protein subfamilies of proton-dependent efflux pumps and the ATPase family of efflux pump in antibiotic resistance. (From Paulsen et al. [1996], with permission.)

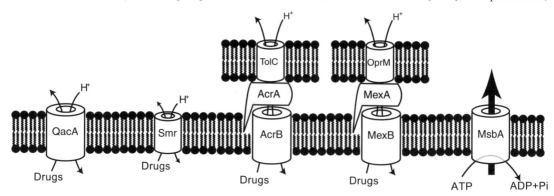

or the RND (resistance/nodulation/cell division) family, based on projected size and the need for partner proteins and subunits. The second major category of efflux pumps, those hydrolyzing ATP, is called the ATP-binding cassette (ABC) family. The schematic orientation of the four classes of efflux pumps in the bacterial cytoplasmic membrane is shown in Fig. 9.1, with counterflow of H^+ or hydrolysis of ATP as the obligate coupling mechanism for efflux. While ATP-driven pumps predominate in eukaryotes, the proton-driven antiporters predominate in bacterial genomes. For example, *Escherichia coli* is predicted to have 18 MFS, 3 to 4 SMR, and 5 to 6 RND members, for a total of 26 efflux pumps driven by counterflow of protons, compared to only 3 to 5 ABC-type ATPase pumps (Borges-Walmsley and Walmsley, 2001; Saier et al., 1998). Further annotation has raised the projected total from 31 to 37 putative drug transporter genes for *E. coli* (Nishino and Yamaguchi, 2001).

The MFS subfamily, represented by QacA (quaternary ammonium compounds [QAC], used as disinfectants and antiseptics, were among the first ligands detected to be substrates for this efflux pump) in Fig. 9.1, has more than 300 predicted members in prokaryotes and eukaryotes and includes the bacterial lactose permease LacY and the GLUT family of human glucose transporters. The use of some bacterial family members for drug efflux is probably a minor variation of a broad range of physiological functions. **Figure 9.2** shows that both N- and C-terminal ends of the MFS pumps are predicted to be on the cytoplasmic face, as exemplified in this prediction for the *Staphylococcus aureus* QacA protein. The N termini of MFS membrane proteins are thought to be involved in energization of transport while the C termini, more variable in sequence, may be involved in specific ligand recognition for export.

Some MFS pumps are predicted to have 14 transmembrane (TM) helices: QacA, EmrB in *E. coli*, TetK from *S. aureus*, TetL from *Bacillus stearothermophilus*, and TcmA from the producer organism *Streptomyces glaucescens* for tetracenomycin. Others have 12 TM domains predicted: Blt and Bmr from *Bacillus subtilis*, EmrD from *E. coli*, NorA from *S. aureus*, and the proteins TetA, TetG, and TetH from a series of gram-negative bacteria (Lomovskaya et al., 2001). Two-dimensional crystals of the TetA pump have been produced, leading to low-resolution structural models (Yin et al., 2000). One hypothesis about the origin of these two MFS subfamilies is evolution by gene duplication from a common six-transmembrane gene precursor. The QacA pump probably functions on its own in the gram-positive *S. aureus* strains, as do the tetracycline pumps TetK and TetL from gram-positive strains. The pumps in the gram-negative strains have partner proteins, in both the periplasm and the outer membrane, indicated in Fig. 9.1 for EmrB, EmrA, and an as yet unidentified outer membrane partner, perhaps the TolC protein.

The SMR family are small 12-kDa proteins, with four predicted transmembrane domains, and may function as oligomers. The RND family of pumps are predicted to have 12 TM domains, again perhaps evolving by gene duplication from a six-TM precursor. In *E. coli* this family includes the AcrB and AcrF pumps (ACR denotes acridine resistance); in *P. aeruginosa* it includes MexB (Fig. 9.1) and MexD; and in clinical isolates of *Neisseria gonorrhoeae* the pump is MtrD.

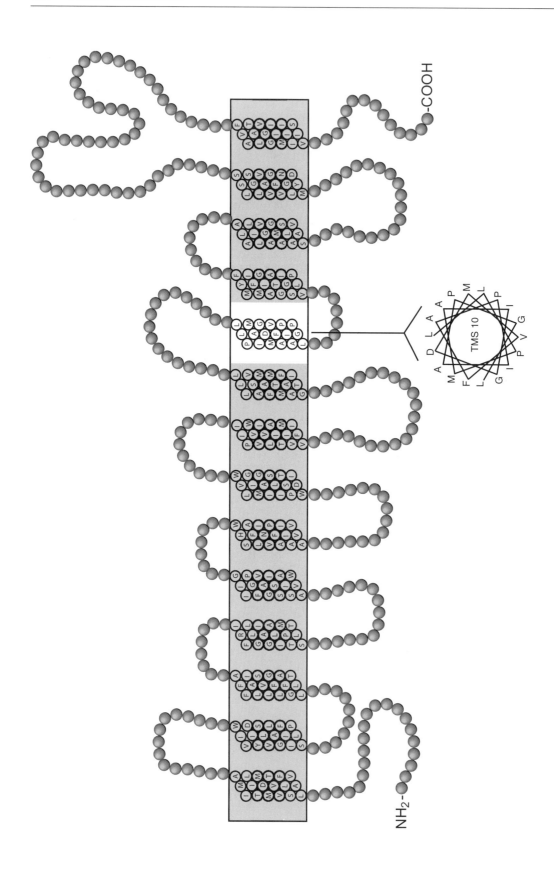

All 30 of the putative *E. coli* proton-driven drug transporter pumps (20 MFS, 3 SMR, and 7 RND family members) have been expressed in multicopy plasmids in an *E. coli* mutant lacking the AcrAB efflux pump (Nishino and Yamaguchi, 2001) and evaluated for increased resistance to 13 antibiotics. Six novel gene products joined 13 known pumps to yield 20 genes that conferred drug resistance of two-fold or more to at least one of the antibiotics. This might make a useful library set for screening new antibiotic candidates for susceptibility to this battery of pumps.

The fourth family is the ABC family of ATPases. It represents a minority of the antibiotic efflux pumps but is an extremely common form of transmembrane transport system. For example, it is estimated that 70 ABC-type ATPases are encoded in the *E. coli* genome, representing almost 5% of the genes. The typical organization of ABC proteins is to be part of multicomponent membrane transport systems, including periplasmic protein components. In *E. coli*, 44 ABC genes are predicted to be part of uptake systems from the periplasm while 13 are predicted to be dedicated for ligand export. The typical domain organization involves two hydrophobic domains, embedded as transmembrane pores, and two hydrophilic domains on the cytoplasmic face of the membrane that serve as ATP binding and hydrolysis sites. Various configurations of the domains are seen, from a four-domain single polypeptide to four separate subunits. The latter configuration occurs in the *E. coli* maltose permease system, $(MalK)_2 \cdot MalF \cdot MalG$, where MalK is the ABC subunit (**Fig. 9.3**). An X-ray structure of the nucleotide binding domain (NBD) of the MalK pump has been reported (Hung et al., 1998), giving a baseline picture of the catalytic ATPase domain but not revealing how the NBD interacts with the transmembrane domains (TMDs), how docking of the MalK-ATP complex to the MalF/MalG membrane subunit triggers ATP hydrolysis, or how the stored energy is utilized for protein conformational changes to transiently open a pore for maltose to be pumped in.

A significant breakthrough in understanding the architecture of an ABC-type transporter has been obtained by crystallization of the MsbA protein from *E. coli*, at a relatively low resolution (4.5 Å) (Chang and Roth, 2001), but sufficient to reveal orientation of NBDs to TMDs and allowing a model for transporter action. MsbA is homologous to human MDR-1 and mouse MDR3, multidrug resistance transporters that are thought to act physiologically as lipid and phospholipid "flippases," moving phospholipid molecules from the inner to the outer layer of the membrane bilayer. *E. coli* MsbA transports lipid A (see chapter 15) through the inner membrane to the outer membrane of the gram-negative envelope, where lipid A is a major structural component. It is proposed that MsbA and homologs act as "hydrophobic vacuum cleaners" to remove lipids and hydrophobic drugs from the inner membrane leaflet (Chang and Roth, 2001; Raviv et al., 1990). MsbA crystallizes as a homodimer, with the transmembrane domain helices (52 Å long) spanning the membrane at a tilt of 30 to 40° from the normal plane of the membrane, creating a chamber between the dimers large

Figure 9.2 Predicted orientation of MFS pumps in the bacterial cytoplasmic membrane. (From Paulsen et al. [1996], with permission.)

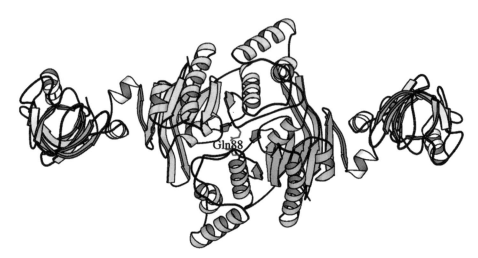

Gln88

Figure 9.3 The *E. coli* maltose transport system: architecture of the MalK dimer. (From Diederichs et al. [2000], with permission.)

enough to bind the lipid A ligand (**Fig. 9.4**). A linking region between the TMD and the NBD, nestled in the aqueous region on the cytoplasmic side of the membrane, is thought to couple conformational changes from ATP binding and hydrolysis in the NBD to the TMD in the membrane. The models proposed by Chang and Roth (2001) allow for recruitment of lipid or drug from the lower (cytoplasmic) leaflet of the membrane bilayer into the chamber as an initial binding/sequestration step (**Fig. 9.4B**). ATP binding to the NBD is sensed by the TMDs that rotate to close the chamber and bring a cluster of charges from the TM helices into the closed chamber. This would destabilize the microenvironment for the hydrophobic ligand, allowing a vectored flipping to an energetically more favorable position in the upper part of the chamber, poised to enter the outer leaflet of the membrane (Chang and Roth, 2001). While the MsbA may not be a good prototype for transporters that move hydrophilic ligands, it is probably a paradigm for ABC transporters that move hydrophobic ones, including antibiotics. Chang and Roth (2001) noted that the chamber could accommodate and transport a wide variety of molecules, consistent with low selectivity for MDR-type transporters, and also that MsbA (and related transporters) is not acting as a pump but as "a molecular machine scanning the lower bilayer leaflet for substrates, accepting them laterally, and flipping them to the outer membrane leaflet."

A second bacterial transporter of the ABC type, in this case the *E. coli* BtuCD protein pair, transporting the hydrophilic ligand vitamin B_{12}, has also recently been solved by X-ray analysis at 3.2-Å resolution (Locher et al., 2002). The functional transporter is the $BtuC_2BtuD_2$ heterotetramer, where the BtuC subunit is membrane spanning, with 10 α-helices per subunit, and the BtuD is the ATPase cassette. Vitamin B_{12} on the periplasmic face is presented to the external face of $BtuC_2$ by the periplasmic binding protein BtuF, initiating a signal across the membrane that leads to ATP hydrolysis and a presumed power stroke that opens the channel between the BtuC subunits to allow passage of vitamin B_{12}. The orientation of the ATPase domains to the membrane-spanning protein por-

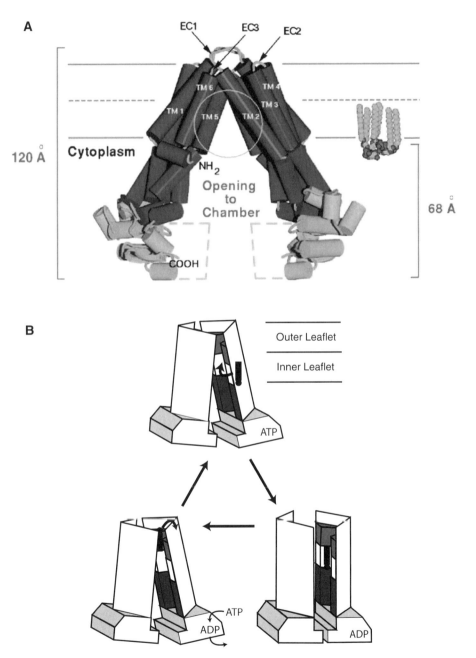

Figure 9.4 Schematic of an ABC transporter. (A) The MsbA dimer and its orientation towards membrane bilayer leaflets. (B) Schematic of lipid A transport by *E. coli* MsbA. (From Chang and Roth [2001], with permission.)

tion and the number and orientation of helices in BtuC are different from the MsbA transporter. The two variants of ABC transporters will create a new platform for design and analysis of alternate ligands and blockers of channel function.

In terms of antibiotic pumps in the ABC family, the resistance to erythromycin in clinical isolates of *Streptococcus epidermidis* (Chu et al., 1996) is due to the *msrA* gene, which encodes such an ATPase subunit for pumping out erythromycins and pristinomycins. Also, the LmrA pump of *Lactococcus lactis* is a broad-spectrum MDR pump. When five candidate ABC-type open reading frames from *E. coli* were expressed and assayed as efflux pumps for the macrolide erythromycin, the *ybjYZ* gene pair was found to encode such a pump and so has been renamed *macAB* (Kobayashi et al., 2001; see also Nishino and Yamaguchi, 2001). MacA is thought to pass through the cytoplasmic membrane once and be mostly in the periplasm, while MacB is thought to be an intrinsic inner membrane protein with the cytoplasmic ATPase domain. As noted in Fig. 9.1 and expounded below, an outer membrane protein is needed to complete ligand efflux across the outer membrane and is provided by the TolC protein. Given X-ray structures for MsbA (Fig. 9.4) and TolC (see Fig. 9.6), we are approaching knowledge of the molecular architecture of multicomponent antibiotic efflux pumps.

Function of the MFS and RND pumps in physiological and antibiotic efflux

The physiologic roles of the various MFS and RND pumps are beginning to be deciphered to give some clue how they may be adapted or taken over for xenobiotic and antibiotic efflux. The Blt pump of *B. subtilis* appears to be used for spermidine efflux and is transcribed with a spermidine acetyltransferase (Paulsen et al., 1996). It is coopted for antibiotic export. The MFS family Ptr pump in *Streptomyces pristinaespiralis* appears to be an autoimmunity pump for this organism when it turns on production of pristinamycins I and II, since both induce ptr transcription. We have noted the OleB efflux pump for glucosyl-oleandomycin in the *Streptomyces antibioticus* producer in chapter 7 as part of the immunity mechanism to its own antibiotic.

In the RND superfamily of pumps, the MexA-MexB-OprM operon (**Fig. 9.5**) has been proposed to be involved in secretion of the nonribosomal peptide siderophore pyoverdin by *P. aeruginosa* in iron-deficient microenvironments.

Figure 9.5 Operon organization of three-component Mex efflux pumps in *P. aeruginosa* and *E. coli acrA-acrB* operon.

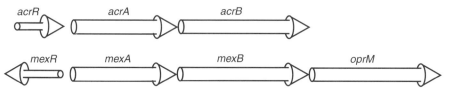

The presence of two membrane barriers in gram-negative bacteria requires a pump component in both the inner and outer membranes and some connecting protein to bridge the periplasm or bring the two membranes transiently into contact (Fig. 9.1). This trio of proteins is conscripted for efflux of tetracyclines, ciprofloxacin, chloramphenicol, and β-lactams. In fact there are four such multicomponent RND family efflux pumps identified in *P. aeruginosa*, with overlapping ranges for pumping out antibiotics such that the total makes this pathogen intrinsically insensitive to most classes of antibiotics. The *E. coli* Acr system probably has a physiological role of pumping out bile acids and fatty acids to lower their toxicity (Paulsen et al., 1996). AcrB is the inner membrane protein component, while AcrA is thought to span the periplasm (Fig. 9.1) and interact with an outer membrane general porin/channel protein, suggested on genetic grounds to be the protein TolC (Fralick, 1996). TolC is also noted below as an outer membrane channel component of the hemolysin secretion system.

The TolC outer membrane protein of *E. coli* (**Fig. 9.6**) can interact with several different inner membrane translocases to form transient conduits across

Figure 9.6 (Left) The architecture of TolC; (Right) models for TolC closed and open states. (Modified from Koronakis et al. [2000], with permission.)

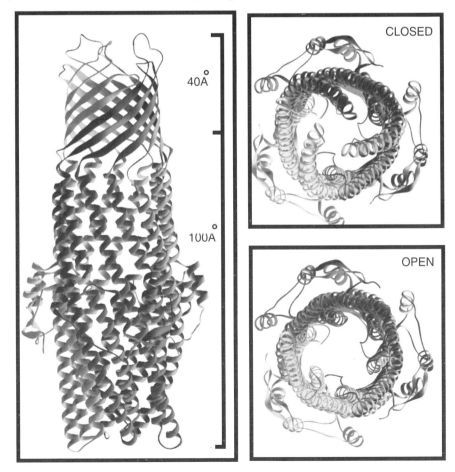

both membranes to produce a tunnel from cytoplasm to external environment that can be traversed by both small molecules and large proteins that get exported (see "Protein secretion machinery in gram-negative pathogens and connection to disease" below) (Koronakis et al., 2000). TolC is thus a prototype for the outer membrane partner proteins of gram-negative efflux pumps. The X-ray structure (Koronakis et al., 2000) of the functional TolC trimer reveals both a 12-stranded β-barrel domain (four per monomer) and an α-helical domain (Fig. 9.6, left panel) contiguous with the barrel domain. It is argued that the β-barrel domain, typical for outer membrane porin structures (Koebnik et al., 2000), delimits the outer membrane portion and the helical region protrudes into and through the periplasm to form interactions, via coil-coil interactions with coiled-coil domains of the inner membrane translocase pair, e.g., AcrAB. As isolated, the channel in the α-helical barrel of TolC is closed, as seen in the top view of Fig. 9.6 (right panels). It is postulated that during small-molecule and protein efflux through this channel, the channel interior is dilated by rotation of the coiled coils, an allosteric untwisting, induced by protein-protein interaction with the inner membrane components of the pump (Koronakis et al., 2000). The open form could produce a tunnel diameter in TolC (bottom panel of Fig. 9.6, right) of 30 Å. When the TolC dissociated again from its inner membrane partners such as AcrAB, it would revert to the closed state to avoid leakage of periplasmic components.

Regulation of efflux pumps

The best studied of the antibiotic efflux pumps are probably the tetracycline pumps, with TetA-L noted above as MFS family members in both gram-negative and gram-positive bacteria. When tetracycline enters such a bacterial cell, it is bound with high affinity to a protein, TetR, that functions as a repressor of the Tet pump gene, *tetA*, in *E. coli*. The Tet·TetR complex relieves the at rest, negative repression of the Tet pump gene expression. The structure of TetR, with and without the tetracycline ligand, bound to Tet operator DNA reveals how binding of the Mg^{2+}-tetracycline complex causes the TetR to lose affinity for its DNA site (Orth et al., 2000) (**Fig. 9.7**). The K_d for binding of the Mg^{2+}-tetracycline complex to TetR is about 10^{-9} M, some thousand-fold tighter than the 10^{-6} M binding to the 30S ribosome, so the relief of *tetA* transcriptional repression kicks in at low levels of drug in the bacterial cell. When Mg^{2+}-tetracycline is bound to TetR, its affinity for DNA upstream of *tetA* drops an estimated nine orders of magnitude (Orth et al., 2000) via ligand-induced, pendulum-like motion of one of the helices in TetR that pries apart the DNA binding domains.

The 42-kDa TetA pump protein is then overproduced, inserts into the cytoplasmic membrane, and acts in antiport mode with entering protons to pump out tetracycline. The Tet efflux pumps may have evolved from such pumps in the tetracycline producers, such as the one encoded by the *otrB* gene in *Streptomyces rimosus* (McMurry et al., 1998). This regulatory circuit logic appears to be generalized for the operons in *P. aeruginosa* for the *mexA, mexB,* and *oprM* genes, controlled by a divergently transcribed repressor *mexR*; for the comparable *mtr* gene system in *N. gonorrhoeae* (**Fig. 9.8**); and for the *AcrF,E,S* operon in *E.*

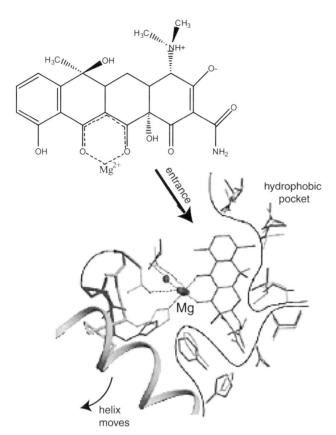

Figure 9.7 Structural basis of relief of repression of *tetA* transcription when Mg^{2+}-tetracycline binds to TetR. (From Orth et al. [2000], with permission.)

coli. The *bmr* pump gene in *B. subtilis* is similarly under transcriptional control by the *bmrR* gene, which encodes a repressor. Bmr functions as an efflux pump for lipophilic cations, such as trimethylphosphonium ions, as well as for fluoroquinolones, chloramphenicol, and doxorubicin. The X-ray structure of the BmrR repressor, free and in complex with triphenylphosphonium, has been solved (Fig. 9.9), indicating that the lipophilic ligand induces selective unfolding and repositioning of an α-helix. This exposes a drug binding pocket that interacts with the ligand by hydrophobic stacking and by electrostatic pairing with a buried glutamate carboxylate anion (see Fig. 4 and 5 in Zheleznova et al., 1999). The helix-to-coil transition and repacking of the BmrR binding domain is req-

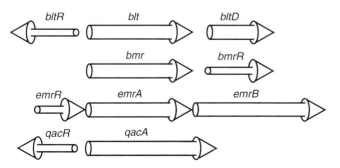

Figure 9.8 Regulatory circuit logic for efflux pump genes.

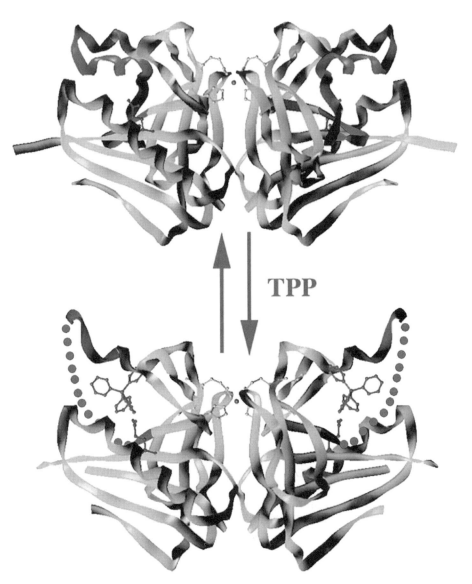

Figure 9.9 Binding of lipophilic cation trimethylphosphonium ion to the BmrR repressor. (From Zheleznova et al. [1999], with permission.)

uisite for high-affinity recognition. Brennan and colleagues have used this observation to propose that this logic may be used for drug binding and recognition by the membrane efflux pump proteins, such as Bmr (Zheleznova et al., 2000), EmrA and B, QacA, and others of the MFS family, many of which have a conserved glutamate in the first transmembrane domain, as do SMR family pumps. They suggest the hydrophobic portions of antibiotics partition into the cytoplasmic membrane at the inner leaflet. If the ligand binding domain of the efflux pump undergoes transient conformational changes via the above helix-to-coil transitions, with one conformation exposing the buried glutamate to bound ligand, the antibiotic will find this site by two-dimensional diffusional encounter.

How the drug-pump complex then senses the ΔpH across the membrane and unidirectionally expels bound antibiotic to the outside in a low-affinity state remains to be analyzed.

The regulation of porin and pump genes is of clinical relevance in carbapenem treatment of *P. aeruginosa* infections (Enne et al., 2001). Point mutations in the *mexR* gene can lead to MexR mutant forms of this repressor protein with lower affinity for promoter targets, allowing relief from repression. This is a common path for upregulation of the *mexA-mexB-oprM* operon noted above. This broad-spectrum, three-component efflux pump provides an exit portal for quinolones, tetracycline, chloramphenicol, and normal β-lactams. Of the two approved carbapenems, imipenem, lacking lipophilic side chains, is not exported. Meropenem, with its heterocyclic side chain, is pumped out and its MICs typically rise from 0.12 to 0.5 mg/liter to 2 to 4 mg/liter. On the other hand, imipenem use selects for *P. aeruginosa* mutants lacking the outer membrane porin OprD; the absence of that pore restricts the drug's entry, and imipenem MICs values rise from 1 to 2 mg/liter to 8 to 32 mg/liter (Enne et al., 2001). Meropenem also has some transit through OprD as its MICs in strains with in this mutant rise an order of magnitude to 2 to 4 mg/liter. Livermore (2000) notes that these observations may favor meropenem use since two mutations (*mexR* and *oprD*), at multiplicatively low frequency, are required to bring the meropenem MIC values out of the useful range. He notes the additional mechanism of the metallo β-lactamases acting as carbapenemases (chapter 8) as an additional resistance determinant.

Reduced outer membrane permeability of *E. coli* O157:H7

We note earlier in this chapter and elsewhere in this book that certain bacteria are better pathogens than others. The gram-negative bacterium *P. aeruginosa* does a good job of keeping intracellular antibiotic concentration low, both by turning on many variants of efflux pumps and also by restricting uptake by expression of outer membrane pore proteins, porins, that restrict inward diffusion of antibiotics and other antibacterial small molecules. Recent studies (Martinez et al., 2001) indicate that the outer permeability barrier of virulent, toxigenic strains of *E. coli* may also be more restrictive for antibiotic permeation. *E. coli* O157:H7, first detected in 1982 in fecal-contaminated undercooked beef, causes up to 75,000 cases of infection annually in the United States, outbreaks of hemorrhagic colitis that can progress to hemolytic uremic syndrome (Mead et al., 1999) (**Fig. 9.10**).

The O157:H7 strain enters through the stomach and colonizes epithelial cells in the intestine, proliferating and producing a toxin. One component of the toxin interacts with a membrane glycolipid, and the other then enters the cells and blocks protein biosynthesis (see Kaper and O'Brien, 1998; Karmali, 1989). *E. coli* O157:H7 exhibits resistance to streptomycin, tetracycline, and sulfa drugs and may do so through reduction of outer membrane permeability for uptake. Martinez et al. (2001) used a kinetic assay for detection of periplasmic alkaline phosphatase activity to calculate that, compared with nonvirulent control strains, *E. coli* O157:H7 has six-fold lower permeability to an anionic substrate small

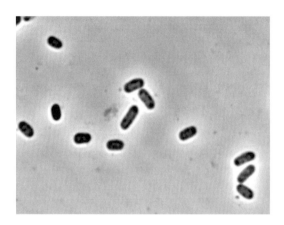

Figure 9.10 Culture of *E. coli* O157:H7. (Courtesy of D. E. Graham.)

molecule and a thousand-fold reduction to phage transformation. The recent sequencing of the *E. coli* O157:H7 genome (Perna et al., 2001) revealed small numbers of changes in the major porins OmpF and OmpC among the 1,387 genes out of 3,500 which are distinct and in strain-specific gene clusters in this pathogenic strain of *E. coli*. Doubtless there will be many contributing factors to the toxicity of the O157:H7 strain, with 15 gene islands of >15 kb encoding putative virulence factors (Perna et al., 2001), but the permeability assay may allow screening for antibiotic agents with more favorable uptake properties in these pathogens.

Protein secretion machinery in gram-negative pathogens and connection to disease

In addition to transporter- and protein pump-mediated export of small molecules, including lipophilic antibiotics, both gram-negative and gram-positive pathogenic bacteria secrete proteins by dedicated protein machinery (see Lee and Schneewind, 2001, for review). Protein secretion through the inner membrane is similar in gram-negative and gram-positive bacteria using the Sec pathway machinery. For gram-positive organisms this allows proteins, such as exotoxins (see chapter 15 for various exotoxins found in the methicillin-resistant *S. aureus* [MRSA] genome), access to the external medium via traverse of the peptidoglycan meshwork. In gram-negative organisms passage across the outer membrane involves several kinds of specialized protein export machinery, termed type I-IV secretion systems, as well as assembly of transmembrane pili involved in attachment of *E. coli* to host cells. These are supramolecular complexes that are assembled in the inner and outer membranes.

Various enteric pathogenic bacteria initiate disease by expression of adherence and sometimes invasin proteins on the outer membranes, assembled via the secretion systems noted below. Adherent but noninvasive pathogens such as *Vibrio cholerae* and the enteropathogenic *E. coli* (EPEC) and enterohemorrhagic *E. coli* (EHEC) make protein-protein contacts to epithelial cells in the small intestine and then turn on signaling pathways in the host cells that activate chloride ion channels for chloride and water efflux to create the watery diarrheal syndromes (Nataro and Kaper, 1998; Prente and Finlay, 2001). *Salmonella* strains and *Shigella dysenteriae* can induce uptake by epithelial cells (see chapter 15) and subsequent passage into extracellular spaces, crossing the epithelial barrier. In typhoid fever this produces bacteria in the blood (bacteremia and septicemia), while *Shigella* invasions are localized to the colonic and rectal mucosa, leading to destructive inflammatory tissue responses and the characteristic dysentery (Sansonetti et al., 2001).

The pore-forming hemolysin protein (HlyA) of uropathogenic *E. coli* that cause 80% of urinary tract infections has multiple repeats of a calcium-binding sequence, inserts into membranes, and is part of a family of repeat toxins (Coote, 1992) that are secreted by the type I machinery. There are three other gene products required to secrete HlyA. HlyC adds C_{14} or C_{16} acyl groups to two lysine side chains in HlyA to increase hydrophobicity. HlyB and HlyD are inner membrane protein components of the type I secretion machinery and TolC, noted above in the Acr efflux system, is the outer membrane partner protein that allows HlyA secretion through the outer membrane into the external medium. HlyB is an ABC-type ATPase, perhaps related to the MsbA transporter noted above, and connects type I protein secretion to ABC-type multidrug resistance transporters. TolC is the 12-stranded outer membrane barrel (Koronakis et al., 2000) with C-terminal α-helices that fill the interior channel at rest to prevent leakage of periplasmic components. Presumably the channel is opened to its full 3.4-nm diameter when complexed with type I secretion partners.

Type II secretion machinery is also known as the general secretory pathway (Lee and Schneewind, 2001) and accounts for the export of some bacterial toxins such as cholera toxin, *E. coli* enterotoxin, the *Shigella dysenteriae* Shiga toxin, and *E. coli* Shiga-like toxins (e.g., in the O157:H7 strains), all with AB_5 oligomeric structures, where the A subunit is enzymatically active when taken up by host cells. The B_5 pentameric component self-assembles in the host membrane and can recognize different glycolipids, globoside Gb3 for the Shiga-like toxin of enterotoxigenic *E. coli* (ETEC) and ganglioside GM1 for cholera toxin. The A component is then dissociated and internalized by the host cell, wherein it carries out some enzymatic step. The Shiga toxin of *Shigella* and *E. coli* O157:H7 is a specific *N*-glycosidase, depurinating a particular residue in 23S rRNA and thereby blocking protein biosynthesis, while the A subunit of the ETEC and of the cholera toxin of *V. cholerae* leads to elevation of cyclic AMP and cyclic GMP, activation of chloride ion channels, and resultant diarrheas (Groisman, 2001).

Also secreted by the type II pathway are exoenzymes, including proteases, elastase, phosphatases, and pectate lysases by such plant pathogens as *Erwinia carotovora*. As many as 12 inner membrane proteins are found in this secretion machine (Russel, 1998), an ATPase at the cytoplasmic face of the inner membrane, a periplasmic chaperone, GspS, and one outer membrane protein, GspD, also known as secretin. Secretin oligomerizes into a dodecameric ring with an inner diameter of 7.6 nm (Nouwen et al., 1999) that is thought to be the channel for protein passage through the outer membrane.

Type III secretion machinery is of particular interest for its central role in the virulence and pathogenesis of *Yersinia* and *E. coli* infections and for invasion of *Salmonella* and *Shigella* into host cells (see Lee and Schneewind, 2001, for review). This topic is discussed further in chapter 15. It is proposed that type III secretion of proteins is induced by physical contact between bacteria and host cells, for example, via specific ion gradients, and serves to directly inject bacterial proteins into the cytoplasm of animal and human cells. The resultant derangement of host cell metabolism can lead to bacterial entry (into epithelial cells by *Salmonella*), neutralization of macrophage killing (by extracellular *Yersinia pestis*), or cell destruction (epithelial cells by EPEC). The type III membrane protein components are analogous to components in assembly of flagella and also build around a secretin dodecamer in the outer membrane and a needle protein (SctF) which grows from the secretin and penetrates the host cell membrane. Proteins being secreted, including 14 *Yersinia* outer proteins (Yops), pass through the secretin channel and the needle directly into the host cell. The substrate recognition signals to determine which bacterial proteins are marked for type III secretion are not yet deciphered (Lee and Schneewind, 2001). The infectivity of *Y. pestis* in causing plague (Perry and Fetherston, 1997) is dramatically decreased when type III secretion is blocked, so this machinery would be a good target for reducing pathogenesis in gram-negative infections.

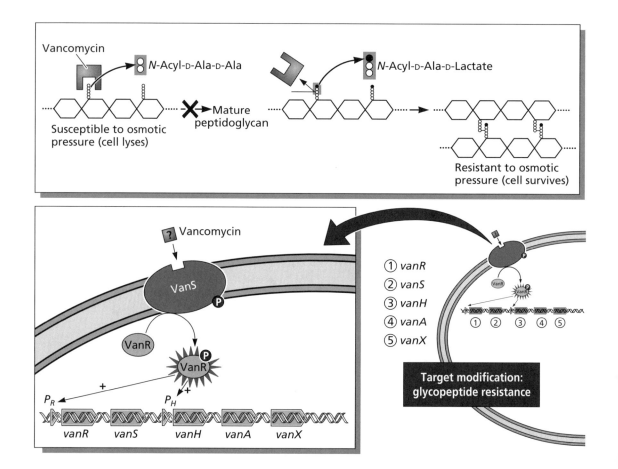

Antibiotic resistance by modification of the target.

chapter 10

Antibiotic Resistance by Replacement or Modification of the Antibiotic Target

The last of the three major routes to clinically important resistance in pathogenic bacteria is the ability of drug-resistant pathogens to modify the drug target to insensitivity while still retaining its essential cellular function. The chapter opening figure is a blowup of that section of Fig. 2.2 that exemplifies the principles of antibiotic resistance arising from replacement or modification of the target to an insensitive form.

This can be achieved by mutation at one or more sites in the target gene or by importation of a gene that specifies a new replacement enzyme that has markedly decreased sensitivity to the drug. β-lactam resistance in the gram-positive *Streptococcus pneumoniae* and *Staphylococcus aureus* strains represent these two variations on a theme. The erythromycin family of macrolides and the streptogramin B family both have decreased affinity in response to methylation of a single adenine in the 23S rRNA in the 50S ribosomal subunit. Finally, we shall note the cell wall reprogramming in vancomycin-resistant enterococci (VRE) phenotypes A, B, and C. Micrographs of *S. aureus*, *S. pneumoniae*, and *Enterococcus faecalis* are shown in Fig. 10.1.

Methicillin resistance in *S. aureus*

Methicillin (**Fig. 10.2**), with a bulky 2,5-dimethoxybenzoyl substituent on the 6-aminopenicillin scaffold, was introduced in 1950 to treat gram-positive bacterial infections that had become resistant to penicillin via inducible β-lactamase hydrolysis of the antibiotic. The bulky side chain substituent in the penicilloyl-O-lactamase acyl enzyme intermediate selectively slows the deacylation hydrolytic step (see chapter 8) and lengthens the lifetime of the covalent acyl enzyme, effectively deactivating β-lactamase during that interval. This strategy was effective for a decade before outbreaks of methicillin-resistant *S. aureus* (MRSA) developed in Europe in 1961, and by the 1980s MRSA was widespread globally.

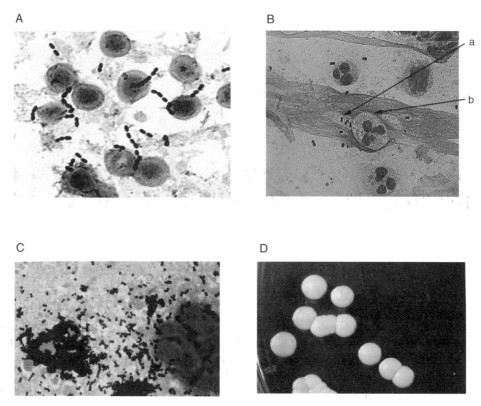

Figure 10.1 Gram-positive pathogens that become drug resistant by target alterations: (A) *Enterococcus faecalis* in a blood culture; (B) encapsulated *Streptococcus pneumoniae*, including (a) gram-positive diplococci surrounded by a capsule and (b) a polymorphonuclear leukocyte with multilobed nucleus; (C) Gram stain of sputum of patient with *Staphylococcus aureus* pneumonia; (D) *Staphylococcus aureus* "golden" colonies on blood agar plates. (From Elliot et al. [1997], with permission.)

MRSA is not elaborating an improved version of β-lactamase that is more efficient at chewing up methicillin, but rather has acquired the *mecA* gene, which encodes a new penicillin-binding protein (PBP), termed PBP2A (also PBP2′), in greater than 90% of the drug-resistant clinical isolates (see Hiramatsu et al., 2001). In hospital environments in the United States, MRSA can reach an incidence of 20 to 40%; in Japan an incidence of up to 60% incidence has been reported (Chu et al., 1996). MRSA can be particularly prevalent in burn centers, but is also present in other long-term care facilities. MRSA poses problems for

Figure 10.2 Structure of methicillin.

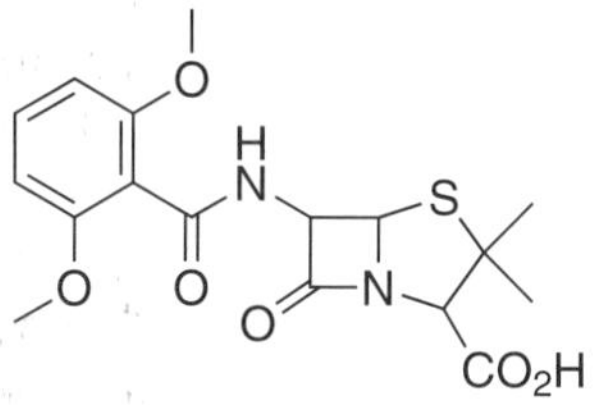

Methicillin

treatment because it is resistant to essentially all β-lactam molecules, including penicillins, cephalosporins, carbapenems, and penems. This pan-β-lactam insensitivity stems from the low binding affinity of the *mecA*-encoded PBP2A, a 76-kDa bifunctional transglycosylase/transpeptidase. In contrast, the normal high-molecular-weight PBPs, PBP1 through 4, may remain sensitive to acylation by β-lactams in methicillin-sensitive *S. aureus* (MSSA).

The molecular basis of the insensitivity of PBP2A to lactams while still carrying out peptidoglycan (PG) cross-linking functions is not yet clear and will probably require an X-ray structure comparison with the sensitive PBPs of the same organism. The origin of the *mecA* gene is also unknown, although horizontal transmission from some other *Staphylococcus* species has been postulated (chapter 7). It is known that the MRSA phenotype arises from transfer of a 30- to 40-kb mobile DNA element with the *mecR1-mecI-mecA* triad of genes at the core of the methicillin-inducible phenotype. We noted in chapter 8 (Fig. 8.12) the close parallel of the logic of the *blaR1-blaI-blaZ* circuitry, in that case for β-lactamase induction, to the *mecR1-mecI-mecA* circuitry for the MRSA phenotype (by a proteolytic two-component gene-activating cascade). The MecR1 protein is a 68-kDa transmembrane sensor/transducer, with a classical PBP exo domain that can be acylated by methicillin, and this covalent occupancy transduced to the endo domain, a zinc protease zymogen, which undergoes autoproteolysis. The released cytoplasmic MecR1 fragment, now an active protease, then cleaves the MecI repressor such that it cannot dimerize and bind DNA. Repression of transcription of the *mecA* gene is relieved and the PBP2A protein is made, is transported to the cell surface, and functions unimpaired for PG cross-linking in the presence of the extracellular methicillin and other lactam antibiotics. The morphology of the PG being synthesized by PBP2A in the absence of the other functional PBPs is somewhat altered but clearly sufficient to allow MRSA growth. There are auxiliary genes in MRSA, the *fem* genes, that add the pentaglycyl cross bridges to PG strands before cross-linking, which also contribute to the phenotype (Berger-Bachi and Tschierske, 1998; Filipe et al., 2000; Scholar and Pratt, 2000). An estimate of the number of PBP molecules has been made for an MSSA cell and the same cell transformed to the MRSA phenotype with the *mec* DNA (Pucci and Dougherty, 2002). The MSSA cell had about 1,100 copies of PBPs (PBP1–4), with PBP2 making up about 45% of the total. The MRSA cell had about 1,900 to 2,000 PBPs per cell, with PBP2A comprising 40% and PBP2 25% of the total.

Intensive medicinal chemistry activity to produce lactams that will target PBP2A and reverse the MRSA phenotype to MSSA have led to some new lactam structures with promising potency. Examples in the carbapenem series are shown in **Fig. 10.3A**, with 2-aryl or 2-carbolinyl substituents, as well as the β-methyl-substituted aryl carbapenem MK-826 (Chu et al., 1996; Lee and Hecker, 1999). MK-826 has pharmacokinetic properties that suggest once-a-day dosing. One carbapenem had been designed at Merck to be active against MRSA by virtue of a large lipophilic side chain. It was observed that such large hydrophobic substituents were antigenic and caused hypersensitivity, so Rosen et al. (1999) devised the carbapenem L-786,392 that, on attack by the active-site serine of PBP2A, underwent chemical fragmentation and expulsion of the antigenic side chain to reduce immunogenicity (**Fig. 10.3B**) (Rosen et al., 1999).

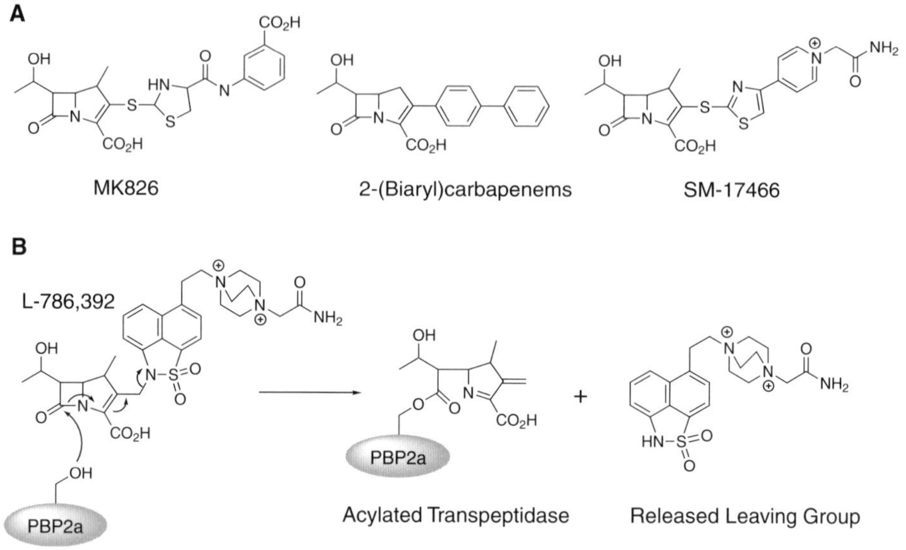

Figure 10.3 Carbapenems with activity against MRSA: (A) molecules with aryl side chain substituents; (B) release of the immunogenic side chain of carbapenem L-786,392 on attack of the β-lactam by the active-site serine of PBP2A.

Such molecules could satisfy a pressing clinical need since MRSA clinical isolates have also gained other drug resistance determinants from the efforts to treat them with varied antibiotics. For example, in MRSA clinical isolates in Japan in 1992, two-thirds had additional drug resistances (Chu et al., 1996). Selection to additional resistance can occur quite rapidly. After the widespread use of the fluoroquinolone ciprofloxacin for treatment of MRSA infections, the incidence of combined MRSA and quinolone resistance went from 5% to >85% in one year.

β-Lactam-resistant *S. pneumoniae*

S. pneumoniae has been an important causative agent in community-acquired pneumonia, meningitis, otitis media, and sinusitis. Unlike the *S. aureus* strains and many other pathogens, *S. pneumoniae* does not use β-lactamases as the major route to penicillin resistance. On the other hand, resistance to penicillin rose 240-fold over the five decades from 1941 to 1991 (see Chu et al., 1996) due to resistance development in the PBP targets themselves. An initial outbreak of lactam-resistant *S. pneumoniae* in South Africa in 1977 has now spread world-wide (Chu et al., 1996). Analysis of transpeptidases/transglycosylases in *S. pneu-moniae* reveal five high-molecular-weight PBPs which contribute to killing by β-lactams: PBP1A, 1B, 2A, 2B, and 2X. A low-molecular-weight PBP3 is not a killing target, whereas PBP2B and 2X are essential. Low-level resistance to pen-icillins involves PBP2X, while cephalosporins elicit a PBP2B of reduced affinity, and these are preludes to further changes in high-resistance phenotypes. In clin-ical isolates with high lactam resistance there are mutations in all five high-molecular-weight PBPs that cause reduced affinities for β-lactams (Nagai et al., 2002). This acquisition of five kinds of mutant proteins would seem to have very low probability if each required independent mutation. There is evidence that at least PBP2B and 2X have undergone homologous recombination in various parts of the encoding genes to create mosaic genes in which resistance is developed by a cassette mechanism (Hakenbeck, 1998; Spratt, 1994). This would represent a natural gene shuffling and could speed evolution of mosaic-resistant PBP proteins.

The X-ray structure of a soluble form of PBP2X has been reported (Pares et al., 1996) after truncation of the N-terminal membrane anchor, revealing a three-domain structure, with the transpeptidase domain in between an amino- and a carboxyl-terminal domain. The gene sequence for *pbp2x* from 35 clinical isolates of penicillin-resistant *S. pneumoniae* (Asahi et al., 1999) has been determined and mapped onto the X-ray structure for the transpeptidase domain, reflecting a clustering of side chain alterations in the penicillin binding site. The modular nature of these proteins may facilitate a gene shuffling strategy to generate diversity and provide an evolutionary route to resistance. In sum, the most remarkable feature in *S. pneumoniae* penicillin resistance is the large number of PBP targets that have been altered to insensitivity to express the phenotype (Hakenbeck et al., 1999). This reflects the remarkably rapid genetic plasticity of bacteria when facing extinction by an antibiotic.

Resistance to macrolides by 23S rRNA methylation

The macrolide class of antibiotics, including erythromycin and the expanded-spectrum agents azithromycin and clarithromycin, have been widely used for respiratory tract infections, but erythromycin resistance has become problematic. Pneumococcal clinical isolates are substantially resistant to erythromycin, and in one study in South Africa in 1992, 70% of MRSA isolates were also resistant to erythromycin (Chu et al., 1996). The major route of resistance is modification of the 23S rRNA in the 50S ribosomal subunit to insensitivity, while efflux, as noted in chapter 9, can also be significant.

The recent X-ray determination of the 50S subunit of the ribosome soaked with erythromycin (Fig. 4.5) visualized the antibiotic bound in the peptidyltransferase cavity, in the vicinity of both A loops and P loops and near A_{2058} (see chapters 4 and 7). It is monomethylation or dimethylation of this N_6 exocyclic amino group of A_{2058} (Fig. 7.6) by an erythromycin ribosome methylation (Erm) modification enzyme that produces the Erm phenotype and reduced affinity of the RNA for the antibiotic, without affecting the role of A_{2058} in peptidyltransferase architecture or function. The cosubstrate is the common biological methyl donor *S*-adenosylmethionine, for both the first and second N-methylations. There are many cellular *N*-methyltransferases known, including RNA *N*-methyltransferases, and evolution of the Erm methyltransferases from such a precursor is likely. More particularly, one such Erm, ErmE, is a constitutively active enzyme in the erythromycin producer *Saccharopolyspora erythraea*, where it provides autoimmunity to the antibiotic producer (chapter 7) and may be a recent progenitor of the Erms in the resistant pathogens. More than two dozen

Erm enzymes have been described in resistant bacteria and an X-ray structure of ErmX (Bussiere et al., 1998) has been reported.

The methyl-A_{2058}-specific enzymatic modification in 23S rRNA not only decreases affinity for macrolide antibiotics of the erythromycin class, but also for those of the lincomycin/clindamycin class, as well as for a third group, the streptogramin B (pristinamycin) family, and this has been described as the macrolide-limcosamide-streptogramin B (MLS_B) phenotype of ribosomal drug resistance (see chapter 4, Fig. 4.5). While the ErmE enzyme in *S. erythraea* is produced constitutively, the MLS_B phenotype is usually inducible by erythromycin in resistant pathogens. The *ermC* gene transcription in *S. aureus* has been well studied (Chu et al., 1996) and indicates that a 141-bp leader sequence just upstream of the *ermC* start codon adopts a secondary structure that sequesters the ribosome binding site so *ermC* transcription is blocked. In the presence of low levels of erythromycin, by mechanisms not yet clear, the secondary structure of the leader is postulated to refold, exposing the ribosome binding site, permitting *ermC* transcription, and producing the ErmC methyltransferase, which methylates A_{2058} and protects the ribosome before lethal concentrations of erythromycin build up in the cell.

One of the goals of medicinal chemistry in developing broad-spectrum erythromycins is to overcome the Erm phenotypes by creating semisynthetic or altered versions of the macrolides that can still bind to methylated A_{2058} versions of the 23S rRNA. Modifications to the expanded-spectrum drug clarithromycin, including oxidation of the 3-hydroxy to a 3-oxo group, produce the ketolide series (**Fig. 10.4**), which are active against erythromycin-resistant *S. pneumoniae* as they do not induce the MLS_B phenotype (Chu et al., 1996). Additional modification of the right-hand side of the macrolactone scaffold and tethered aryl substituents provide sufficient affinity for methylated ribosome 50S subunits to make ketolides promising new drugs. Telithromycin has recently been approved for human use and ABT-773 is in advanced clinical evaluation.

VRE reprogramming the peptidoglycan termini

The increasing use of vancomycin to treat infections caused by the gram-positive MRSA in the 1980s and 1990s selected for drug-resistant enterococci, less potent pathogens than staphylococci but opportunistic in the space vacated by other

Figure 10.4 Structure of 3-ketolides telithromycin and ABT-773, broad-spectrum erythromycin derivatives.

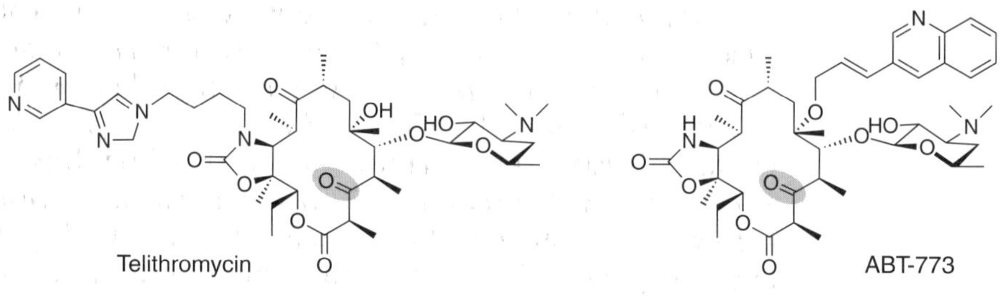

bacteria and in patients with compromised immune systems. *E. faecalis* species account for about 90 to 95% of vancomycin-resistant clinical isolates and *E. faecium* another 5%, with minor species accounting for the rest. Enterococci are the leading causes of endocarditis and are common pathogens in patients with indwelling catheters, including dialysis patients and those undergoing cancer chemotherapy who have chemotherapy-induced white cell depletion in the middle of treatment cycles (Murray, 2000). **Figure 10.5** shows a rise in VRE incidence from below 0.5% in 1989 to 26% in 1994 in hospital wards and in intensive care units, where enterococci can contaminate and multiply in surgical wounds (see Poole, 2001, and references therein). There had been few therapeutic choices for VRE treatment, but the recent approvals of both the Synercid combination and the oxazolidinone linezolid (chapter 4) have come with indications of efficacy against VRE.

The first major clinical phenotype of VRE was termed VanA, followed by the closely related VanB, which has essentially the same molecular mechanism but differs in the continuing sensitivity to teicoplanin (**Table 10.1**) (see Fig. 7.8 for teicoplanin structure). The VanC phenotype has been found in *Enterococcus gallinarum*, and subsequent variations of these three phenotypes have been reported (Cetinkaya et al., 2000).

The VanA and VanB phenotypes are plasmid borne and the relevant genes are often found on transposable elements that account for their rapid spread through enterococcal populations. Five tandemly arranged genes have been found to be necessary and sufficient for both VanA and VanB phenotypes (**Fig. 10.6**), with three enzymes, VanH, VanA, and VanX, involved in reprogramming of the PG termini from *N*-acyl-D-Ala-D-Ala to *N*-acyl-D-Ala-D-lactate (**Fig. 10.7**) and two proteins, VanS and VanR, comprising a two-component regulatory pair that are sensor and response regulator for inducible reprogramming to vancomycin resistance. The switch from D,D-dipeptide to D,D-depsipeptide at the uncross-linked PG terminus effects a thousand-fold decrease in the binding constant for vancomycin (Bugg et al., 1991) and mirrors the thousand-fold increase in vancomycin MICs seen in VRE (**Fig. 10.8**). The affinity loss is in large part due to the loss of the middle hydrogen bond from the peptide carbonyl on

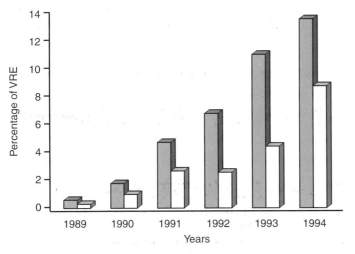

Figure 10.5 Incidence of VRE in intensive care units (shaded bars) and nonintensive care units (unshaded bars) in the early 1990s. (From Hughes and Tenover [1997], with permission.)

Table 10.1 Phenotypes of glycopeptide-resistant enterococci

Phenotype	Sample species	MIC (mg / liter)		Transferable resistance	Induction
		Vancomycin	Teicoplanin		
VanA	E. faecium	64–>1,000	16–512	Yes	Yes
	E. faecalis				
	E. avium				
	E. gallinarum				
VanB	E. faecium	4–1,024	0.25–2	Yes	Yes
	E. faecalis				
VanC	E. gallinarum	2–32	0.12–2	No	Some
	E. casseliflavus				

the underside of the cup-shaped vancomycin molecule to the amide N-H of the D-Ala-D-ala terminus, along with probable ground state repulsions between the depsipeptide lone pair electrons on the ester oxygen of D-Ala-D-Lac.

VanH is a pyruvate reductase (D-lactate dehydrogenase in the reverse direction) using NADH to reduce the C_2 ketone to the C_2-OH in lactate, with chirality control to produce D-lactate. The availability of this D-hydroxy acid in substantial amounts now allows the VanA enzyme to function as a D-Ala-D-lactate depsipeptide ligase, with a 150-to-1 preference at pH 6 for making D-Ala-D-Lac over D-Ala-D-Ala (Lessard et al., 1999). Meanwhile, the native D-Ala-D-Ala ligase has been working to produce its product, D-Ala-D-Ala, so there will be both D,D-dipeptide and D,D-depsipeptide (Fig. 10.6) in the VRE cell. These would normally compete with each other for elongation by MurF, the D-Ala-D-Ala-adding enzyme which converts UDP-muramyl tripeptide to UDP-muramyl pentapeptide to conclude the cytoplasmic phase of peptidoglycan biosynthesis (chapter 3). The presence of the third enzyme, VanX, is required for high-level VRE phenotypes, and VanX acts specifically as a D,D-dipeptidase while sparing the D-Ala-D-lactate from hydrolysis (Lessard and Walsh, 1999). The selectivity on a k_{cat}/K_m basis is almost 10^{10}, a staggering difference that ensures only D-Ala-D-lactate persists in a cell expressing VanH, VanA, and VanX. Then MurF has no competition from D-Ala-D-Ala when it uses D-Ala-D-lactate to make the UDP-muramyl-L-Ala-D-Glu-L-Lys-D-Ala-D-lactate. The subsequent enzymes in the PG

Figure 10.6 A five-gene cluster is necessary and sufficient to confer the VanA and VanB phenotypes of VRE.

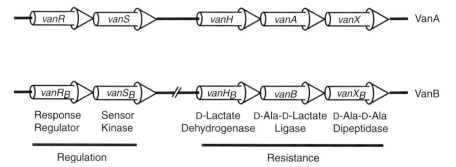

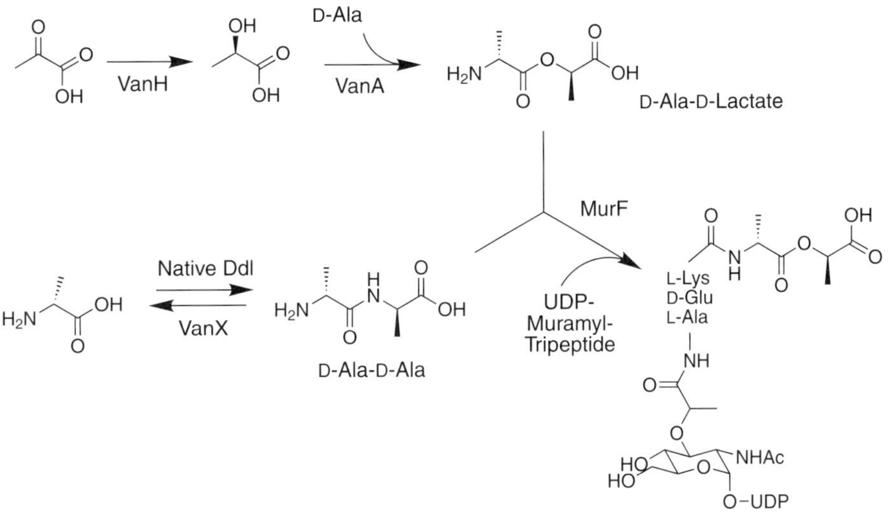

Figure 10.7 Reprogramming of the PG termini from D-Ala-D-Ala to D-Ala-D-lactate by the three-enzyme cassette VanH-VanA-VanX; role of VanX and MurF in partitioning of D-Ala-D-Ala versus D-Ala-D-Lac for destruction or elongation.

pathway take the depsipeptide through to the lipid II stage. This analog is a good substrate for transpeptidase cross-linking (**Fig. 10.9**), enabling the covalently cross-linked, mechanically sound PG layer to be produced such that VRE are not labile to osmotic lysis.

We noted in chapter 7 that the glycopeptide antibiotic producers use a similar strategy to switch on VanH, VanA, and VanX homologs to reprogram their PG layers and create protective self-immunity to the actions of the glycopeptide

Figure 10.8 Loss of one hydrogen bond between vancomycin and D-Ala-D-lactate provides a 1,000-fold drop in binding affinity.

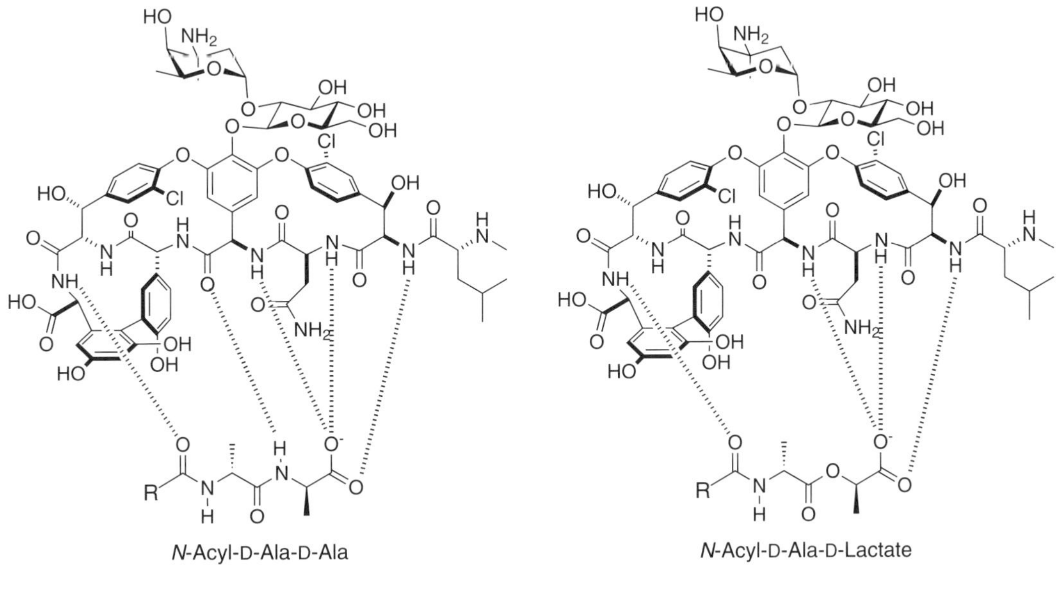

N-Acyl-D-Ala-D-Ala   *N*-Acyl-D-Ala-D-Lactate

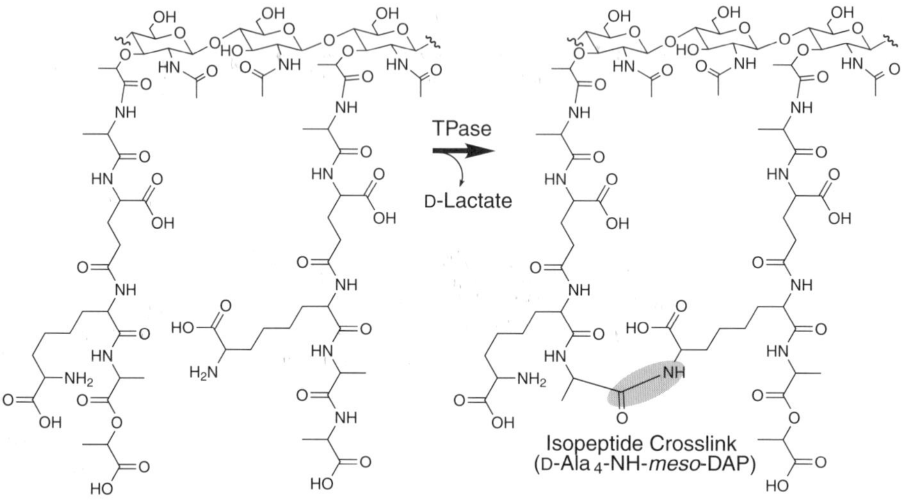

Figure 10.9 PG-D-Ala-D-Lac termini are substrates for transpeptidase-mediated crosslinking.

antibiotics they are making and exporting (Fig. 7.9). Such producer genes may be the source of the three-enzyme cassette in the opportunistically pathogenic VREs. The X-ray structures of a D-Ala-D-Ala ligase from *Escherichia coli* (Fan et al., 1994), a D-Ala-D-lactate ligase from the soil bacterium *Leuconostoc mesenteroides* (Kuzin et al., 2000) that has innate immunity to vancomycin, and the VanA ligase from VRE (Roper et al., 2000) have been determined, validating their close architectural homologies and indicating changes in the active site from a Tyr_{216} to a Phe_{216} to a His_{216} as one progresses through the three enzymes (**Fig. 10.10A**) and gains increasing selectivity for D-Ala-D-lactate over D-Ala-D-Ala formation. All three of the X-ray structures have a phosphinophosphate inhibitor bound, produced from the phosphinate reacting with ATP in the active site (**Fig. 10.10B and C**). The phosphinates are potent against the D-Ala-D-X ligases in vitro, but these charged molecules do not penetrate into bacterial cytoplasms and so are not active against whole bacteria.

Extending the hypothesis that VRE phenotypes reflect molecular reprogramming of D-Ala-D-Ala ligases is the VanC ligase from *E. gallinarum* (Navarro and Courvalin, 1994). This enzyme is a D-Ala-D-Ser ligase, showing about 350-fold selectivity for D-Ser in place of $D-Ala_2$ in the ligase active site (Park et al., 1997). The carry forward of D-Ala-D-Ser by MurF and subsequent PG biosynthetic enzymes yields a PG terminus with D-Ala-D-Ser where the CH_2OH side chain of the D-Ser interferes with the recognition by vancomycin compared to its complementary surface fit of the smaller CH_3 group of the terminal D-Ala. The affinity drop is more modest, about 10-fold.

The VanB operon has a comparable five-gene cluster—$VanS_B$, $VanR_B$, VanH, VanB, and $VanX_B$—and the molecular logic of the PG reprogramming enzymes is identical to that of the VanA operon. What differs is the observation that while both vancomycin and teicoplanin induces the transcription of the five genes of the VanA operon, only vancomycin but not teicoplanin induces the VanB operon (Table 10.1), explaining why VanB strains remain sensitive to teicoplanin (Arthur

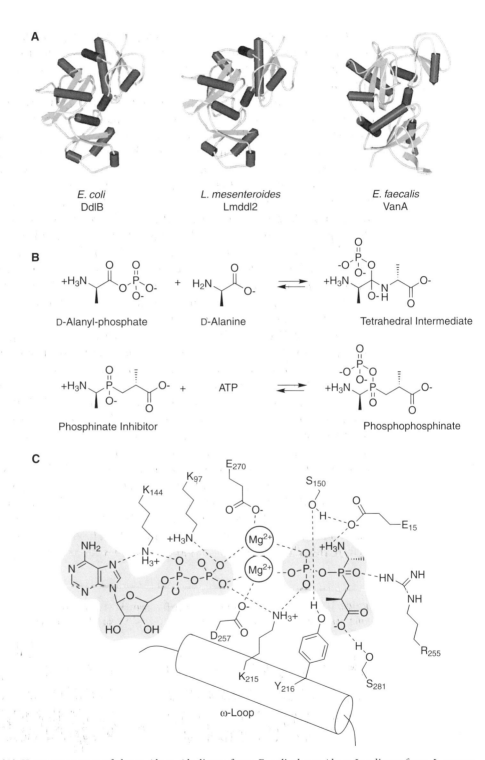

Figure 10.10 (A) X-ray structures of the D-Ala-D-Ala ligase from *E. coli*, the D-Ala-D-Lac ligase from *L. mesenteroides*, and the VanA D-Ala-D-Lac ligase from *E. faecalis*. (B) The phosphorylation of the dialkylphosphinate analog in the active site of the ligase produces a transition-state analog that behaves like a slow, tight-binding inhibitor. (C) Active-site architecture of *E. coli* DdlB with ADP and phosphophosphinate bound. (From Shi and Walsh [1995], with permission.)

and Courvalin, 1993). These results suggest that the glycopeptide antibiotic(s) are the inducers for VanA or VanB (vancomycin only) and indeed, mutants in the $VanS_B$ sensor protein can convert it to respond to extracellular teicoplanin. The two-component VanS-VanR logic seems typical of these bacterial sensor/ transducer systems (Walsh et al., 1996b). Vancomycin in the extracellular microenvironment is sensed by the exo domain of VanS, whether directly or indirectly by some PG fragment as in the AmpC-sensing system (see chapter 8). This signal is transduced across the membrane to the cytoplasmic histidine kinase domain of VanS, which is now autoactivated to phosphorylate its dimeric subunit partner in *trans* (**Fig. 10.11**). The phospho-His form of VanS can transfer the $-PO_3$ group to the specific response regulator protein VanR, a two-domain transcription factor, to an Asp side chain in the N-terminal domain. The phospho-Asp form of the N-terminal domain of VanR communicates this change in phosphorylation state to the C-terminal DNA binding domain, and transcriptional activation of *vanH*, *vanA*, and *vanX* occurs to start the PG reprogramming. There is some evidence that in the default state in VanA phenotypes, the VanS acts in net fashion as a VanR kinase, while the $VanS_B$ may act at rest mostly as a phosphatase for phospho-Asp $VanR_B$.

Given that VanA and VanB phenotypes of VRE collect five genes to make a PG reprogramming that alters one hydrogen bond to vancomycin, there are several approaches for reversing the phenotype. One approach is to use VanS, VanR, VanH, VanA, and VanX as targets for molecules that inactivate them, and some inhibitors of VanX have been reported (Araoz et al., 2000). Such an inhibitor in combination with vancomycin would mimic the Augmentin strategy for β-lactam antibiotics (see chapter 8). A second strategy has been to screen against VRE for glycopeptides that retain antibiotic activity. This has led to semisynthetic versions of lipoglycopeptides such as LY333328 (see chapter 15, Fig. 15.6) that are 80- to 100-fold more active than the parent glycopeptides that lack the lipid chain, restoring two of the three logs of activity lost against the VRE phenotype. This compound is in clinical development under the name ortavancin. The hydrophobic chlorobiphenyl moiety can be moved around the disaccharide chain (Ge et al., 1999) and retain VRE activity, suggesting the lipid

Figure 10.11 Proposal for the VanS-VanR sensor kinase/response regulator to turn on the *vanH*, *vanA*, and *vanX* genes to reprogram peptidoglycan biosynthesis.

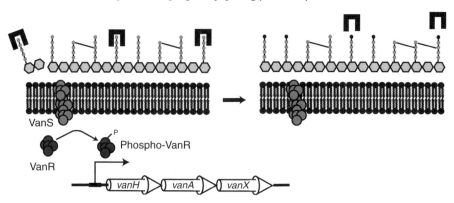

is a membrane anchor to preconcentrate the lipoglycopeptide and provide a higher effective concentration at the external surface of the membrane where the PG cross-links occur. It has been proposed that such hydrophobic derivatives of glycopeptides are selectively inhibiting transglycosylases in VRE, redirecting these drug candidates from transpeptidase inhibition to new targets (Ge et al., 1999; Sun et al., 2001).

Antibiotic Biosynthesis

I N THIS SECTION OF THE BOOK WE EXAMINE strategies for biosynthesis of major classes of antibiotics. The logic and machinery for polyketide-derived aromatic and modular antibiotics is discussed in chapter 12. Chapter 13 examines the parallel assembly-line strategy for nonribosomal peptide antibiotics including the penem, oxapenem, and carbapenem classes. Chapter 14 takes up the biosynthetic pathways of other classes of antibiotics, including the aminocoumarins and the aminoglycosides. The biosynthesis of terpene and alkaloid natural products, some of which have antibiotic activity, is not discussed. Readers are directed to the multivolume set *Comprehensive Natural Products Chemistry* (Barton et al., 1999) for those topics and a broader context of the molecules of chapters 12 to 14.

We introduce this section with chapter 11, which summarizes what is known about the genes and proteins that control the timing of synthesis of antibiotics in producer organisms. This is a complement to chapter 7, in which the defense mechanisms of antibiotic producers were examined at the protein level. The *Actinomycetales* order of bacteria, and specifically the *Streptomycetes* family within that order, are prolific generators of chemical weaponry against their neighbors, producing an estimated 8,400 of the 12,000 known natural antibiotics (Champness, 2000). The molecular signaling pathways that have begun to be deciphered in streptomycetes, in particular in *Streptomyces coelicolor*, are likely to be of general utility for analysis of the logic of other antibiotic producers.

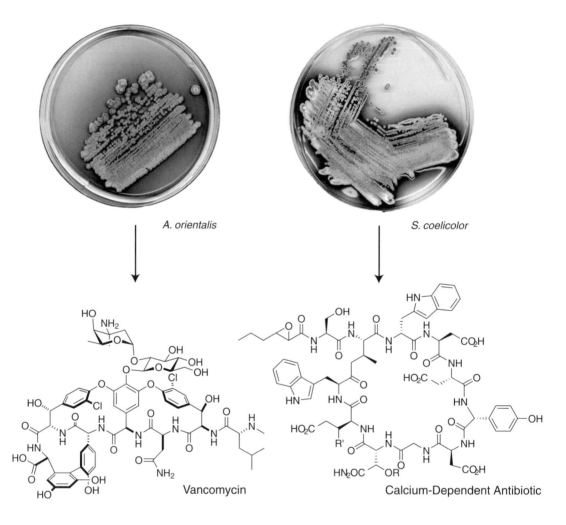

A. orientalis

S. coelicolor

Vancomycin

Calcium-Dependent Antibiotic

Amycolatopsis orientalis, the vancomycin producer, and *Streptomyces coelicolor*, the producer of calcium-dependent antibiotic.

chapter 11

Regulation of Antibiotic Biosynthesis in Producer Organisms

Regulation of antibiotic production in streptomycetes

Of the circa 12,000 known antibiotics, it has been estimated that some 160 are or have been in human clinical use. Streptomycetes, gram-positive filamentous bacteria, account for the production of about 55% of these commercially significant antibiotics (Champness, 2000).

Table 11.1 summarizes 26 examples, including both macrocyclic and aromatic polyketides, nonribosomal peptides, β-lactams, hybrid polyketide-peptide structures, coumarins, and polypyrroles, which differ in structures and modes of antibacterial action. Many of the compounds in this table are discussed in detail in other chapters of this book. These streptomycete and actinomycete antibiotics share a common feature that their biosynthesis is often temporally coordinated with other changes in colony morphology, in particular the developmental changes that include aerial mycelia and spore formation (e.g., see Bibb et al., 2000, and references therein; Chakraburtty and Bibb, 1997). A variety of conditions, including nutrient limitation, can start both the developmental and the antibiotic production programs, and it has become clear that there are networks of regulatory signals and systems that intersect and also run in parallel. Understanding the machinery of antibiotic gene regulation would increase the chances for rational enhancement and control of antibiotic levels and aid in getting combinatorial biosynthetic pathways to function in vivo.

Figure 11.1 shows micrographs of cultures of *Streptomyces avermitilis*, the avermectin producer; *Streptomyces clavuligerus*, the clavulanate producer; *Amycolatosis orientalis*, the vancomcyin producer; and *Streptomyces coelicolor*, the host organism for many of the recombinant approaches to combinatorial biosynthesis, described in chapters 12 and 16.

Several different antibiotic-producing streptomycetes have been valuable in elucidating some of the molecular logic that controls timing and amounts of antibiotic production, using genetic screens for effects on antibiotic production as a fruitful route to define gene identity and function. At present there is some

Table 11.1 Selected actinomycete antibiotics

Antibiotic	Producer	Class[1]	Target[2]	Application
Avermectin	*Streptomyces avermitilis*	Macrolide(PK)	Chloride ion channels	Antiparasitic
Bleomycin	"*Streptomyces verticillus*"	Glycopeptide	DNA strand breakage	Antitumor
Chloramphenicol	*Streptomyces venezuelae*	N-dichloroacyl phenylpropanoid	Ribosome binding	Antibacterial
Chlorotetracycline	*Streptomyces aureofaciens*	Tetracycline (PK)	Ribosome binding	Antibacterial
Clavulanic acid	*Streptomyces clavuligerus*	β-lactam	β-Lactamase inhibitor	Combined with β-lactam as antibacterial
Daptomycin	*Streptomyces roseosporus*	Lipopeptide	Lipoteichoic acid?	Antibacterial
Daunorubicin (daunomycin)	*Streptomyces peucetius*	Anthracycline (PK)	DNA intercalation	Antitumor
Erythromycin	*Saccharomyces erythraea*	Macrolide (PK)	Ribosome binding	Antibacterial
FK506 (tacrolimus)	*Streptomyces hygroscopicus*	Macrolide (PK)	Binds to FK protein	Immunosuppressant
Fosfomycin	*Streptomyces* spp.	Phosphonic acid	Peptidoglycan	Antibacterial
Gentamicin	*Micromonospora* spp.	Aminoglycoside	Ribosome binding	Antibacterial
Kanamycin	*Streptomyces kanamyceticus*	Aminoglycoside	Ribosome binding	Antibacterial
Mitomycin C	"*S. caespitosus*," "*S. verticillatus*"	Benzoquinone	DNA cross-linking	Antitumor
Nocardicin	*Nocardia uniformis*	β-Lactam	Peptidoglycan	Antibacterial
Nosiheptide	"*S. actuosus*"	Thiopeptide	Ribosome binding	Growth promoter
Novobiocin	*Streptomyces niveus*	Coumarin glycoside	DNA gyrase (β subunit)	Antibacterial
Oleandomycin	*Streptomyces antibioticus*	Macrolide (PK)	Ribosome binding	Antibacterial
Oxytetracycline	*Streptomyces rimosus*	Tetracycline (PK)	Ribosome binding	Antibacterial
Pristinamycin	"*S. pristinaespiralis*"	Peptidic macrolactone + polyunsaturated macrolactone (PK)	Ribosome binding	Antibacterial
Rifamycin	*Amycolatopsis mediterranei*	Ansamycin (PK)	RNA polymerase	Antibacterial (tuberculosis and leprosy)
Teicoplanin	*Actinoplanes teichomyceticus*	Glycopeptide	Peptidoglycan	Antibacterial

Table 11.1 (*continued*)

Antibiotic	Producer	Class[1]	Target[2]	Application
Tetracycline	*Streptomyces aureofaciens*	Tetracycline (PK)	Ribosome binding	Antibacterial
Thienamycin	"*S. cattleya*"	β-Lactam	Peptidoglycan	Antibacterial
Tylosin	*Streptomyces fradiae*	Macrolide (PK)	Ribosome binding	Growth promoter
Vancomycin	*Amycolatopsis orientalis*	Glycopeptide	Peptidoglycan	Antibacterial
Virginiamycin	*Streptomyces virginiae*	Macrocyclic lactone (PK) + macrocyclic peptidolactone	Ribosome binding	Growth promoter

[1] PK, polyketide
[2] Ribosome binding will inhibit protein synthesis.
Adapted from Kieser et al. (2000), with permission.

understanding of two layers of regulatory networks, the first using two-component sensor kinase/response regulator machinery for global regulation and the second using quorum-sensing molecules that travel between cells and have been termed streptomycetes "hormones" for pathway-specific regulation (Takano et al., 2000; Yamada and Nihara, 1999).

The sequence of the *S. coelicolor* genome has recently been determined (Bentley et al., 2002) and found to contain 7,825 predicted genes, almost double the gene content of *Escherichia coli* (4,289) and *Bacillus subtilis* (4,099). Consistent with the large genome and selective gene expression in distinct soil environments are an enormous number of regulatory genes, 965 genes representing more than 12% of the genome. These include 65 σ factors that control the promoter recognition specificity of the core subunits of RNA polymerase to enable selective transcription of sets of genes and at least 53 two-component pairs of transmembrane sensor kinases/response regulators for gene transcription in response to external signals. Twenty gene clusters are predicted to encode enzymes acting in secondary metabolic pathways, including some for the antibiotics of Fig. 11.2. Many of these secondary natural product biosynthetic gene clusters are out on the periphery of the linear *S. coelicolor* chromosome and are thought to have been added on to the core chromosome-encoded functions (Bentley et al., 2002). The peripheral regions of other streptomycete chromosomes may be loci for additional antibiotic biosynthetic genes.

A second example of a bacterium that uses quorum signals for antibiotic gene biosynthesis is the plant pathogen *Erwinia carotovora*, which regulates carbapenem assembly, as will be noted at the end of the chapter (Swift et al., 1996).

Global regulators of antibiotic production in *S. coelicolor*: two-component regulators

From the sequence of the genome of *S. coelicolor,* one can identify gene clusters for the four known antibiotics of this bacterium: actinorhodin (polyketide), un-

A

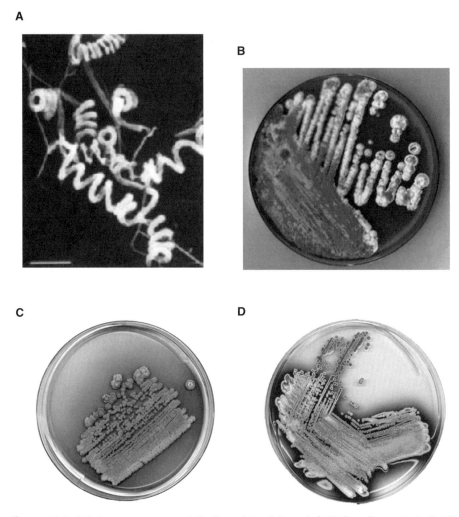

B

C

D

Figure 11.1 (A) *Streptomyces avermitilis* (from Miyadoh et al. [1997], with permission); (B) *Streptomyces clavuligerus* (from www.cbs.umn.edu/asirc, © 1997, with permission); (C) *Amycolotopsis orientalis*; (D) *Streptomyces coelicolor.*

decylprodigiosin (hybrid polyketide-polypyrrole), calcium-dependent antibiotic (CDA) (nonribosomal peptide), and methylenemycin (polyketide) (**Fig 11.2**). Genetic screens have turned up mutants at the *abs* locus that are deficient in production of all four antibiotics, as though a global regulatory network were blocked. Mapping and sequence analysis indicated two Abs proteins, Abs1 and Abs2, that are close to the CDA biosynthetic gene cluster (see Bibb, 1996). The Abs1-Abs2 pair has all the predicted sequence hallmarks of a standard two-component regulatory system, with Abs1 a transmembrane histidine kinase and Abs2 the aspartate-containing response regulator that gets phosphorylated by the phospho-His form of Abs1. The phospho-Asp form of Abs2 is a negative regulator of target genes, which include the antibiotic pathway-specific transcription factors to be discussed below. So in the absence of some signal to the contrary, the default position is that Abs2 is phosphorylated and keeps the transcription

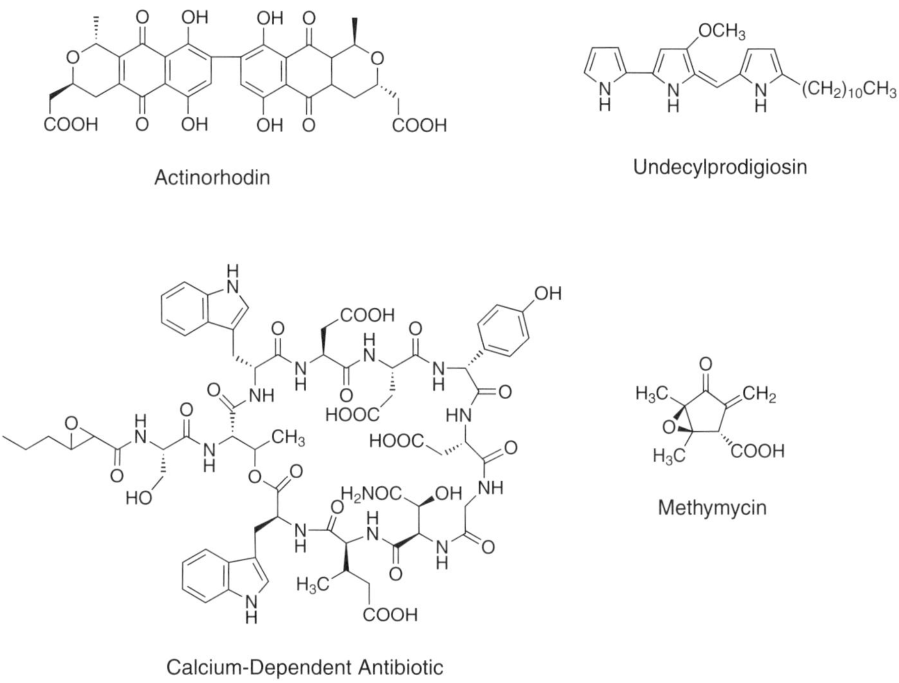
Actinorhodin
Undecylprodigiosin
Calcium-Dependent Antibiotic
Methymycin

Figure 11.2 Structures of secondary metabolites produced by *S. coelicolor*.

of target genes controlling the antibiotic biosynthetic cluster genes turned off (Fig. 11.2). The identity of the signal is not yet known; possibly it is a ligand for the extracellular or transmembrane domain of Abs1 that converts this two-component system from off to on and relieves the gene repression. A reasonable speculation, based on other two-component system logic, is that the response to the unknown signal is that Abs1 switches from a kinase mode to a phosphatase mode, inducing hydrolysis of the P-Asp-Abs2 to the dephospho form (**Fig. 11.3**), with loss of binding affinity to target gene promoter regions; release of dephospho-Abs2 would allow target gene transcription to proceed.

Figure 11.3 Two-component regulatory logic for antibiotic gene transcriptional control by Abs1 and Abs2 in streptomycetes.

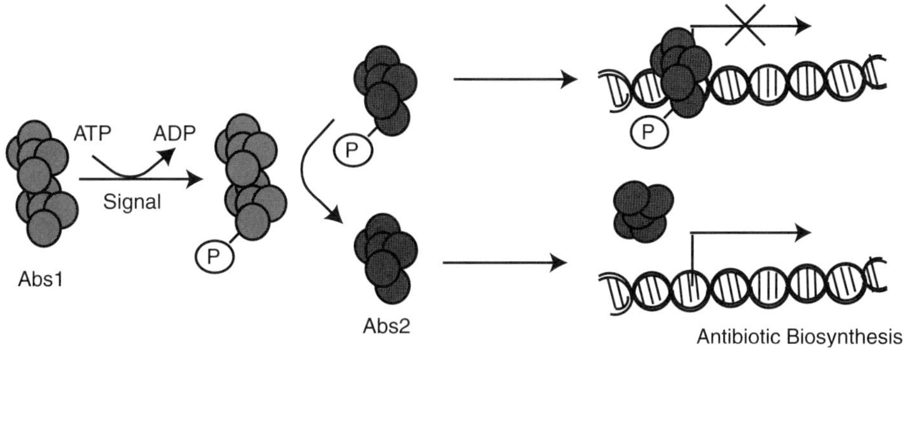
ATP
ADP
Signal
P
Abs1
Abs2
Antibiotic Biosynthesis

The Abs1-Abs2 pair is probably not the only global regulator that controls the timing of antibiotic biosynthetic gene expression in this and other streptomycetes. For example, there is an Abs2 homolog, RedZ, in the undecylprodigiosin cluster. Also, overexpression of another two-component pair, AfsQ1-AfsQ2, will substitute. The Abs knockout leads to precocious production of all the *S. coelicolor* antibiotics in hours to days and in amounts up to 60-fold higher than normal, dependent on the culture conditions. There has been speculation that control of the timing of antibiotic production by the mycelial mat may be important not to interfere with successful execution of the development program, e.g., spore production by the aerial hyphae. Delay of production of the pore-forming CDA lipopeptide, for example may be important to avoid autotoxicity. A third two-component system, the *cutR* and *cutS* genes, also acts in negative regulation of antibiotic production (Chang et al., 1996), suggesting several intersection points for environmental sensing and the expression of antibiotic biosynthetic genes. The availability of the *S. colelicolor* genome sequence will now allow systematic analysis of the role of each of the 53 two-component systems in antibiotic production.

Antibiotic pathway-specific regulation in *Streptomyces* by butaneolides

The most extensive analysis of regulation of a specific antibiotic pathway, one step down from the Abs global regulators, is probably in *Streptomyces virginiae* in production of the two antibiotics virginiamycin M1 and virginiamycin S1 (**Fig. 11.4**). Virginiamycins have been isolated multiple times and virginiamycin M1 has also been known as pristinamycin IIA and streptogramin A. The M1 molecule is a macrolactone that is a hybrid of a polyketide with a dipeptide-derived oxazolyl-proline moiety. The S1 component is a cyclic hexapeptide with a lactone or depsipeptide linkage between Thr_1 and $PheGly_6$. Thr_1 has an aryl-*N*-cap typical of chain initiation strategies in nonribosomal peptide antibiotics. The gene cluster for a homologous pristinamycin pair that comprise the antibacterial combination Synercid (see chapter 4) has been elucidated (Bozdogan and Leclercq, 1999; Soltani et al., 2001). The enzymatic logic for biogenesis of such peptide and mixed polyketide/peptide antibiotics is examined in chapter 13.

Figure 11.4 Structures of virginiamycin antibiotics.

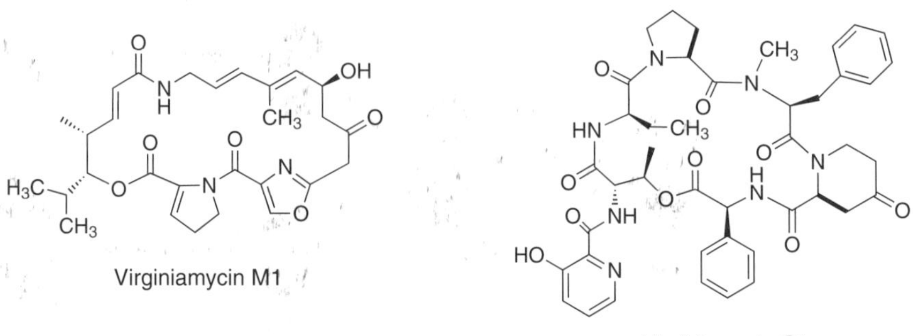

Virginiamycin M1

Virginiamycin S1

Butaneolide signaling molecules

The control of production of the virginiamycins in *S. virginiae*, the nucleoside antibiotics showdomycin and minimycin in *Streptomyces lavendulae*, the four antibiotics of *S. coelicolor* (see "Regulation of antibiotic production in strepto-mycetes" above), daunorubicin in *S. peucetius*, and doubtless many other of the streptomycete antibiotics of Table 11.1 is mediated by interaction of specific transcriptional repressor proteins with cell-permeable small ligands, the buta-neolides. Later in this chapter and elsewhere in this book (e.g., chapter 15) we note that gram-negative bacteria use *N*-acylhomoserine lactones (*N*-acyl-HSLs) as cell-permeant signaling molecules whose concentrations reflect bacterial cell density and so act as quorum sensors. The molecules that most likely serve as equivalent quorum sensors in the gram-positive streptomycete bacteria are γ-butyrolactones, five-ring lactones analogous to the acyl-HSLs but lacking the amino group (**Fig. 11.5**). The hydrophobic side chain of the butyrolactones, known generically also as butaneolides, is in the same locus as the N-acyl moiety of the gram-negative quorum molecules. There is variation in the side chain length and in particular in the oxidation state and stereochemistry of the six-oxo substituent of butaneolides between streptomycete species (Yamada and Nihara, 1999). In the A-factor butaneolide of *Streptomyces griseus*, it is a ketone; in the Im2-type butaneolide of S. *lavendulae*, it is a 6-β-OH, while in *S. virginiae*, it is a 6-α-OH (**Fig. 11.6**). The biosynthesis of these substituted butyrolactones is likely to arise by enzymatic condensation of the primary three-carbon metab-olite dihydroxyacetone-P, where the C_1-OH attacks the activated carbonyl group of a β-keto-acyl-*S*-CoA or β-keto-acyl-*S*-ACP (acyl carrier protein) thioester. This intermediate would then undergo intramolecular aldol condensation, de-hydration, and enone reduction, to yield the 6-keto oxidation state found in the *S. griseus* A-factor (**Fig. 11.7**). Stereospecific reductases would control subsequent production of the 6-α- and 6-β- stereochemical variants (Yamada and Nihara, 1999).

These small molecules produced by one cell can diffuse into a neighboring streptomycete cell in a manner that is cell density dependent and can complex with an intracellular receptor protein with nanomolar affinity. In S. *lavendulae* the partner protein for the 6-β-butaneolide is the FarA receptor, in S. *griseus* the A-factor binds to the ArpA receptor, while in *S. virginiae* the 6-α-hydroxybutyrolactone binds the corresponding BarA receptor (Fig. 11.6).

The FarA, ArpA, and BarA antibiotic pathway-specific transcription factors are transcriptional repressors in the absence of the butaneolide ligands. For ex-ample, BarA sits on the promoter regions of target genes and keeps them off.

Figure 11.5 Comparison of quorum-sensing molecules.

Acyl Homoserine Lactones
(Gram-Negative)

Butyrolactones
(Gram-Positive)

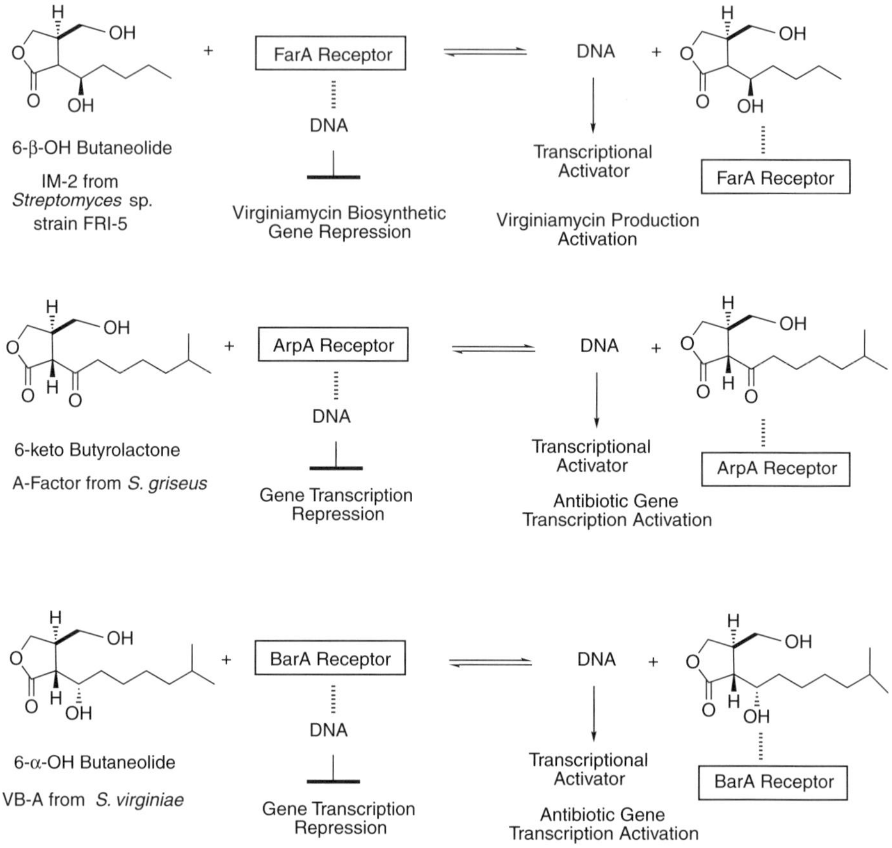

Figure 11.6 Different redox states at C_6 of butaneolide quorum-signaling molecules and differential interaction with streptomycete transcriptional repressors ArpA, FarA, and BarA.

The negative regulation is relieved on binding of the butaneolide because the complex has a lower affinity for DNA and falls off; then repression ceases and gene transcription can begin.

Integrating the regulatory circuitry for antibiotic production in streptomycetes

Genetic analysis had identified one of the targets of the BarA repressor protein as the *vmsR* gene. *vmsR* has homologs in other antibiotic-producing strepto-mycete pathways: *dnrI* for daunorubicin, *actII-orf4* for actinorhodin, and *redD* for the undecylprodigiosin cluster (Kawachi et al., 2000). The protein products of these target genes have been termed SARPs (*Streptomyces* antibiotic regulatory proteins) (Champness, 2000) and are all homologs of the *E. coli* transcription factor and DNA binding protein OmpR (**Fig. 11.8**). OmpR belongs to a large family of transcription factors called the "winged helix-turn-helix" family (Martinez-Hackert and Stock, 1997; Martinez-Hackert et al., 1996). With its companion sensor protein EnvF, OmpR is the gene regulatory component of the

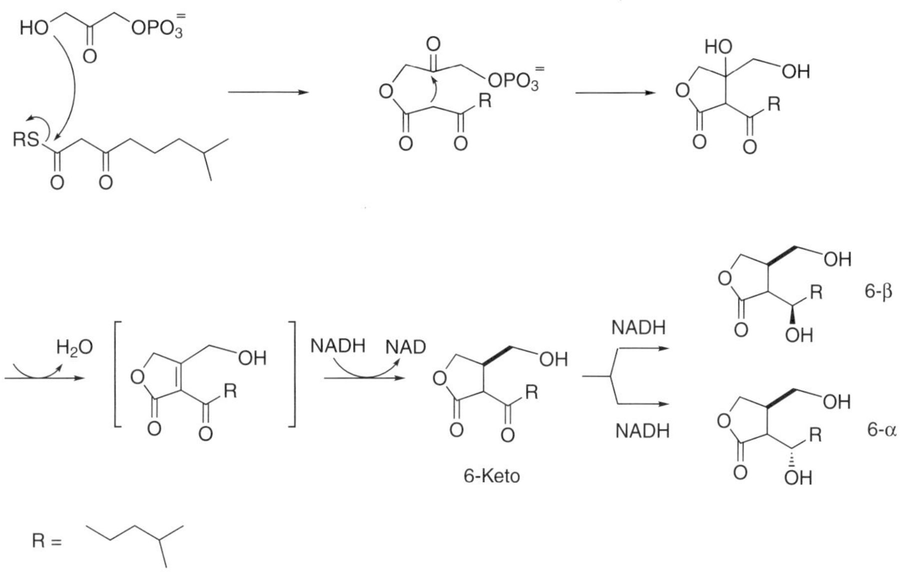

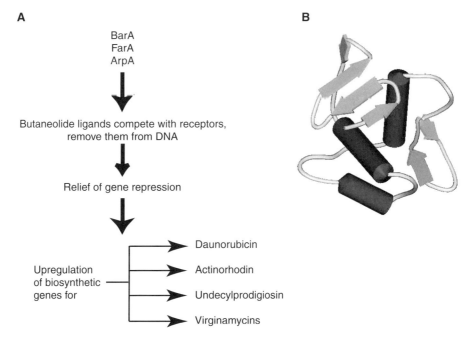

Figure 11.7. Proposed biosynthetic pathway for the quorum-sensing butaneolides.

Figure 11.8 (A) SARP are homologs of OmpR; (B) structure of the OmpR transcription factor.

EnvF-OmpR two-component system that controls the expression of bacterial outer membrane porins in response to changes in external osmolarity. Phospho-OmpR increases with increased osmolarity and binds more tightly to the promoter of its target genes, repressing transcription of *ompF* and activating transcription of *ompC*. It is likely that the SARP have architectures comparable to those of OmrR and recognize target gene promoters in similar fashion, by the action of an N-terminal domain phosphorylated by the phospho form of the partner sensor kinase and a C-terminal DNA binding domain whose affinity for target DNA is modulated by the phosphorylation state of the N-terminal domain.

When the VmsR protein is produced by increased *vmsR* gene transcription, the net result is increased synthesis of both virginiamycins M1 and S1. Whether VmsR acts directly on the nonribosomal peptide synthetase and polyketide synthase genes that directly encode the enzymes for antibiotic assembly or whether there is yet a third layer of regulatory protein circuitry is not yet known. *vmsR* is specific to the antibiotic pathway and not any of the contemporaneously regulated developmental pathways since the phenotype of a knockout is specific to virginiamycin production (Kawachi et al., 2000). Analogously, the ArpA protein of *S. griseus* in the absence of 6-keto butaneolide ligand represses expression of several genes. When the quorum-signaling ligand titrates ArpA off DNA promoter sequences, among the downstream genes transcribed are the biosynthetic gene clusters for the aminoglycoside antibiotic streptomycin (Yamada and Nihara, 1999) (see chapter 14).

It is likely that the two layers of antibiotic gene regulation in streptomycetes, the global level effected by two-component sensor/regulators and the pathway-specific SARP for each antibiotic cluster, will be generalizable and use comparable molecular logic to receive cues from the environment about when to turn on antibiotic production. In chapter 7 we noted several examples of mechanisms by which antibiotic producers provide immunity to themselves, including the coordination of synthesis with export of antibiotics to keep the intracellular concentration of the antibiotic below the growth inhibitory threshold.

The temporal regulation of antibiotic production and export is exemplified also in the *S. virginiae* BarA context. Just downstream of *barA* and *barB* are the two genes *varS* and *varR*. The VarS protein appears to be a virginiamycin efflux pump, imparting self-resistance to the antibiotic producer by keeping intracellular concentration of this ribosome-targeting antibiotic low. This capacity is acquired just in time by increased transcription of *varS* by relief of repression by the adjacent gene product VarR, an analog of the TetR repressor (see chapter 9). In the absence of small-molecule ligands (the Vb butaneolide for BarA and virginiamycin S for VarS), the BarA and VarR proteins dimerize and bind to the promoter regions of *barB* and *varS*, keeping transcription at low to negligible levels. When the Vb butyrolactone concentration is elevated (increased cell density) to saturate BarA and the virginiamycin S molecule can bind to VarR, both repressor-ligand complexes fall off their DNA promoter regions and transcription of *barB* and *varS* goes up. BarB is required for virginiamycin biosynthesis, while VarS is the efflux pump that will facilitate export of the antibiotic as it is produced (**Fig. 11.9**).

Studies on the *Streptomyces fradiae* biosynthetic cluster for the 16-membered macrolide tylosin (see chapter 4 for mechanism of action and Fig. 4.3 for struc-

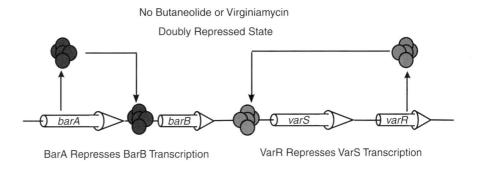

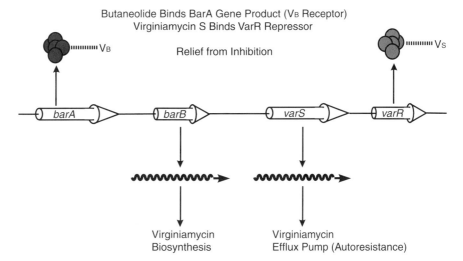

Figure 11.9 Butaneolide and virginiamycin S in coordinate regulation of virginiamycin biosynthesis.

ture) (Stratigopoulos and Cundliffe, 2002) indicate that this 43-gene cluster, encompassing 85 kb of DNA, has five identified regulatory genes, *tylP, tylQ, tylR, tylS,* and *tylT,* that fit the paradigm for streptomycete regulation noted above for the virginiamycin class. The TylP protein is thought to be the quorum-sensing butaneolide receptor and the ligand-receptor complex is thought to bind at a DNA sequence just in front of the *tylQ* gene, turning TylQ production off. The drop in TylQ relieves repression of transcription of the TylR protein, which is a global regulator. This activates expression of the *tylS* and *tylT* genes to produce the TylS and TylT proteins, which are SARPs that turn on transcription of some of the *tyl* polyketide synthase genes and the *tyl* deoxysugar biosynthesis genes, required for tylosin assembly to begin. The novel feature in the tylosin gene cluster regulation is the discovery that TylQ is a repressor that is at high levels in *S. fradiae* cells before tylosin is produced and is turned off as a key signal for the global regulator and the SARP gene transcriptions to begin. The signal for transcriptional shutdown of *tylQ* is not yet determined.

A schematic for regulation of biosynthetic gene expression for the major classes of streptomycete antibiotics (polyketides, nonribosomal peptides, and aminoglycosides) is thus beginning to take shape. The availability of the full *S. coelicolor* genome sequence will facilitate a detailed understanding of the full regulatory network with hierarchy and nodal points of signal integration in the near future. For now one can say that external signals, including nutrient limitation and concomitant growth slowing or cessation on the one hand and cell density-dependent levels of butaneolide signaling molecules on the other, impinge on a set of global regulatory genes, some of which will encode two-component sensor/response regulator systems (Fig. 11.9). In turn, these will control transcriptional activation of antibiotic pathway-specific transcription factors that will upregulate the transcriptional expression of clusters of biosynthetic enzymes to produce the palette of varied antibiotic structures (**Fig. 11.10**) (Bibb, 1996). One also expects that regulation of expression of the many σ subunit genes (65 in *S. coelicolor*) of RNA polymerase will be part of the integrated response. Studies in *Streptomyces lividans* indicate rifampin-resistant RNA polymerase mutants in the β subunit become activated for actinorhodin and undecylprodigiosin biosynthesis by upregulation of *redD* and *actII-orf4* transcription. These results suggest the mutations stabilize a β subunit conformer that mimics the RNA polymerase form induced by signals that initiate

Figure 11.10 Schematic for signal input and regulatory networks controlling antibiotic production in streptomycetes. (From Bibb [1996], with permission.)

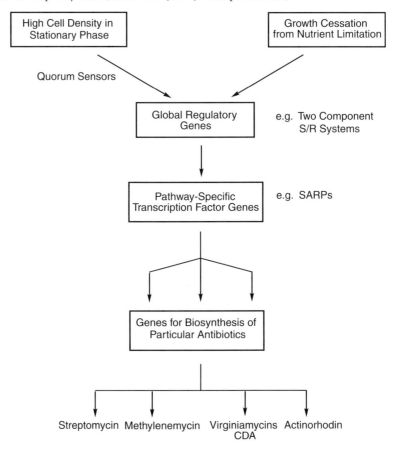

the onset of antibiotic production in response to environmental cues (Hu et al., 2002).

Regulation of virulence factors and antibiotic biosynthesis in gram-negative bacteria by quorum-sensing *N*-acyl homoserine lactones

Analogous gene regulatory logic can be detected in control of virulence factors and antibiotic production in gram-negative bacteria that produce and secrete acyl-HSLs instead of the gram-positive butaneolides as diffusible cell density-dependent quorum-sensing and -signaling molecules. We note two examples below.

Plant pathogenic bacteria often secrete enzymes (exoenzymes) with hydrolytic capacity to destroy the components of plant cell walls to release the nutrients that can then be utilized by the pathogens. *E. carotovora* is one such phytopathogen that uses the population density-driven pheromone/quorum-signaling systems to upregulate exoenzyme production and secretion to digest plant cell walls to make nutrients available to the resource-limited bacteria (Swift et al., 1996). These *Erwinia* also use the same signaling logic to coordinately upregulate the genes for carbapenem biosynthesis (**Fig. 11.11**). The β-lactam antibiotic kills off neighboring bacteria that would otherwise compete for the released plant cell nutrients and sterilizes the microenvironment except for the producing *Erwinia*. Figure 11.11 shows a schematic for the production of the 3-keto-octanoyl homoserine lactone (OHHL) by the CarI enzyme of *E. carotovora* and its binding to the CarR transcriptional repressor protein, releasing the OHHL-Car complex

Figure 11.11 Regulation of exoenzyme and carbapenem antibiotic production in *Erwinia carotovora* by the acylhomoserine lactone OHHL.

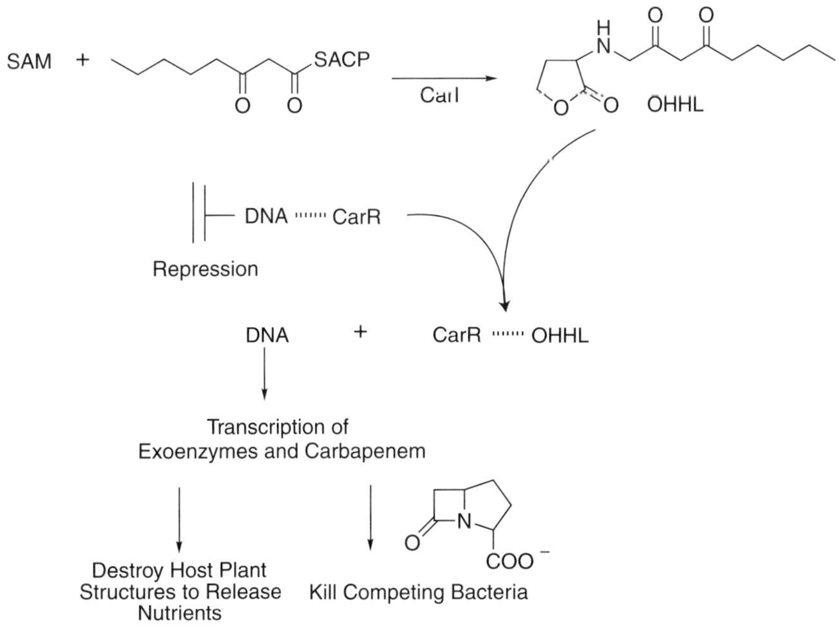

from promoter regions of target genes and relieving transcriptional repression. Exoenzyme synthesis and secretion destroys the host plant cell structures, releasing nutrients. Concomitantly the carbapenem (see chapter 13 for biosynthetic pathway) kills competing bacteria. There are some bacterial competitors that have learned to strike back: *B. subtilis* strains can secrete an acyl-HSL lactonase that hydrolyzes the extracellular signal molecules, rendering *E. carotovora* incapable of making antibiotics (Dong et al., 2000).

A second example is provided by the pathogenic bacterium *Pseudomonas aeruginosa* and its quorum-sensing biology. At least two HSLs are known in this gram-negative organism, a 3-keto-dodecanoyl-HSL 3-oxo-dD-HSL and an *N*-acyl-HSL where the chain is shorter and saturated, the *N*-butyryl-HSL (BHL) (**Fig. 11.12**) (Winzer et al., 2000). It has been proposed that the two quorum-signaling systems act in a hierarchical cascade (Swift et al., 1996) for production

Figure 11.12 A double cascade of quorum-signaling *N*-acylhomoserine lactones in *P. aeruginosa*.

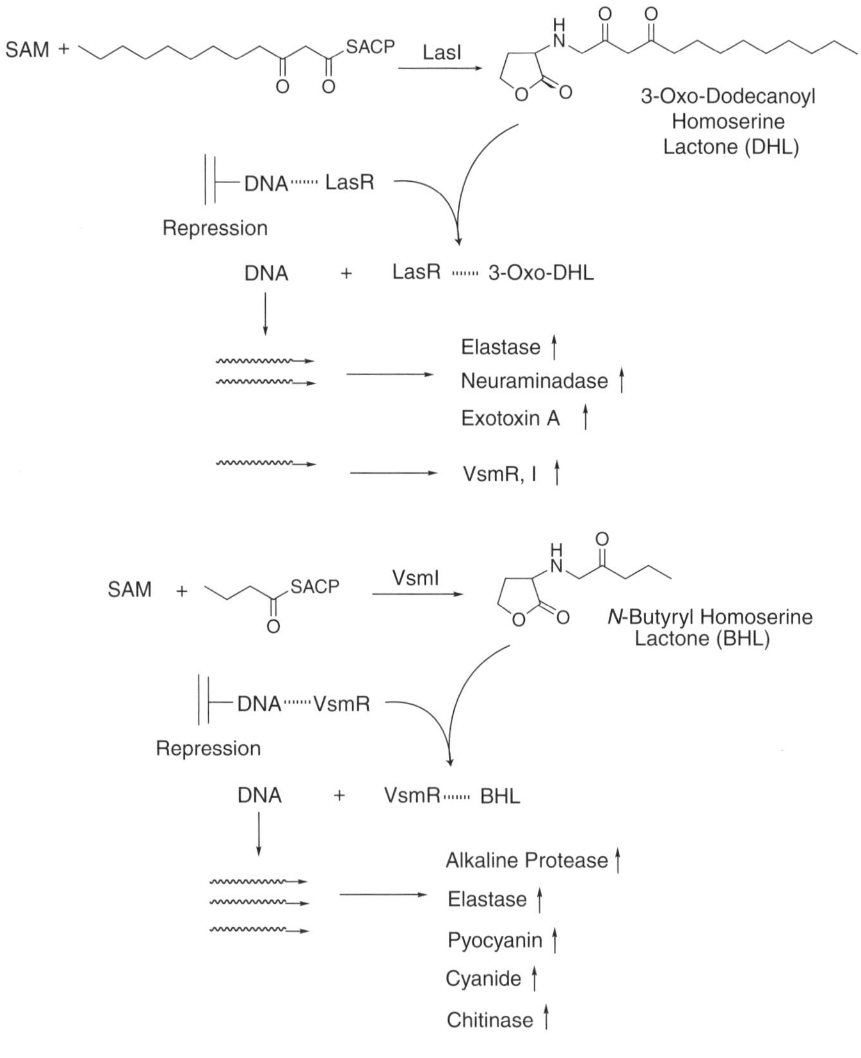

of virulence factors. As shown in Fig. 11.11, the 3-oxo-dD-HSL is generated first by action of the LasI synthase at a specified cell density. This binds with high affinity to the LasR repressor and allows transcription of genes that make such enzymes as elastase and neuraminidase and the protein exotoxin A. The repression of the transcription of the *vsmR* gene is also relieved. The VsmI protein is also an acyl-HSL synthase, this time of BHL, the short-chain quorum sensor, which is a specific ligand for the VsmR repressor. The BHL-VsmR complex falls off DNA and activates transcription of more elastase and of alkaline protease, chitinase, pyocyanin, and cyanide.

A third quorum-sensing molecule in *P. aeruginosa* has recently been characterized as a structurally distinct entity, 2-heptyl-3-hydroxy-4-quinolone, arising from anthranilate and a 3-keto-decanoyl acyl donor (Calfee et al., 2001). This pseudomonal quinolone is part of the quorum-sensing hierarchy and controls multiple virulence factor biosynthesis, so interdiction of its biosynthesis or action might be an antipseudomonal strategy.

Summary

The *N*-acylhomoserine lactones of *Erwinia, Pseudomonas*, and many other bacteria (Schauder and Bassler, 2001) and the γ-butyrolactones of streptomycetes, noted above, serve equivalent purposes, as low-molecular-weight pheromones, for communicating population density-dependent signals between bacteria of the same species. They share membrane permeability and actions as activating ligands for specific transcription factors, while specificity is built in at the ligand-receptor recognition level. We will note a third set of extracellular ligands, small peptides in *Staphylococcus aureus* strains, in chapter 15 that exemplify a comparable logic for communication of external circumstances to the developmental and antibiotic-producing circuitry of bacteria. These signaling systems account for control of essentially all the major classes of antibiotic biosynthetic genes.

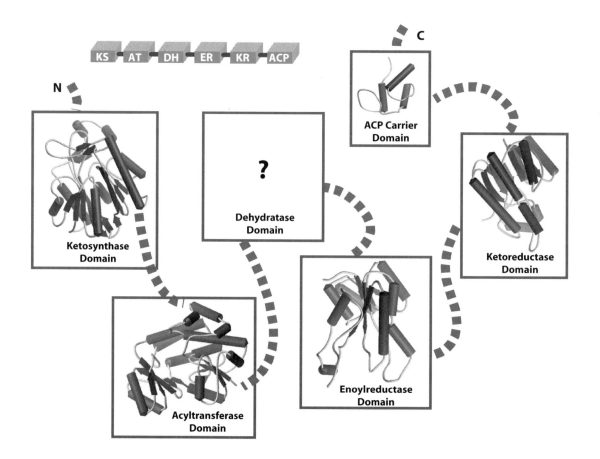

Structural motifs in the catalytic and carrier domains of polyketide synthase assembly lines.

chapter 12

Polyketide Antibiotic Biosynthesis: Assembly-Line Enzymology

General characteristics of polyketide synthases and comparison to fatty acid synthases

The genes encoding polyketide natural products are found in clusters, presumably to facilitate coordinate regulation and induction of expression of all the protein components required for the many steps in these specialized biosynthetic pathways when an appropriate signal, of the types noted in chapter 11, is received and transduced. The biosynthetic genes are also congregated with export pumps and any other resistance-conferring genes, as noted in chapter 7, to turn on the self-protection mechanisms at the same time. Extensive reviews by Rawlings (Rawlings, 1999; Rawlings, 2001a; Rawlings, 2001b) are recommended for a thorough analysis of both type I and type II polyketide synthases. These reviews also allow entry to the massive literature in which the chemical pathways for biosynthesis of the natural product classes discussed in chapters 12 to 14 are worked out, providing the framework that allowed interpretation of function of each protein domain with particular chemical steps in the multimodular assembly lines once the gene sequences became available.

The chemistry practiced by polyketide synthases (PKSs) is closely parallel to that of fatty acid synthases (FASs), which have been extensively studied for decades to decipher mechanisms and organization and have provided precedents for understanding PKS logic. Both PKSs and FAS enzymes convert short-chain acyl-*S*-CoA thioesters into long-acyl-chain products by a series of iterative elongation cycles that add two (FAS, PKS) or three carbon units (PKS) per elongation cycle (see Shen, 2000). The building block used for chain initiation in FAS is typically acetyl-CoA, while the building block for elongation is often malonyl-CoA. The acyl starter units for PKS can be a more diverse set of acyl groups, including acetyl, malonyl, malonamyl, propionyl, butyryl, cyclohexyl, benzoyl, and 3-hydroxy-5-amino benzoyl (**Fig. 12.1**). During chain extension, FAS complexes use malonyl-CoA while PKS catalysts usually make one of two choices for building blocks in each elongation cycle, malonyl- or methylmalonyl-CoA

A

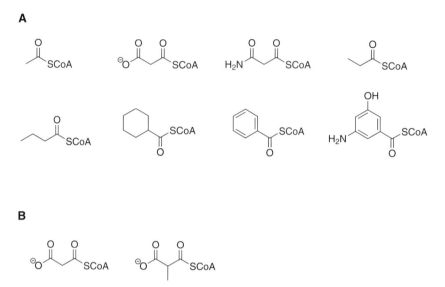

B

Figure 12.1 Building blocks for (A) initiation and (B) elongation cycles by PKS assembly lines.

(Fig. 12.1). Rarely, ethylmalonyl and methoxymalonyl CoAs can also serve as extender units. As noted below, decarboxylation of malonyl or methylmalonyl extender units is mechanistically obligate for chain elongation, so malonyl-CoAs lead to chain extension by two carbons while methylmalonyl-CoAs add a C_3-methyl branched unit.

In FAS and PKS catalysts there are multiple domains or subunits that participate in specific chain initiation, elongation, and termination steps. When the domains are gathered in *cis* as part of large, multidomainal subunits, the FAS and PKS systems are called type I. When the catalytic and carrier protein domains are scattered as separate subunits, in *trans*, that associate transiently and dissociate in each catalytic cycle, these are termed type II synthases. We will examine the type II synthases first, in the next section, since they come in discrete pieces and give insights into the role of the individual domains that are collected in the modular assembly lines of the type I synthases.

The central feature of both FAS and PKS catalysis is that the thermodynamically activated acyl-CoA monomers that serve both in chain initiation and chain elongation are converted to acyl-S-enzyme intermediates and the C-C bond-forming chemistry in each cycle of chain elongation (**Fig. 12.2A**) occurs on covalently tethered acyl-S enzymes. After the appropriate number of elongation cycles when the full-length acyl chain has been produced, its covalent connection to the S enzyme is broken by a specialized chain termination catalytic domain (type I) or separate subunit (type II) called a thioesterase (TE) (**Fig. 12.2B**). The thiol tether on the enzyme in all the acyl-S-enzyme intermediates is provided by a 20-Å-long phosphopantetheine prosthetic group introduced posttranslationally onto a specific serine side chain in an 8- to 10-kDa domain/subunit called an acyl carrier protein (ACP) (see **Fig. 12.3A and B**). The ACP domain is thus the noncatalytic carrier protein for the growing acyl chain, surrounded by a set of

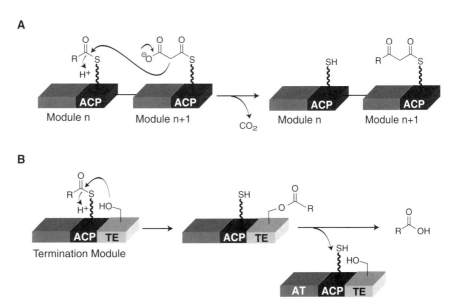

Figure 12.2 (A) Chain elongation and (B) chain termination chemical steps in PKS assembly lines.

dedicated catalytic domains, either in *cis* (type I) or in *trans* (type II). Before phosphopantetheinylation, by a modifying enzyme known as a phosphopantetheinyltransferase (PPTase) (Lambalot et al., 1996), the carrier protein is in an inactive, apo form (**Fig. 12.4A**). After modification the HS-pantetheinyl (HS-pant) arm of the holo ACP is chemically competent to serve as the docking site for the acyl groups being brought in as acyl-CoA thioesters by transthiolation

Figure 12.3 Structure of acyl carrier protein domains from (A) holo ACP domain of *Bacillus subtilis* FAS, with phosphopantetheinyl prosthetic group shown in ball and stick representation; (B) apo ACP form of *S. coelicolor* actinorhodin synthetase.

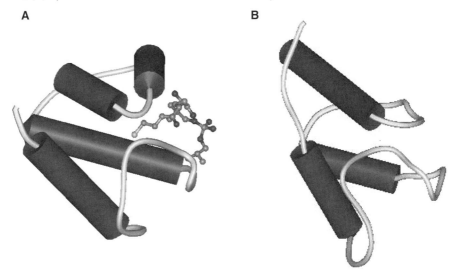

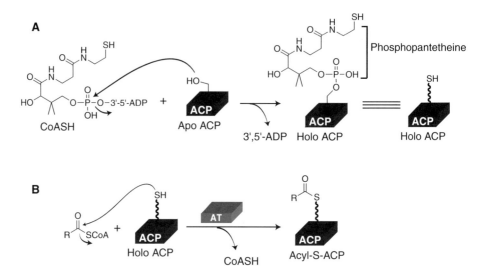

Figure 12.4 Acyl carrier protein domain: (A) apo to holo conversion by posttranslational priming with phosphopantetheine; (B) loading of holo HS-ACP with acyl groups by transthiolation via AT domain catalysis.

via acyltransferase (AT) domain catalytic action (**Fig. 12.4B**) during chain initiation and for the growing chain during elongation cycles.

In the type I FAS and PKS complexes there will be multiple holo ACP domains in the assembly line, and chain elongation involves translocation of the growing acyl chain from upstream to downstream modules, with each holo ACP serving as the docking station (**Fig. 12.5A**). In the type II FAS and PKS complexes, there is one ACP subunit, and the elongating acyl chain is built up by iterative cycles of elongation while remaining covalently tethered to the same ACP protein scaffold (**Fig. 12.5B**).

The chemical steps carried out by FAS and PKS arrays are the same. First a malonyl- or methylmalonyl-CoA monomer is loaded onto the HS-pant-holo ACP domain by transthiolation under the aegis of an AT domain to produce the malonyl- or methylmalonyl-S-ACP (**Fig. 12.6A**). This acyl-S-ACP will serve as the carbon nucleophile, when it undergoes decarboxylation to give the C_2-stabilized carbanion equivalent, enabled by the thioester linkage (**Fig. 12.6B**) in the C-C bond-forming step. The electrophilic acyl donor for the C-C bond is provided by an acyl group that is transiently docked as an acyl-S-enzyme intermediate at the active site of the ketosynthase (KS) domain or subunit (**Fig. 12.6C**). This covalent acyl intermediate is tethered to the active-site cysteine of the KS domain and arose via a similar transthiolation reaction. The C-C bond-forming step is catalyzed by the KS domain, which induces the decarboxylation of the malonyl- or methylmalonyl-S-ACP and transfers the acyl chain from the active-site cysteine to the attacking C_2 carbanion/enolate (**Fig. 12.6D**). Whether decarboxylation occurs first or is coupled in the same transition state to C-C bond formation is not fully established. The result is a β-keto-S-ACP product (hence the name ketosynthase) where the upstream acyl chain has translocated to the downstream acyl-S-ACP during chain elongation.

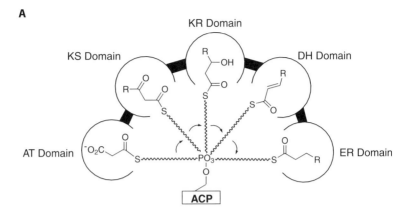

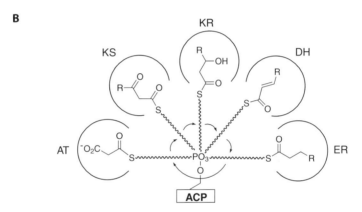

Figure 12.5 ACP interactions (A) in type I PKS and FAS, within each module; (B) in type II PKS and FAS, between separate subunits.

The next three enzymatic steps, provided in *cis* (type I) or in *trans* (type II), involve a net four-electron reduction of the β-keto all the way to a β-methylene group in fatty acid biosynthesis. In FAS catalysis this was established to occur by sequential action of the ketoreductase (KR), dehydratase (DH), and enoyl-reductase (ER) domains/subunits, respectively (**Fig. 12.7**). The KR catalytic domain uses NADPH to reduce the ketone to the β-hydroxy substituent. The acidic α-hydrogen of the β-OH-acyl-S-ACP can be readily abstracted in the DH active site to initiate elimination of the OH group and yield the αβ-enoyl-S-ACP. This conjugated double bond can then be reduced by a proton-hydride addition from a reduced flavin coenzyme, FADH$^-$, in the active site of the enoyl-S-ACP reductase, with the hydride adding to C_β to produce the fully saturated $C_\alpha H_2$-$C_\beta H_2$ two-carbon extender unit.

With the reaction sequence of an FAS elongation cycle as a guide, the PKS cycles can be analyzed analogously. The type 1 modules offer more functional group variety in the final product structures by incomplete maturation of the extender units when a KR, DH, or ER domain is nonfunctional. Chain elongation occurs, but the intermediate redox states persist and can be translocated to

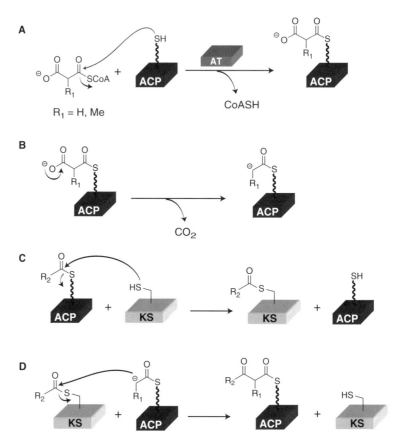

Figure 12.6 Four stages to the C-C bond-forming chain elongation steps of PKS and FAS assemblies: (A) malonyl- or methylmalonyl-S-ACP formation; (B) decarboxylation to generate the carbon nucleophile; (C) the acyl-S-Cys-KS donor; (D) the product, β-keto-acyl-S-ACP.

the next downstream module. As shown in **Fig. 12.8** for a hypothetical three-module type I PKS, a defect in the KR domain of module n will leave the β-carbon in the keto oxidation state. In module $n + 1$ a defect at the active site of the DH domain leaves the β-carbon of the C_2 unit introduced in that cycle as the β-OH. Finally, a defect in the ER domain of module $n + 2$ will allow the $\alpha\beta$-ene to survive. Hydrolytic action of the TE domain to cause release of the eight-carbon acyl chain from ACP_{n+2} will yield the highly functionalized polyketide chain. Thus the main difference between FAS and type I PKS assembly lines is the loss of function in one or more of the tailoring domains in a given PKS module. Where three cycles of elongation by a FAS assembly line will yield the fully saturated octanoate, the PKS natural products have been arrested at intermediate stages of reduction of the β-keto groups arising in each condensation cycle, thereby permitting subsequent chemistry and molecular recognition characteristic of this natural product class.

The type II PKS complexes can also show dramatic variation in both the redox states of the extender units and the number of ring structures when the final polyketide product is released. As we shall note in the next section, it is

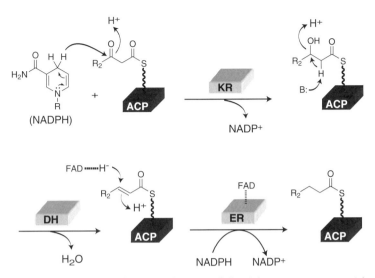

Figure 12.7 Three-stage four-electron reduction of the β-keto group: sequential action of KR, DH, and ER domains.

likely that the multiple ring structures of the aromatic polyketides occur from polyketonic intermediates without substantial reduction of the multiple β-keto groups in the acyl-S-ACP intermediates.

Type II organization of polyketide synthases: tetracycline, tetracenomycin, and daunorubicin biosynthetic clusters and the action of cyclases

The four rings of the tetracycline family of antibiotics, such as oxytetracycline and chlortetracycline (**Fig. 12.9**), and also of tetracenomycin and the antitumor antibiotic doxorubicin (Fig. 12.9) are produced by type II polyketide synthases along with some partner aromatases and cyclases also expressed in the clusters (Fig. 12.10) (see Shen, 2000, for recent review of aromatic PKSs). The oxytetracycline cluster differs from the canonical assembly by having two clusters of genes, the minimal PKS three subunits KS_α, KS_β, (KS_β are also known as CLF [chain length factor] subunits), and ACP in tandem, and then a KR and a

Figure 12.8 Proposal for incomplete redox adjustment in three cycles of a PKS assembly line.

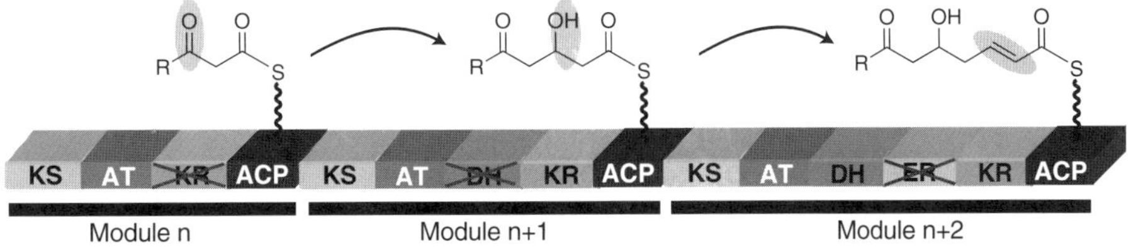

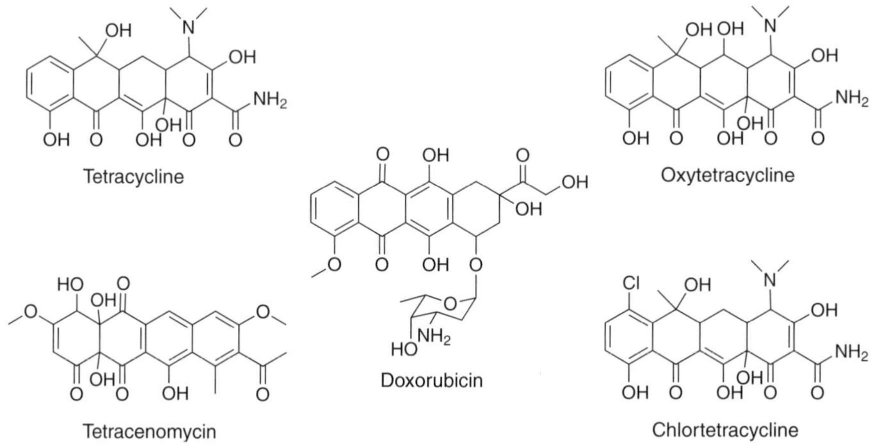

Figure 12.9 Tetracyclic aromatic polyketide antibiotics generated by type II PKS: tetracycline, oxytetracycline, chlortetracycline, tetracenomycin, and doxorubicin.

bifunctional aromatase/cyclase some 10 kb away (see Petkovic et al., 1999). The minimal type I PKS in this and related systems, e.g., actinorhodin biosynthesis by *Streptomyces coelicolor* (Hopwood, 1997; Khosla, 1997), is thought to use the KS_α/KS_β pair of subunits as a functional dimer, perhaps with the catalytically defective β subunit serving in part as a CLF, modulating the number of chain extension cycles before cyclization occurs. The holo form of the HS-pant-ACP

Figure 12.10 Modular organization of PKS producing the aromatic tetracyclic antibiotic doxorubicin.

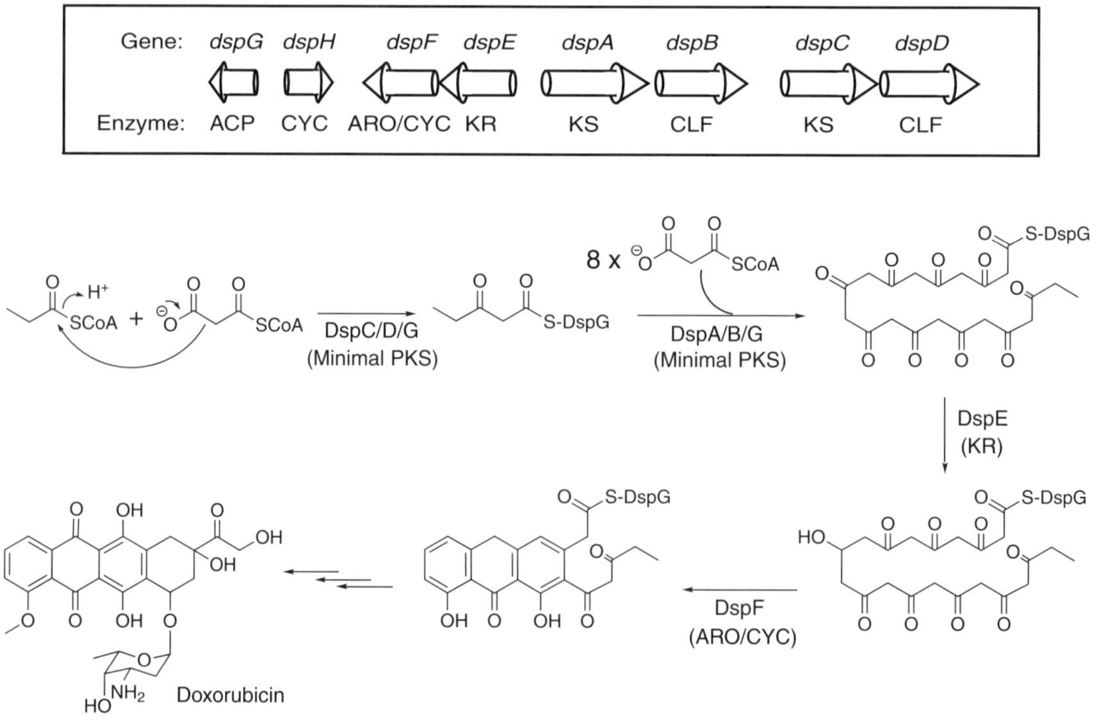

provides the thiol on which a first malonyl-*S*-ACP is assembled while the starter acyl unit is loaded onto the active-site cysteine thiol of the KS_α subunit. The acylated KS then catalyzes malonyl decarboxylation and acyl transfer to the developing enolate anion to yield the β-keto-acyl-S-ACP and regenerate the KS cysteine thiolate for the next cycle of elongation (**Fig. 12.11**). Chain transfer back to the KS active-site cysteine must occur to enable another iteration of this catalytic C-C bond formation and elongation cycle (shown by malonyl-S-ACP addition in the center of the figure).

In biosynthesis of daunorubicin or doxorubicin, the starter unit is propionyl-CoA and all extender units are malonyl-CoA. After nine condensation cycles a decaketidyl-*S*-ACP is built up (**Fig. 12.12A**), in which all 10 of the β-ketone groups are thought to persist without reductive modification in the acyl chain. Analogously, the oxytetracycline synthase uses the half amide of malonyl-CoA, malonamyl-CoA, as the starter unit and eight malonyl-CoAs as extender units to build up a 19-carbon-chain nonaketidyl-*S*-ACP as the full-length acyl chain prior to cyclization (**Fig. 12.12B**). The tetracenomycin starter unit is acetyl-CoA, and after nine malonyl-CoA extender units are added, a 20-carbon nonaketidyl-*S* enzyme (**Fig. 12.12C**) undergoes two rounds of cyclase-mediated ring closures. The first cyclase, TcmN, closes three rings to make TcmF2, and TcmI closes the last ring to give the fused four-ring system analogous to the tetracycline skeleton. The post-PKS/cyclase tailoring enzymes methylate one of the phenolic OH groups and the COOH group and then use an oxygenase, TcmG, to introduce the three hydroxyl groups in tetracenomycin C, probably arising from monooxygenation of the A ring and then epoxidation and hydrolytic opening of the epoxide at the A/B ring junction (see Hutchinson, 1997, for review) (Fig. 12.12C).

When the aromatase and cyclase genes in these type II PKS clusters are knocked out, defective, or otherwise absent, then aberrant cyclization patterns ensue as the reactive polyketonic acyl enzymes condense nonenzymatically to a variety of cyclic products that are released from the ACP scaffold. None of the nonenzymatic routes give the natural tetracyclic systems, indicating the cyclases are important in both setting a productive folding conformer of the acyclic

Figure 12.11 The iterative chain elongation cycles of type II PKS and FAS.

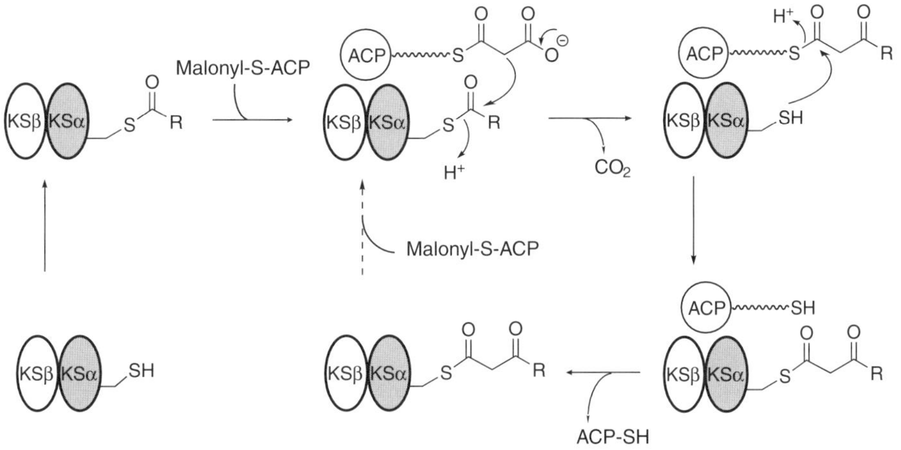

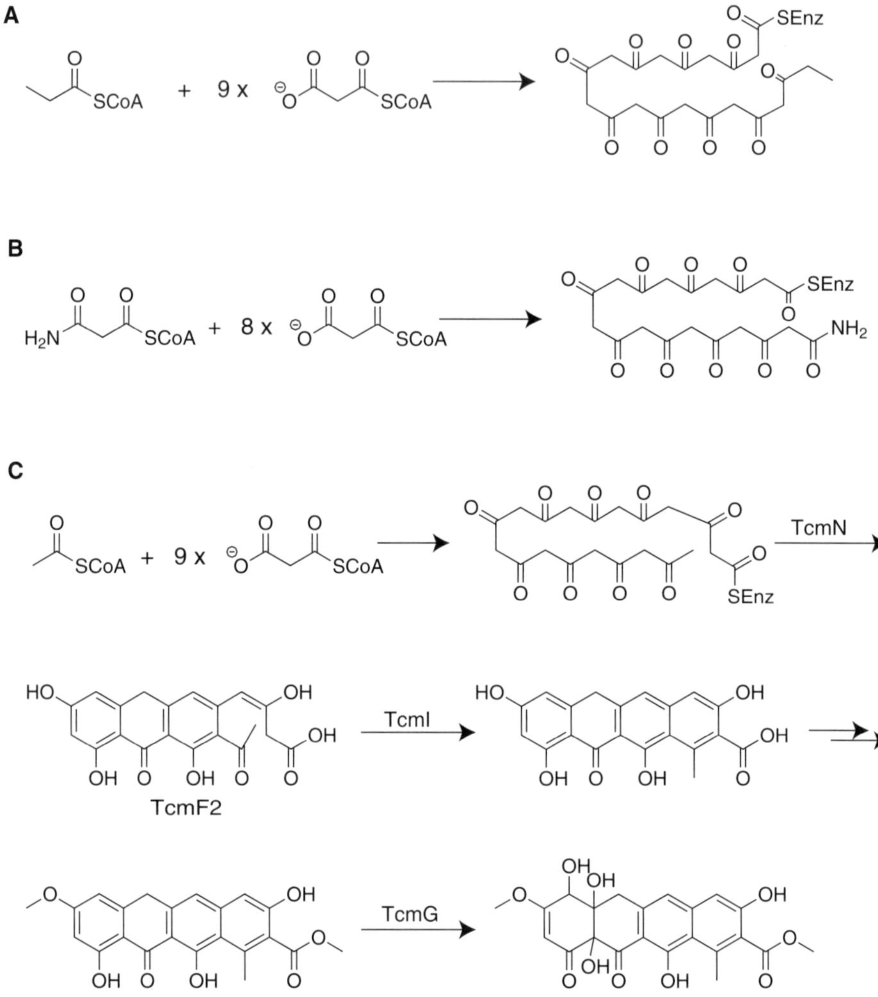

Figure 12.12 Polyketidyl-*S* enzyme intermediates: (A) daunorubicin synthase; (B) tetracycline synthase; (C) tetracenomycin synthase.

polyketonic acyl chain and then catalyzing regiospecific cyclizations and dehydrations to the natural product connectivity patterns. Some type II clusters contain multiple cyclases, e.g., TcmN and TcmI in the tetracenomycin cluster (Fig. 12.12) and DpsF and DpsH in the daunorubicin cluster (Fig. 12.10), and they are presumed to recognize different acyclic substructures and catalyze distinct partial cyclizations (see Hutchinson, 1997, for review). The broad outlines of the C-C bond-forming strategies and points of cyclization are clear, but the timing and details of steps are not well studied as yet. For example, in creating the four rings of the tetracycline skeleton, the nonaketidyl enzyme is presumed to be folded in a conformer such that carbon-carbon bonds are created between C_2 and C_{19}, C_4 and C_{17}, C_6 and C_{15}, and C_8 and C_{13} (**Fig. 12.13**), with C_2, C_4, C_6, and C_8 acting as carbanion equivalents (enolate resonance forms) to attack the ketones at C_{19}, C_{17}, C_{15}, and C_{13}, respectively, to generate the fused four-ring aromatic system (6-methylpretetramid). Subsequent dehydrations and aromati-

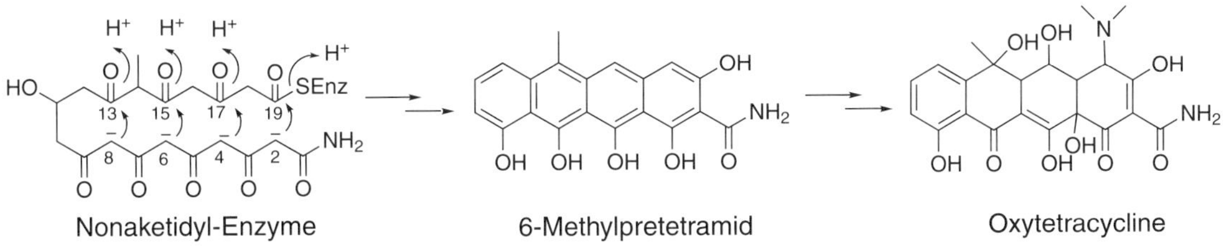

Figure 12.13 Bond-forming reactions in the polyketidyl-*S*-tetracycline synthase acyl enzyme.

zation of the left-hand ring, hydroxylations, redox adjustment, amination, and dimethylation must occur via a series of tailoring enzymes to produce the final oxytetracycline from this tetracyclic precursor (Hutchinson and Fujii, 1995).

In doxorubicin biosynthesis there are two additional carbons in the 21-carbon decaketidyl-*S*-ACP acyclic precursor, and while it also undergoes cyclase-mediated closure of four rings, the connectivity established is distinct (**Fig. 12.14A**), suggesting a different folding conformation of this reactive acyclic acyl chain. The carbanion equivalents at C_3, C_6, C_8, and C_{10} are induced to attack with regiospecificity the four ketones at C_{20}, C_{19}, C_{17}, and C_{15}, respectively, while all nonenzymatic side reaction cyclizations are suppressed. It appears the DpsF cyclase makes the first three rings (**Fig. 12.14B**), probably before disconnection

Figure 12.14 Doxorubicin biosynthesis: (A) C-C bond-forming steps from an enzyme-bound conformer; (B) DpsF-mediated cyclization of the first three rings; (C) DpsH action and postsynthase tailoring reactions.

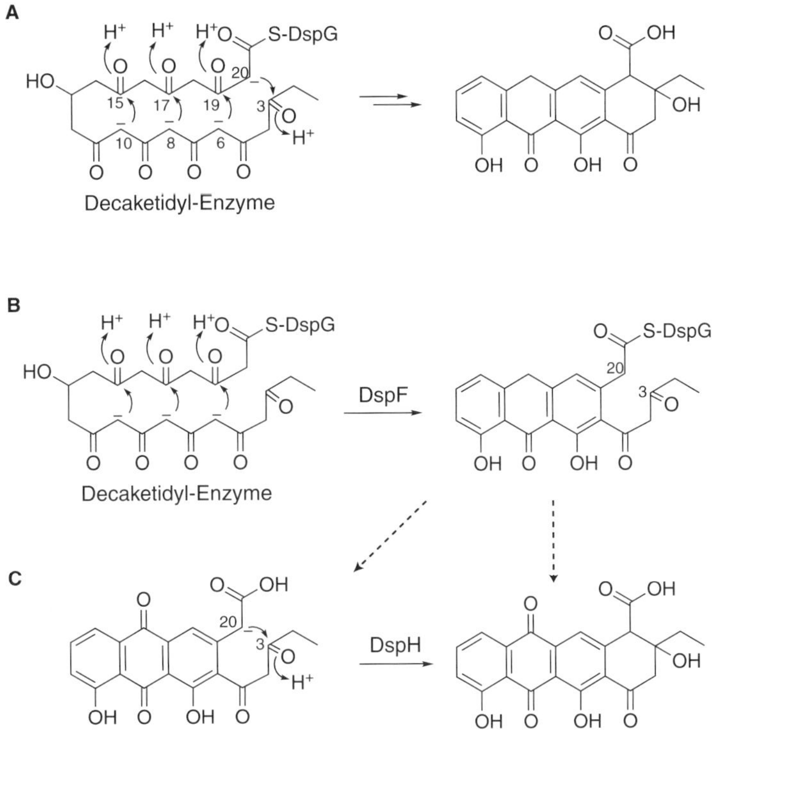

of the acyl chain from the ACP scaffold. Subsequently, DpsH (**Fig. 12.14C**) may cyclize the last ring, making the C_3-C_{20} linkage and releasing the acyl chain from the ACP. Completion of the doxorubicin antitumor antibiotic involves oxygenation at C_{16} and C_{18} to create the tandem quinone-hydroquinone system in the two middle rings and glycosylation of the OH at C_5 with the unusual aminodeoxy sugar daunosamine (Hutchinson, 1997) by tailoring enzymes encoded by contiguous genes of the biosynthetic cluster.

While the minimal subunits of a type II PKS appear to be a KS_α, KS_β, and ACP, the doxorubicin cluster has two sets of KS_α and KS_β, DpsC/DpsD, and DpsA/DpsB (Fig. 12.10), which are thought to do the first condensation cycle (C/D) and then the next eight cycles (A/B). When KR subunits are encoded in the clusters, as in doxorubicin and tetracycline clusters, the KRs will act regio- and stereospecifically. In the doxorubicin pathway, reduction of the C_{13} ketone to the C_{13}-OH is thought to occur prior to cyclization and may be important for conformer population, directed cyclization, and/or subsequent dehydration and aromatization. How the growing polyketone-containing acyl chain is protected and sequestered as it grows on the ACP subunit is not well understood but will be important for rational redesign of cyclizations in type II PKS combinatorial biosynthesis efforts. Hybrid type II polyketides can be made by interchanging the core PKS subunits and cyclases (see Khosla, 1997).

Type I polyketide synthases: modular assembly lines for erythromycin and tylosin

In contrast to the separate subunit logic of the type II PKS and FAS complexes, the type I FASs and PKSs are modular, with several catalytic and carrier protein domains connected together into very high-molecular-weight subunits. The macrolides of the erythromycin class contain 14-membered macrolactone rings while the tylosins have 16-membered rings (**Fig. 12.15**); they reflect six and seven elongation cycles, respectively. The prototypic organization for the macrolide synthases was revealed when the genes encoding the aglycone deoxyerythronolide B (DEB) were sequenced (Cortes et al., 1990; Donadio et al., 1991) and revealed three polypeptides in the 200-kDa molecular weight range which together comprise the DEB synthase (DEBS) catalytic activity, converting the starter propionyl-CoA and six methylmalonyl-CoA extender molecules into DEB (**Fig. 12.15A**). Inspection of the DEBS1, DEBS2, and DEBS3 subunits shows that each contains two modules for elongation (for the six cycles of methylmalonyl additions), that DEBS1 starts with an additional loading module, and that DEBS3 has a chain termination TE domain at its C terminus. The loading module at the N-terminal start of DEBS1 has an AT and an HS-ACP domain for installing the propionyl starter unit as propionyl-S-ACP.

The core domains in a type I PKS module engaged in chain elongation are the KS, AT, and ACP, usually placed in that order, with the AT loading a malonyl or methylmalonyl group from the acyl-CoA substrate onto the holo HS-ACP. In DEBS1, 2, and 3 the AT domains in modules 1 to 6 are methylmalonyl specific. The KS active-site cysteine thiol self-acylates with the donor acyl group, while the methylmalonyl-S-ACP on decarboxylation is the carbon nucleophile

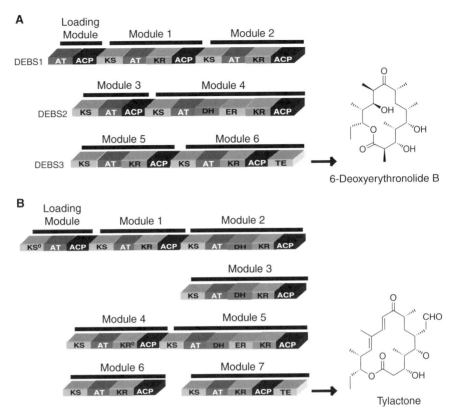

Figure 12.15 Modular organization of the synthases for erythromycin and tylosin: (A) the assembly line for the erythromycin aglycone 6-DEB; (B) the assembly line for the 16-membered aglycone tylactone.

for β-keto-acyl-S-ACP formation, the same logic as seen above for the type II C-C bond formations. Unlike the aromatic polyketide natural products, which undergo a series of cyclizations to form fused-ring systems via the polyketonic groups in the full-length acyl chain, the β-ketone group may be reduced in each cycle of a type I PKS by additional domains. Thus the KS, AT, and ACP core domains of a PKS module may be joined by a KR domain (modules 1 and 2), a DH domain (module 4), and an ER domain (module 4). Since modules 1 and 2 have KR domains, but not DH or ER domains, the triketide acyl chain that accumulates on the ACP_2 of DEBS1 has C_3 and C_5-OH substituents (**Fig. 12.16**). The growing acyl chain moves from DEBS1 to the DEBS2 subunit, passes along modules 3 and 4, and reaches the HS-ACP docking station at the end of DEBS2. Module 3 has only the core KS-AT-ACP, so the ketone persists, while module 4 has the DH-ER-KR domain triad, so there the newly introduced β-keto is reduced all the way to β-CH_2. In DEBS3 module 5 and module 6 both have only the KR domain as optional domain, so again β-OH groups persist in these two elongation cycles. From the order and placement of the 28 domains (10 in DEBS1, 9 in DEBS2, 9 in DEBS3) in the three-subunit assembly line, one can predict the length and functionalization of each carbon in the 15-carbon-long acyclic acyl chain and the patterns of methylation at $C_{2,4,6,8,10,12}$ from the six

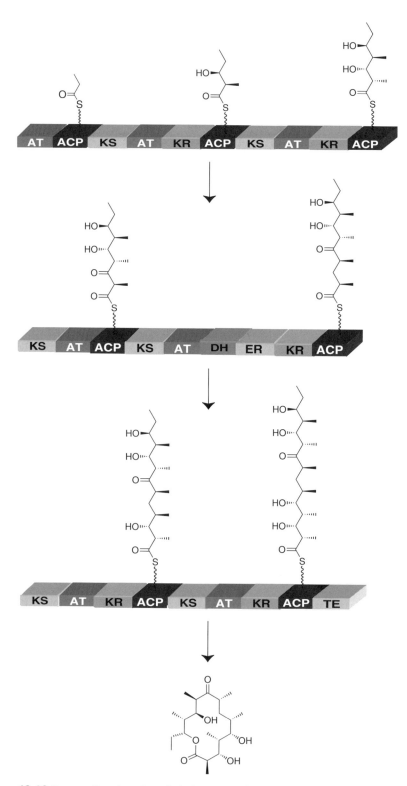

Figure 12.16 Intermediate-length acyl chains accumulating on the DEBS assembly line.

methylmalonyl groups. The stereochemistry of the four hydroxy substituents is controlled by KR stereochemistry in modules 1, 2, 5, and 6.

The remaining task for DEB synthase is to disconnect the mature full-length acyl group covalently docked at the seventh and most terminal ACP waystation, in module 6. Just downstream of that ACP is the 28th and last domain of the assembly line, the TE domain. It acts as a cyclase, catalyzing intramolecular capture of the C_1 thioester carbonyl by the C_{13}-OH group, producing the 14-membered macrolactone 6-DEB as the free HS-ACP is generated and the DEBS assembly line is freed for another catalytic cycle (**Fig. 12.17**). We shall note below the subsequent enzymatic tailoring steps for 6-deoxyerythronolide, devoid of antibiotic activity, to be converted into the oxygenated, glycosylated antibiotic.

There is interest in engineering PKS assembly lines to give macrolactone rings of different sizes. In the pikromycin PKS (Xue and Sherman, 2001), release of both the normal 14-membered macrolactone (narbonolide) and a shorter 12-membered lactone (10-deoxymethynolide) is observed (**Fig. 12.18**), reflecting a competition between cyclization from module 6 (to the 14 ring) and premature cyclization of the growing chain on module 5 (12 ring). An additional distinction between the 12-ring and 14-ring lactones is that the last module, which installs carbons 1 and 2, has no KR and therefore leaves C_3 as the unreduced β-ketone that becomes the C_3 ketone in narbonolide and in its 10-hydroxy-5-desosaminyl product, pikromycin. This persistent 3-keto group makes pikromycin a naturally occurring ketolide, an analog of the broad-spectrum macrolides in clinical development (Fig. 10.4). Pikromycin does not induce the Erm rRNA methyltransferases and so does not induce the macrolide-lincosamide-streptogramin B resistance phenotype (chapter 10) (see Xue and Sherman, 2001).

Analogously, a mutant of *Saccharopolyspora erythraea* has been reported to make some 16-membered ring product along with the normal 14-ring deoxyerythronolide B in a mutant. The extra elongation cycle is attributed to a slow transfer of the growing chain from module 4 to module 5, allowing time for an extra elongation on module 4 (Wilkinson et al., 2000). Whether such side reactions can be engineered to become major fluxes to products remains to be determined. Insertion of a PKS module from rapamycin synthase into DEBS1 to make a three-module extended subunit, followed by expression in *S. erythraea*

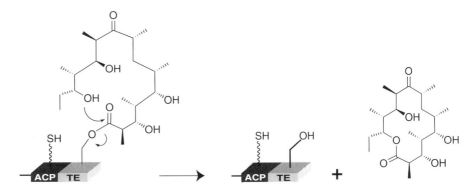

Figure 12.17 Release of the mature acyl chain from the last module by the DEBS3 TE domain acting as a cyclase to yield the macrolactone 6-DEB.

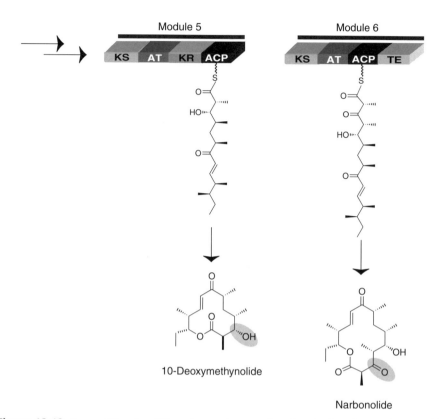

Figure 12.18 Competition for different macrolactone ring sizes in the pikromycin assembly line: the 14-ring narbonolide and 12-ring 10-deoxymethynolide by cyclization from module 5 or from module 6; note the presence of the C_3-keto group in pikromycin.

led to production of an octaketide with a 16-membered ring, albeit at 3 to 5% efficiency compared to normal polyketide levels from wild-type DEBS1-3 (Rowe et al., 2001).

Note that in contrast to the nonaketidyl-S-ACP and decaketidyl-S-ACP acyl enzymes in the tetracycline and doxorubicin synthases, where eight and nine ketones accumulate, unreduced, through the chain elongation cycles, the DEBS full-length heptaketidyl-acyl-S-ACP$_7$ has only one ketone, dramatically reducing the options for Claisen couplings and transannular cyclization pathways. The optional KR, DH, and ER domains in this and other related modular PKS assembly lines, acting in *cis* in tightly coupled fashion, reroute the fate of the acyl chains into hydrolysis or macrolactonization (Fig. 12.17 and 12.18) rather than carbocyclic ring formations.

A second contrast between type I and type II PKSs is the number of ACP domains and the translocation patterns of the growing chain. In type II FASs and PKSs, a single ACP subunit is used and the growing β-keto acyl chain produced in each cycle of condensation/elongation, is translocated back to the KS active-site cysteine to be used as a donor in the next cycle (Fig. 12.11). The growing acyl chain is always on the KS active-site cysteine thiol when it acts as a donor for the next elongation cycle and the (methyl) malonyl-S-ACP is always the carbon nucleophile on decarboxylation. In the type I modular PKS, there is one HS-ACP per module and the growing chain is transferred unidirectionally from N terminus to C terminus through a cascade of acyl-S-ACP intermediates (Fig. 12.16). The (methyl) malonyl-S-ACP again acts as carbon nucleophile under KS-mediated decarboxylation.

Post-assembly-line modifications: monooxygenases and glycosyl transferases

As we noted in chapter 4, many of the macrolide antibiotics are glycosylated, to provide hydrogen bond interactions with the ribosome 23S rRNA, highlighted by the contacts of the desosamine sugar of erythromycin to A_{2058} (Fig. 4.5). In fact, the most common of the post-assembly-line tailoring reactions for poly-ketides made both by type I and type II PKSs are oxygenation, glycosylation, and methylation of heteroatoms. We noted dimethylation and trioxygenation to finish the tetracenomycin pathway in the type II systems above.

The post-assembly-line methylations use S-adenosylmethionine (SAM) as the cosubstrate methyl donor, providing a CH_3^+ equivalent to a nucleophilic nitrogen, oxygen, or carbon (carbanion) atom in the nascent polyketide product. Some of the C methylations via SAM occur while the growing chain is still on the PKS assembly line.

In the maturation of 6-DEB to erythromycin A there are five enzymatic steps: two hydroxylations at C_6 (EryF) and C_{12} (EryK), two glycosyltransferases that install L-mycarose (EryBIV) at the C_3-OH of the macrolactone to produce the 3-α-mycarosylerythronolide B and then D-desosamine (EryCII) at the C_5-OH to produce erythromycin D. Finally, O methylation (EryG) at the 3-OH of the mycarosyl sugar completes the biosynthesis of erythromycin A (**Fig. 12.19**) (Katz, 1997). The EryF hydroxylase acts on 6-DEB while the EryK monooxygenase acts at C_{12} only after both sugars have been added. Each hydroxylase is a member of the heme-containing cytochrome P450 monooxygenase family, typical for many antibiotic oxygenation catalysts. The above five genes for these tailoring enzymes are in the erythromycin biosynthetic gene cluster, signaling their dedicated metabolic function and enabling coordinate regulation. In pik-romycin, where the 3-position is the ketone, there is no glycosylation at that locus. There are only two maturation enzymes in the cluster: a cytochrome P450 PikK that is the 10-hydroxylase and the desosaminyltransferase (Xue and Sherman, 2001). In other polyketides a wide range of post-assembly oxidative chemistry ensues, including aromatic ring phenolic couplings and halogenations.

The presence of the sugars on the macrolactone ring is required for anti-biotic activity as a consequence of providing key binding determinants for 23S rRNA recognition on the 50S ribosome subunit. Analogously, in the daunorubicin/doxorubicin pathway, the L-daunosamine sugar (Fig. 12.9) is a key constituent for bioactivity. The sugars attached to these polyketide antibiotics and also to the peptide-based antibiotics discussed in the next chapter are often unusual deoxy and/or amino sugars that are found only as components of the antibiotics (Liu and Thorson, 1994). In turn, the genes that encode their bio-synthesis are also found clustered with the rest of the antibiotic biosynthesis and

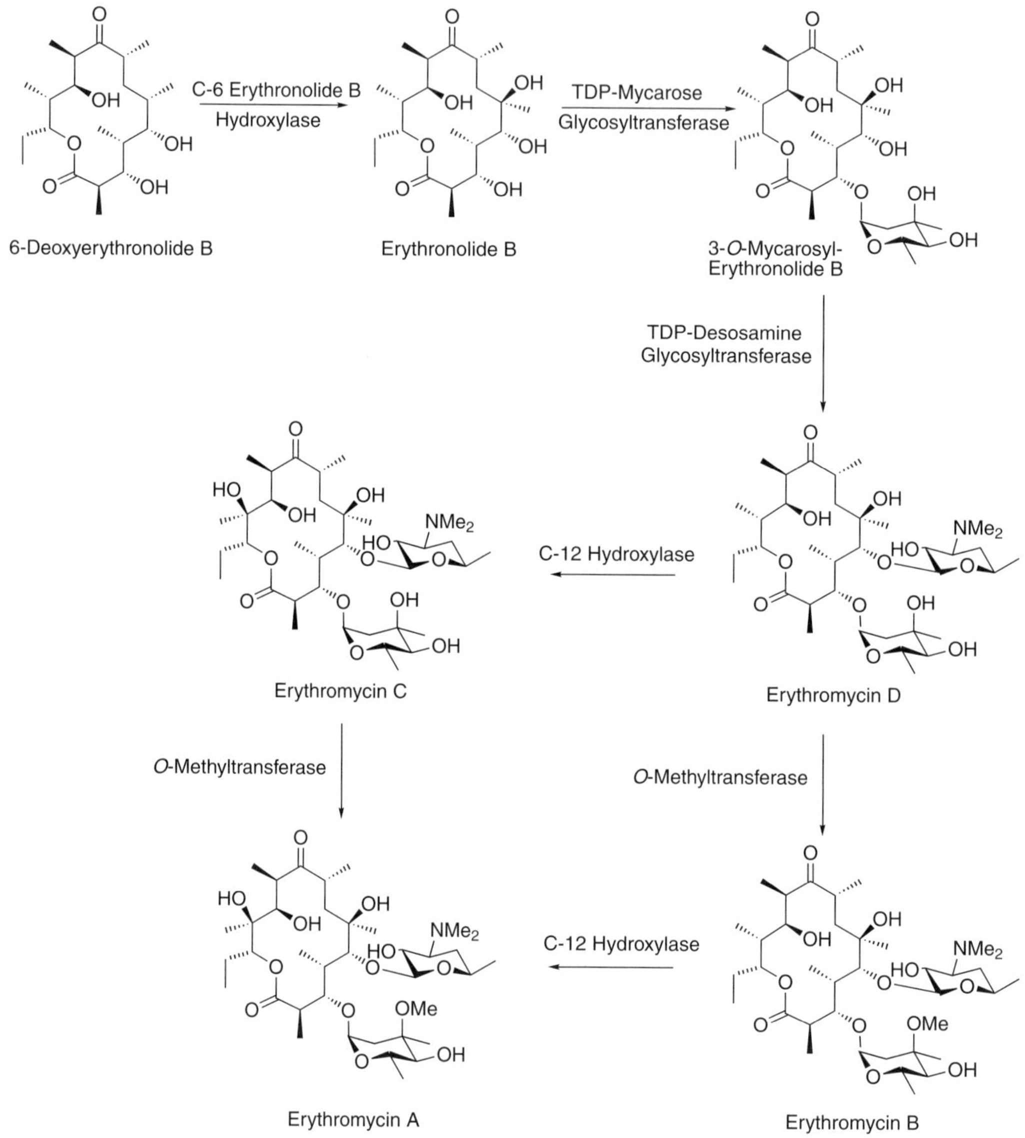

Figure 12.19 Five enzymatic steps to convert 6-DEB to erythromycin A.

resistance genes along with the specific glycosyltransferases (see Thorson et al., 2001, for review).

The biologically active form of sugars that serve as substrates for glycosyl transfer enzymes are nucleoside diphospho (NDP) -sugars, activated at C_1 by the NDP linkage (**Fig. 12.20**) for transfer to some cosubstrate nucleophile. In the antibiotic NDP-sugars, the nucleosides are typically the pyrimidine TDP or the corresponding UDP. Thus the biosynthetic pathways for these deoxy sugars produce TDP-L-mycarose or TDP-D-desosamine, starting from the TDP glucose, in turn produced from the primary metabolites TTP and glucose-1-P (Thorson et al., 2001).

The general outline of these deoxy sugar pathways is to convert TDP-glucose to TDP-4-ketoglucose, then eliminate water to the 4-keto-glucose-6-ene and re-

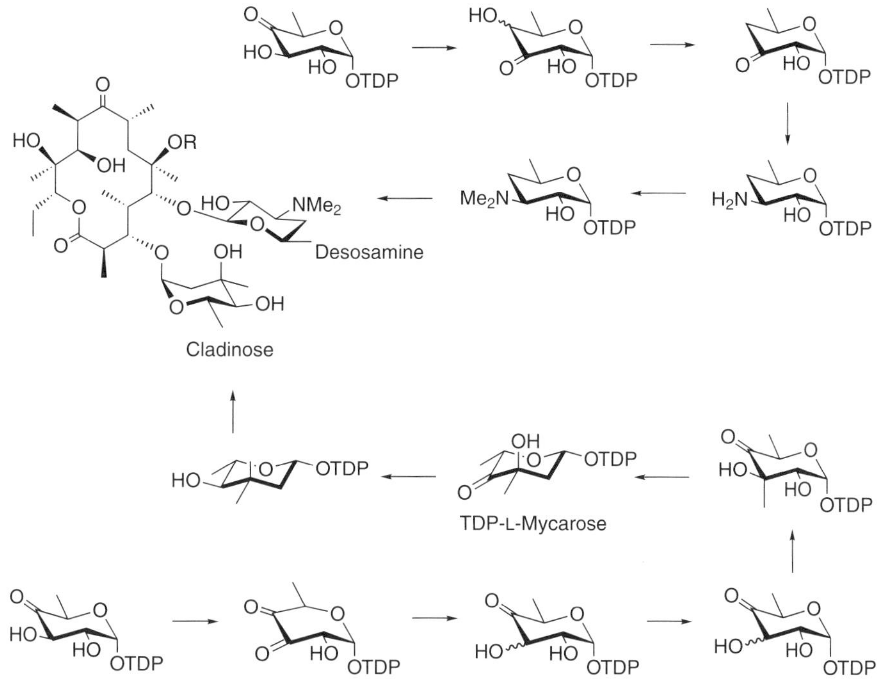

Figure 12.20 Transformations to produce TDP-D-desosamine and TDP-L-mycarose from TDP-4-keto-6-deoxyglucose in erythromycin assembly.

duce the conjugated double bond to create the 4-keto-6-deoxy glucose as an early common intermediate (Fig. 12.20). From this 4-keto-6-deoxy NDP-sugar there are specific enzymes that epimerize both C_3 and C_5; one can eliminate the −OH at C_2 to effect net deoxygenation and reductively aminate at C_3 or C_4. The C_5 epimerization provides entry into the TDP-L-sugar series. N and C methylation can occur at carbanionic sites adjacent to the 4-keto group. Chiral reductions of the 4-ketone groups produce the finished TDP-deoxy sugars such as daunosamine, desosamine, and L-mycarose in the macrolides or L-vancosamine in vancomycin. For example, in TDP-desosamine (Fig. 12.20), the C_3-OH has been converted to the amine (by reductive amination of a C_3,C_4-diketo intermediate) and *N,N*-dimethylated by SAM, and C_4 has been reduced from alcohol to CH_2 and C_6 reduced to the CH_3 state. The TDP-L-mycarose (Fig. 12.20) has been deoxygenated at C_2 and C_6, C-methylated at C_3, and epimerized at C_5 before transfer to the macrolactone scaffold by EryBIV. Thus, there is extensive enzymatic machinery dedicated to producing the deoxy and amino substitutions on the normal hexoses derived from primary metabolism for post-assembly-line glycosylations of polyketides.

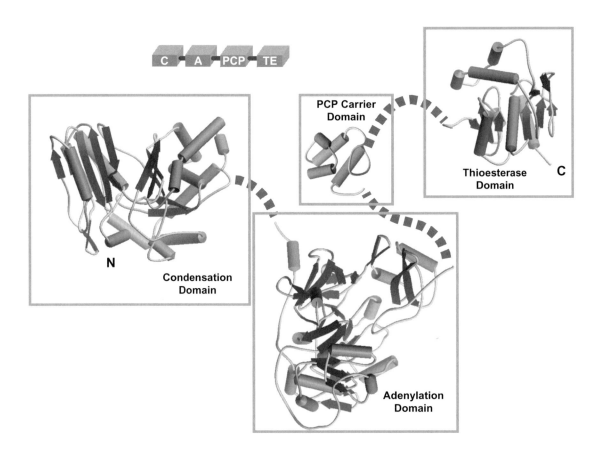

Structural motifs in the catalytic and carrier domains of nonribosomal peptide synthetases.

chapter 13

Enzymatic Assembly Lines for Nonribosomal Peptide Antibiotics

As noted in earlier chapters (chapters 3, 6, and 10), a large percentage of the peptidic natural products that have antibiotic activity are produced by nonribosomal peptide synthetases (NRPSs) (**Fig. 13.1**) (for review, see Konz and Marahiel, 1999; Marahiel et al., 1997; and von Dohren et al., 1997). These include the ACV (L-aminoadipyl-L-cysteinyl-D-valine) tripeptide precursor to the β-lactam families of antibiotics, the channel-forming tyrocidine and gramicidin S, and the topical antibiotic bacitracin. Additionally, the glycopeptides of the vancomycin group are generated on NRPS assembly lines, then heavily modified, as noted later in this chapter. Similarly, lipopeptide antibiotics such as ramoplanin and daptomycin are made this way. Finally, the two-component pristinamycins of the Synercid complex are hybrids of nonribosomal peptide and polyketide synthase assembly lines.

Initiation, elongation, and termination modules: core domains and additional domains

The NRPS catalysts have organizational analogies to the type I polyketide synthases (PKSs) as multidomainal catalysts organized into modules, with multiple modules collected in one or more protein subunits. The extreme example is the fungal enzyme cyclosporin synthetase, which assembles the cyclic undecapeptide immunosuppressant drug cyclosporin A on a single polypeptide of molecular weight 1.5 MDa, with 43 domains in the 11 modules, one for each amino acid that is selected, activated, and incorporated into the growing chain. The ACV synthetase has three modules in a polypeptide of 450 kDa (**Fig. 13.2**), while the heptapeptide scaffold of vancomycin or chloroeremomycin (Fig. 13.2) is assembled by three subunits with three, three, and one module, respectively.

As in the type 1 PKS assembly lines, the NRPS assembly lines have a chain initiation module at the N terminus, then tandemly arrayed elongation modules

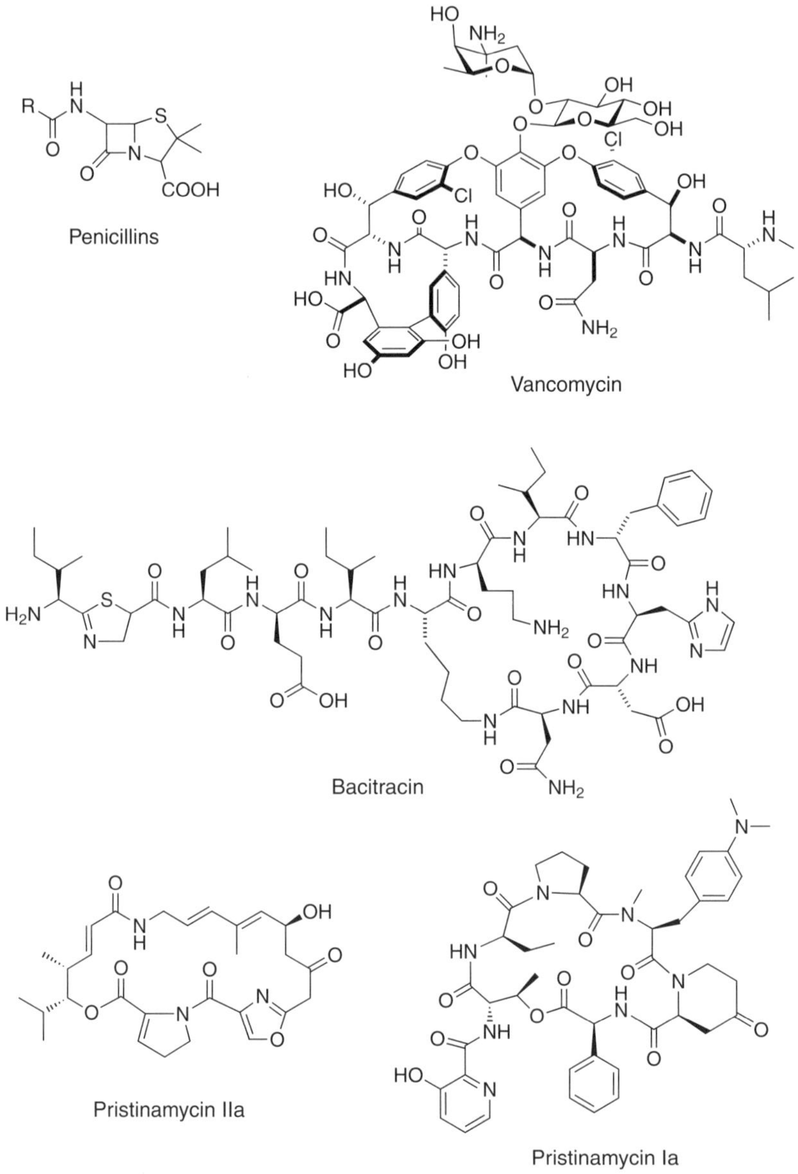

Penicillins
Vancomycin
Bacitracin
Pristinamycin IIa
Pristinamycin Ia

Figure 13.1 Examples of antibiotics made on nonribosomal peptide synthetase assembly lines.

Figure 13.2 NRPS assembly line organization: the three modules of ACV synthetase.

SH
SH
SH
A Aad
PCP
C
A Cys
PCP
C
A Val
PCP
E
TE

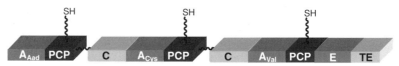

before a termination module at the C terminus of the protein assembly line. The core domains of the elongation modules are analogous to those in the type 1 PKS assembly lines (see chapter 12) but in NRPS modules are termed condensation (C), adenylation (A), and peptidyl carrier protein (PCP) domains. Each 8- to 10-kDa PCP domain is structurally and functionally analogous to ACP domains (chapter 12), undergoing the same posttranslational modification of a serine side chain on the inactive, apo PCP to the HS-pantetheinylated (HS-pant) holo PCP by dedicated partner phosphopantetheinyltransferase (PPTase) enzymes (Lambalot et al., 1996). The HS-pant-PCP domain in each module serves as the docking site for covalent attachment of an amino acid monomer that will be incorporated into the growing chain (**Fig. 13.3**).

Each A domain in a C-A-PCP module selects and activates the amino acid to be tethered on the adjacent HS-PCP. The selection of an amino acid occurs by binding in the active site of the A domain, and the code for recognition has been deciphered by a combination of X-ray analysis on the Phe-activating A domain of gramicidin S synthetase, bioinformatics analysis of >150 A domains, and mutagenesis to change selection (Stachelhaus et al., 1999). The bound amino acid is converted to aminoacyl-AMP as ATP is cleaved (**Fig. 13.4**) and PP_i released. This first half-reaction of A domains is the same as that of the aminoacyl-tRNA synthetases that activate amino acids for ribosome-dependent peptide bond formation, but X-ray analysis suggests convergent evolution for A domains and aminoacyl-tRNA synthetases. While the aminoacyl-tRNA synthetases transfer the thermodynamically activated aminoacyl group to bound cognate tRNAs, the A domains transfer the aminoacyl group to the in *cis* HS-pant-PCP domain, to generate the covalent aminoacyl-*S*-PCP in each module (Fig. 13.4).

The specificity of the A domains and their order and placement in the modules of an NRPS assembly line provide the instructions for thiotemplated peptide synthesis. In contrast to ribosomal peptide synthetase, where the collection of cellular aminoacyl-tRNA synthetases activates only the 20 proteinogenic amino acids, over 100 amino acids have been found in nonribosomal peptide natural products, indicating great diversity in amino acid monomer recognition, including activation of β-, γ- and δ-amino acids, such as β-alanine, γ-aminobutyrate, and δ-aminoadipate (Konz and Marahiel, 1999) (**Fig. 13.5**).

The third of the core domains in an NRPS elongation module, the C domains, are the peptide bond-forming condensation catalysts, using the imme-

Figure 13.3 Core domains of an NRPS elongation module: C-A-PCP and conversion of Apo PCP to Holo PCP domains by posttranslational phosphopantetheinylation.

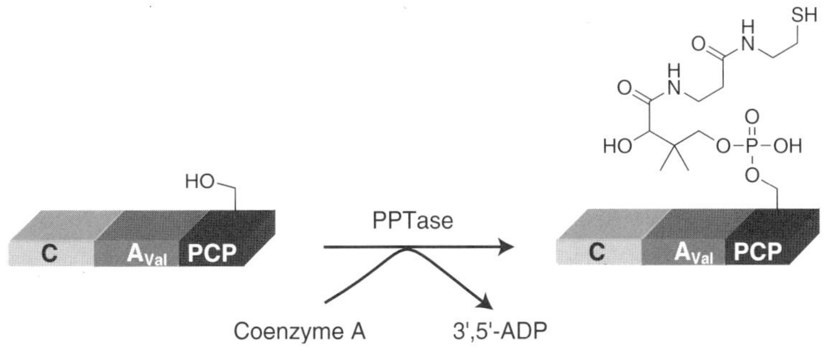

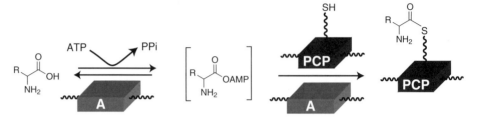

Figure 13.4 Two steps of NRPS adenylation domain catalysis: selection and activation of amino acid as tightly bound aminoacyl-AMP; aminoacyl group transfer to generate the covalent aminoacyl-*S*-PCP intermediate.

diate upstream intermodular peptidyl-*S*-PCP as acyl chain donor and the intramodular aminoacyl-*S*-PCP as the nucleophilic acceptor (**Fig. 13.6**) through its free amino group. Peptide bond formation is unidirectional and the growing peptidyl chain moves from upstream to downstream HS-PCP domain. The C domain is functionally analogous to the ketosynthase domain in the type 1 PKS assembly lines, but, rather than making C-C bonds, makes the C-N connection in peptide bond formation.

Chain initiation modules tend to lack a C domain and instead have an A-PCP two-domain structure to activate and load the first amino acid onto the first HS-PCP domain (**Fig. 13.7A**), as exemplified in the ACV synthetase discussed below. Chain termination modules have the general structure C-A-PCP-TE, where the C-terminal thioesterase domain (TE) has the same role as in the

Figure 13.5 Representative nonproteinogenic amino acids selected for chain incorporation by NRPS A domains.

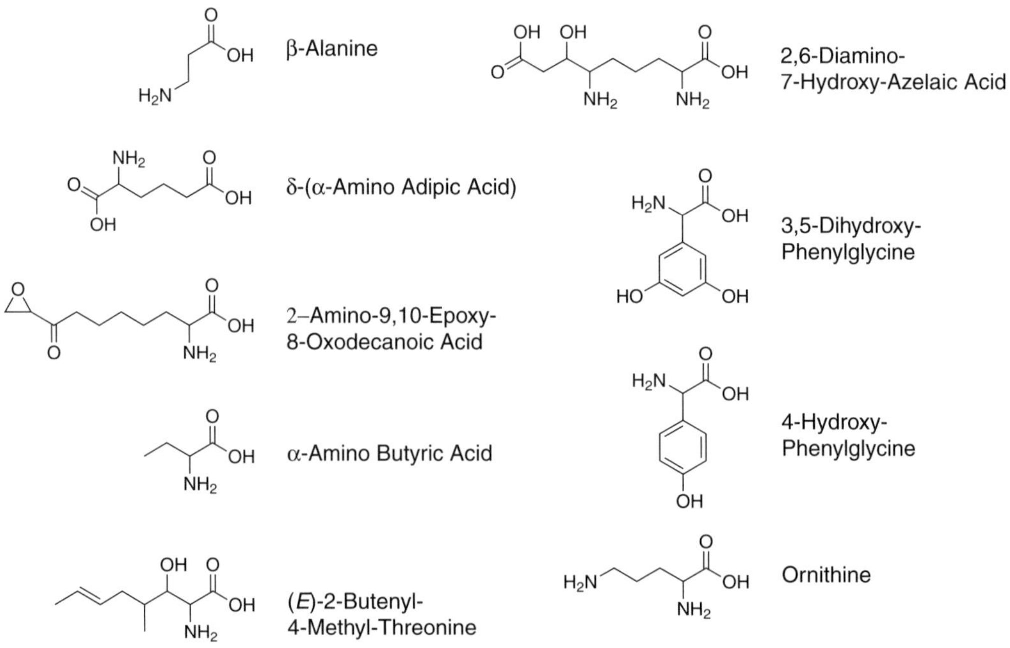

β-Alanine

2,6-Diamino-7-Hydroxy-Azelaic Acid

δ-(α-Amino Adipic Acid)

3,5-Dihydroxy-Phenylglycine

2–Amino-9,10-Epoxy-8-Oxodecanoic Acid

α-Amino Butyric Acid

4-Hydroxy-Phenylglycine

Ornithine

(*E*)-2-Butenyl-4-Methyl-Threonine

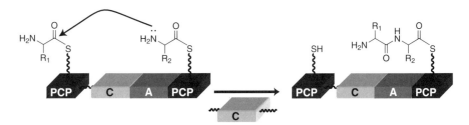

Figure 13.6 C domain action in NRPS catalysis: peptide bond condensation and elongation via peptidyl chain transfer to the downstream PCP domain.

Figure 13.7 (A) A-PCP two-domain chain initiation modules; (B) C-A-PCP-TE four-domain chain termination modules and three different pathways of chain termination.

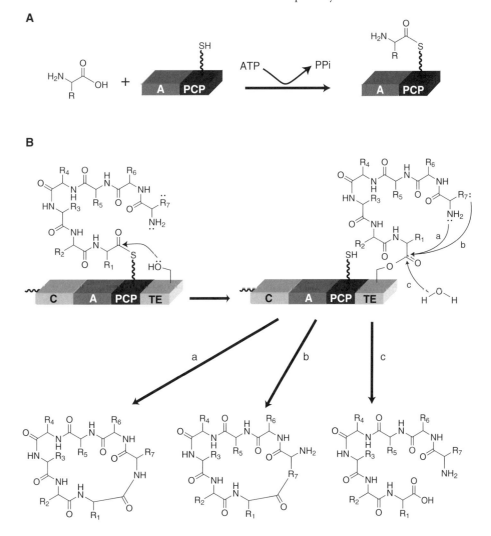

type 1 PKS assembly lines, for disconnection of the covalent thioester linkage between the full-length peptidyl chain and the most downstream PCP domain. As for the PKS assembly lines, NRPS TE domains can function as hydrolytic catalysts or macrocyclization catalysts (**Fig. 13.7B**) (Trauger et al., 2000).

In addition to the core C-A-PCP domains in NRPS modules, particular assembly lines may carry out additional chemical steps during chain elongation, and additional domains are placed in those modules where chemical tailoring of the growing chain occurs. For example, the cyclic undecapeptide immunosuppressant cyclosporin A has *N*-methyl groups on seven of the peptide bonds, and there are seven *S*-adenosylmethionine-utilizing *N*-methyltransferase domains embedded in the seven modules of the cyclosporin synthetase assembly line (von Dohren et al., 1997). We shall note below epimerization domains in the ACV, vancomycin, and tyrocidine assembly lines and a heterocyclization domain in the second module of bacitracin synthetase as additional tailoring domains placed in *cis* in the assembly lines.

Assembly lines for ACV, the vancomycin heptapeptide, tyrocidine, and bacitracin: epimerization, macrocyclization, and heterocyclization

ACV synthetase

The enzyme that assembles the acyclic tripeptide precursor of the penicillins and cephalosporins in *Acremonium chrysogenum*, the β-lactam producer organism, is a single-polypeptide NRPS. As shown in Fig. 13.2, ACV synthetase has 10 domains in the 450-kDa protein to carry out the thiotemplated assembly of ACV. There are three amino acids that have to be selected and activated as aminoacyl-AMPs, so there are three A domains, with Aad, Acys, and Aval arranged in that order in the three modules of the enzyme. There are three holo HS-PCP domains, created by posttranslational phosphopantetheinylation of the apo PCPs, for covalent tethering as aminoadipyl-*S*-PCP$_1$, cysteinyl-*S*-PCP$_2$, and valyl-*S*-PCP$_3$. Two peptide bonds are formed, the first between aminoadipate and cysteine catalyzed by the C domain in module 2, and the second, between Aad-Cys-*S*-PCP$_2$ as donor and Val-*S*-PCP$_3$ as acceptor, by the C domain in module 3, generating a tripeptidyl-*S* enzyme docked at PCP$_3$. This accounts for eight of the 10 domains.

The ninth domain is an epimerization (E) domain in module 3, where it could epimerize the L-Val-*S*-PCP$_3$ to D-Val-*S*-PCP$_3$. The epimerization passes through the planar, resonance-stabilized Cα-carbanion and this is accessed more readily in the valyl-thioester, Val-*S*-PCP$_3$, than in free valine. It is not yet clear if the valyl residue is epimerized to a D,L-mixture before or after condensation (as the L,L,L-tripeptidyl-*S*-PCP). If this occurs before, then the C domain in module 3 should be D-specific for the acceptor Val-*S*-PCP$_3$. If epimerization is effected on the tripeptidyl-*S*-PCP$_3$ after condensation, then the TE domain may be D-specific (**Fig. 13.8A**). The 10th and most C-terminal domain, the TE domain acts in this assembly line as a simple hydrolase. The TE domain is a member of the superfamily of active-site serine α,β-hydrolases. It uses the active-site Ser side chain as nucleophile to attack the tripeptidyl thioester and transfer the chain to make a tripeptidyl-*O*-Ser-TE acyl enzyme intermediate (**Fig. 13.8B**).

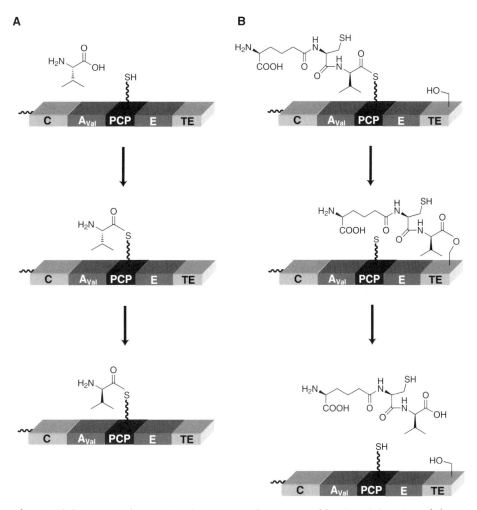

Figure 13.8 Domain function in the ACV synthetase assembly Line: (A) action of the E domain to make D-Val-S-PCP₃; (B) chain termination by the TE domain through deacylation of a tripeptidyl-O-Ser-TE acyl enzyme intermediate.

This is the species that is then hydrolyzed in a deacylation step that frees up the NRPS assembly line for the next catalytic cycle, releasing the L,L,D-tripeptide-COOH. The logic and order of all 10 domains in ACV synthetase is thus clear and illustrates the modularity of the thiotemplate peptidyl chain assembly process.

Two features of amino acid selection are worth noting in ACV synthetase's use of aminoadipate. Not only is it a nonproteinogenic amino acid, but also the Aad-specific A domain in module 1 activates the C_6-COOH, not the C_1-COOH, of aminoadipate as the acyl-AMP. Thus, the amide bond in the Aad-Cys-S-PCP₂ intermediate formed by the C domain of module 2 is an isopeptide bond, carried forward to the released tripeptide. In the next section of this chapter we will turn to the post-assembly-line enzymatic tailoring to convert the acyclic ACV into the fused four/five-ring system of penicillins.

Enzymatic assembly of the heptapeptide for vancomycin and chloroeremomycin

Vancomycin and chloroeremomycin have the identical cross-linked heptapeptide scaffold. The biosynthetic gene cluster for chloroeremomycin, but not yet for vancomycin, has been reported and contains a cluster of some 30 genes (van Wageningen et al., 1998) (**Fig. 13.9**). Notable in this cluster are three very large open reading frames, ORFs 4 to 6, that encode the three subunits, CepA, CepB, and CepC, of the NRPS heptapeptide synthetase. Inspection of the predicted domain order from bioinformatic analysis (**Fig. 13.10**) indicates 24 domains distributed over the three subunits, with CepA containing modules 1 to 3, CepB modules 4 to 6, and CepC the seventh module. The logic utilized for the ACV tripeptide synthetase is transposable to this NRPS assembly line. Seven amino acids in the heptapeptide mandate seven A domains and seven coupled PCP domains in HS-pantetheinyl holo form to be functional. There are six peptide bonds to be made and six C domains. There are four D-amino acids in the final D,D,L,D,L,L-acyclic heptamer. Epimerization domains are found in modules 2, 4, and 5 but not module 1. Finally, the heptapeptide scaffold in the natural product is the free acid and the TE domain is presumably a heptapetidyl-S-PCP$_7$ hydrolase. The source of D-Leu at the first residue is still unclear, but the A

Figure 13.9 Thirty genes clustered for chloroeremomycin biosynthesis.

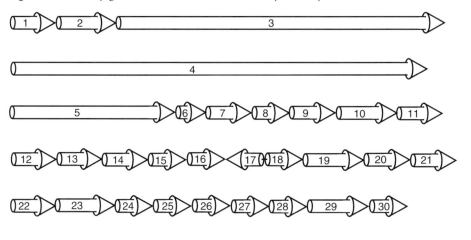

Function	ORF	Function	ORF
Nonribosomal Peptide Synthetase	3-5	HPG Synthesis	1, 17, 21, 22
Oxidative Crosslinking	7-9	DHPG Synthesis	27-30
N-Methylation	16	β-OH Tyr Synthesis	18-20
Halogenation	10	Transport	2
Glycosyl Transfer	11-13	Regulation	6
Sugar Synthesis	14, 23-26	Epimerase	15

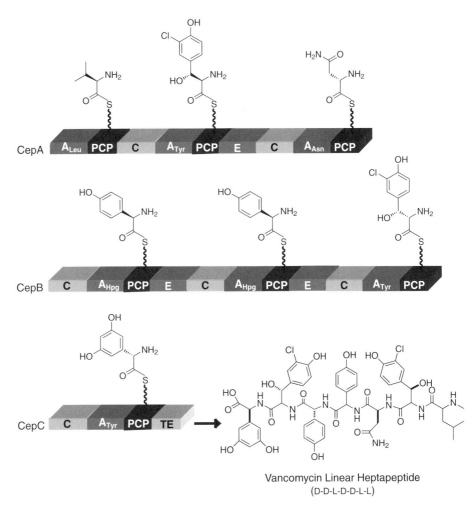

Figure 13.10 A 24-domain, seven-module assembly line for the heptapeptide backbone of chloroeremomycin or vancomycin synthetase.

domain can activate both L-Leu and D-Leu and install D-Leu on the adjacent HS-PCP of module 1 (Trauger and Walsh, 2000). If the C domain of module 2 is D-specific for the Leu$_1$ donor, then the issue could be resolved. Presumably the C domain in module 3 is specific for a D,D-dipeptidyl donor but an L-Asn-S-PCP$_3$ acceptor, while the C domain in module 5 would be predicted to recognize a D,D,L,D-tetrapeptidyl-S-enzyme donor and a D-4-OH-PheGly-S-PCP acceptor. The chiral specificity of the C domains has not yet been verified experimentally.

The last feature of note in this heptapeptide assembly line is the utilization of two nonproteinogenic amino acid monomers, D-4-OH-PheGly at positions 4 and 5 and 3,5-(OH)$_2$-PheGly at position 7. All three electron-rich aryl side chains participate in post-NRPS assembly-line cross-linking reactions, to be described below. The 4-OH-PheGly and 3,5-(OH)$_2$-PheGly monomers are synthesized as the L-isomers by enzymes also encoded in the biosynthetic cluster (Fig. 13.9). A four-enzyme pathway from chorismate via *para*-hydroxyphenylpyruvate and *para*-hydoxymandelate leads to the 4-OH-PheGly (ORFs 1, 17, 21, 22), while the 3,5-dihydroxy isomer instead derives from a type III PKS followed by three enzymes of the crotonase superfamily (ORFs 27 to 30 in Fig. 13.9), using acyl-CoAs in iterative Claisen condensations to build up the eight-carbon amino acid incorporated at residue 7 (Chen et al., 2002). These eight ORFs emphasize the coordinate regulation and commitment to produce the nonproteinogenic amino acid monomers on a just-in-time basis and validate the versatility of the NRPS A domains to introduce variation in these thiotemplated peptide assembly lines.

Bacitracin and tyrocidine assembly lines: macrocyclizations by TE domains

The tyrocidine synthase and bacitracin synthase assembly lines from *Bacillus brevis* and *Bacillus licheniformis*, respectively (**Fig. 13.11**), comprise three subunits that contain 10 and 12 modules, respectively, for the deca- and dodecapeptide antibiotics. Both are cyclic peptides connected with differing regiochemistry of cyclization. Tyrocidine is cyclized head to tail, the amino group of D-Phe₁ at-

Figure 13.11 The NRPS assembly line of tyrocidine synthetase.

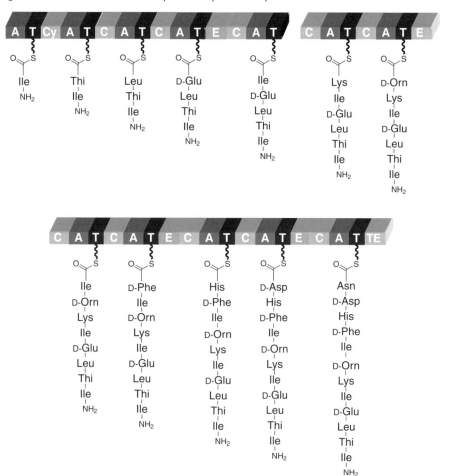

tacking the Leu_{10} carbonyl to make the cyclic amide (see Trauger et al., 2000), but bacitracin has cyclized to give a lariat primary structure with the side chain amino group of Lys_7 attacking the carbonyl of the terminal residue Asn_{12} (**Fig. 13.12**). The distinct cyclizations are catalyzed by the TE domains at the end of these NRPS assembly lines, functioning as macrolactamizing cyclases rather than as hydrolases. The acyl-O-TE intermediates must be kinetically sequestered from water and folded into an active-site conformation such that the Leu_{10}-COO-TE and the Asn_{12}-COO-TE ester bonds can be captured intramolecularly by the amine nucleophiles in the peptidyl chains. In the case of the tyrocidine synthetase, it has been established that the TE domain has all the information needed to induce chain folding and cyclization since the excised TE domain autonomously retains catalytic competency for decapeptidyl-thioester cyclization and, when presented with a D-phenylactyl substitution at D-Phe_1, will create the macrolactone. The distinction between hydrolyzing and cyclizing TE domains in type I PKS and in NRPS assembly lines is not yet clear but will be of relevance in combinatorial approaches to macrocyclizations.

Figure 13.12 Bacitracin chain release by intramolecular macrolactamization by the TE domain of bacitracin synthetase: making the Lys_7-Asn_{12} isopeptide bond.

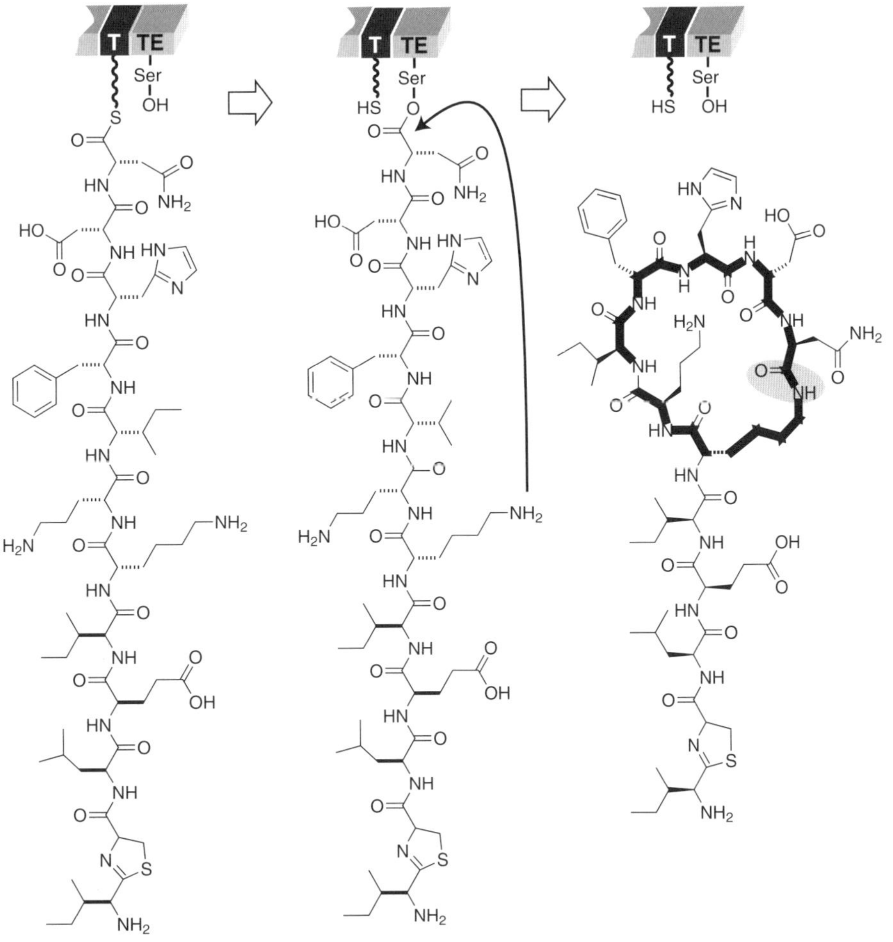

In addition to its lariat type of macrolactam structure, bacitracin has an additional structural feature of note: residues 1 and 2, Ile_1-Cys_2, are converted to a five-ring dihydrothiazole, a thiazoline, during the chain elongation step in module 2 (**Fig. 13.13**). Analysis of the condensation domain in module 2 of bacitracin synthetase reveals it is a variant and a member of a cyclization (Cy) domain subfamily (Keating and Walsh, 1999). In addition to behaving as typical C domains and catalyzing the amide bond formation, these Cy domains, also found in bleomycin synthetase (see Du et al., 2001), catalyze first cyclization of the thiolate side chain of cysteine onto the just-formed peptide bond carbonyl and then dehydration to generate the cyclic imine double bond and drive the cyclization equilibrium to the thiazoline ring. This modification changes the connectivity of the acyl chain. Also, the thiazoline ring is a good divalent metal ion chelator, which is thought to be relevant to the Mg^{2+}-mediated coordination of undecaprenyl phosphate in its antibiotic action (chapter 3).

ACV post-assembly-line enzymology: ACV to penicillins to cephalosporins—comparison with carbapenem and clavulanate biosynthesis

The enzymatic transformation of the acyclic ACV tripeptide to the bicyclic β-lactam structure of penicillins is catalyzed by a single nonheme Fe^{II} enzyme, isopenicillin N synthase (IPNS), that reduces cosubstrate O_2 by four electrons to two molecules of water (**Fig. 13.14**). In turn the β-lactam ring is expanded from the five-ring thiazolidine to the six-ring dihydrothiazine ring of the cephalosporin antibiotics, again by a single nonheme Fe^{II} dioxygenase (**Fig. 13.15**)

Figure 13.13 Action of the cyclization domain of bacitracin synthetase to create the thiazoline ring from Cys_1-Leu_2.

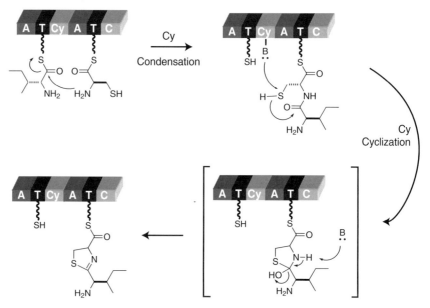

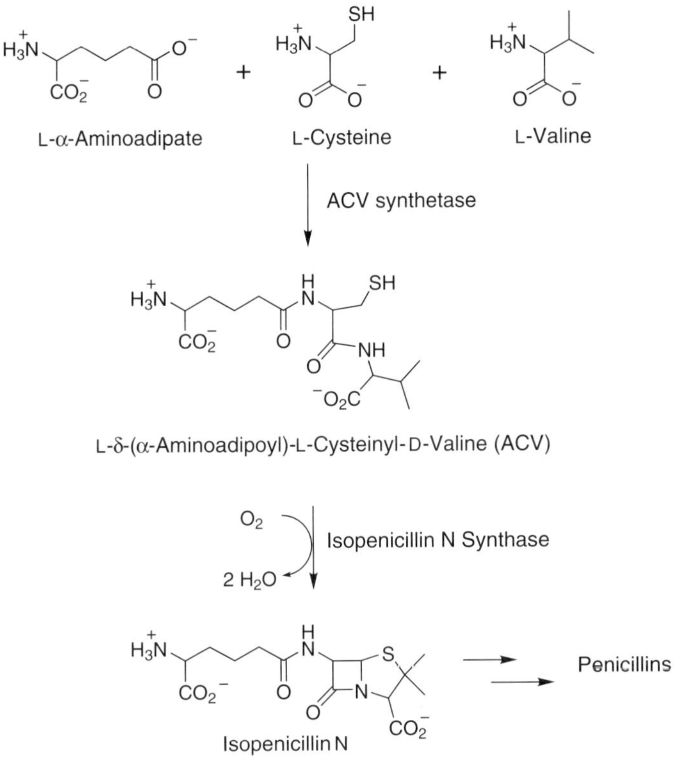

Figure 13.14 Double cyclization of ACV to the β-lactam skeleton of penicillins by isopenicillin N synthase.

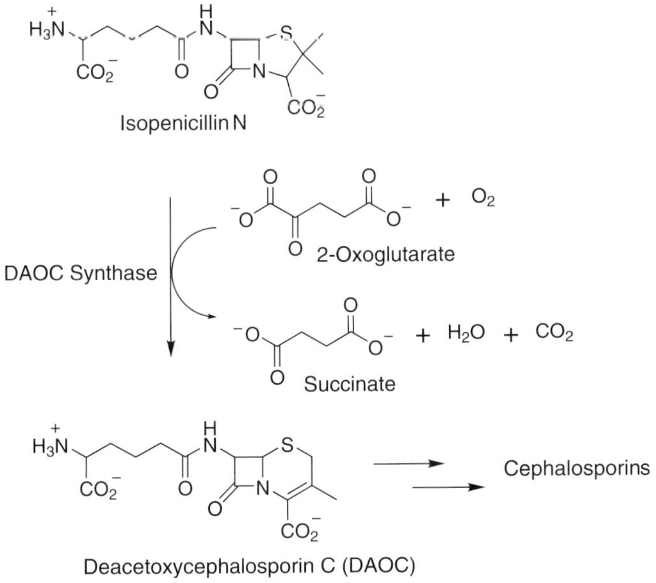

Figure 13.15 Expansion of the five ring of penicillins to the six ring of cephalosporins by expandase (deacetoxycephalosporin C synthase).

which acts after an epimerase has converted isopenicillin N to penicillin N, by equilibration of the L-aminoadipyl C_2 center to the D,L-mixture. The expandase, also known as deacetoxycephalosporin C synthase (DAOCS), works only on the D-aminoadipyl-penicillin, requires a molecule of α-ketoglutarate as cosubstrate, and decarboxylates it to succinate and CO_2 while O_2 is reduced to H_2O and the second oxygen atom is incorporated into the succinate carboxyl.

The X-ray structures of both IPNS, from *Aspergillus nidulans* (Roach et al., 1997) (**Fig. 13.16**), and of DAOCS, from *Streptomyces clavuligerus* (Valegard et al., 1998), have been solved and reveal the two enzymes are members of a superfamily (**Fig. 13.17**) of nonheme ferrous iron dioxygenases. They use two His and one carboxylate (Asp/Glu) as scaffolding ligands (see Que, 2000) for the Fe^{II}, as does a third enzyme in β-lactam oxidative metabolism, clavaminate synthase (CAS) (Zhang et al., 2000), noted below.

While DAOCS and CAS show typical α-keto acid-decarboxylating dioxygenase stoichiometry from this common ferrous iron active-site scaffold, IPNS diverges, by not requiring an α-keto acid cosubstrate and by the number of electrons removed from substrate. IPNS oxidizes ACV by four electrons as it creates the fused four/five-ring system of the penicillin skeleton, funneling all four electrons to O_2 as it is reduced to two molecules of H_2O. By contrast, DAOCS and CAS perform two-electron oxidations of bound substrate in each catalytic cycle. Clearly the same architectural platform for ferrous iron can be guided into diverse but selective oxygen-based chemistry by ligation of oxidizable substrate. All three of these enzymes are thought to generate a high-valent $Fe^{IV}=O$ ferryl species as the key oxidant for the two-electron redox cycle. The DAOCS and CAS generate the ferryl oxidant from the oxidative decarboxylation of bound α-ketoglutarate, while IPNS is believed to generate the $Fe^{IV}=O$ oxidant by two-electron oxidation of ACV as it cyclizes, with C-N bond formation, to

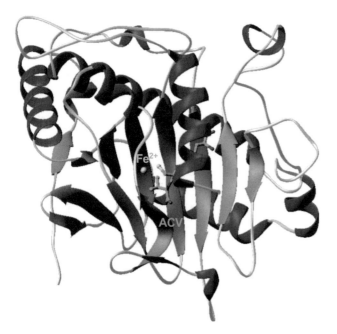

Figure 13.16 X-ray structure of IPNS with active-site iron and bound ACV substrate.

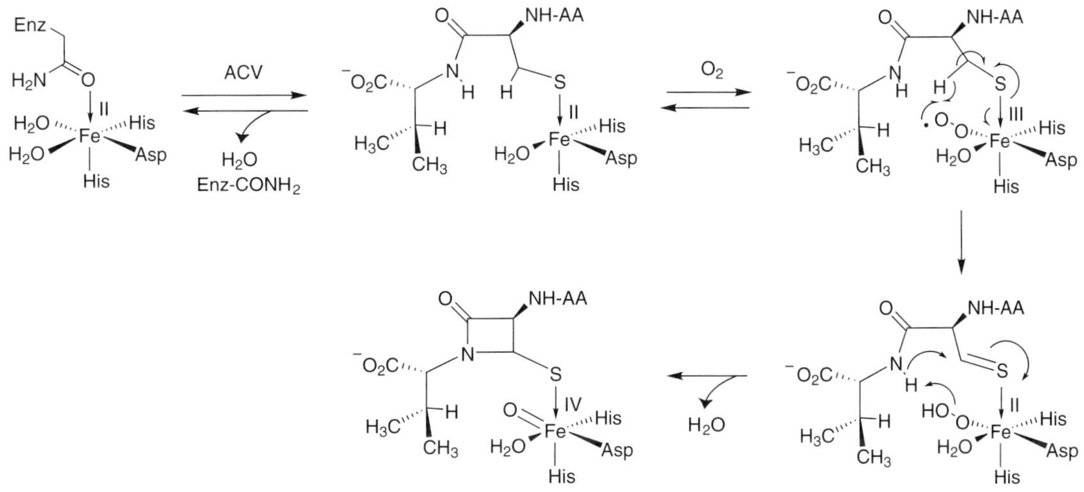

Figure 13.17 Proposed mechanisms for the formation of the first ring (β-lactam) by IPNS.

the iron-coordinated monocyclic β-lactam intermediate (Fig. 13.17) (Roach et al., 1997).

The second half of the IPNS reaction is the two-electron oxidation G/cyclization of the thiol-coordinated mono lactam to the thiazolidine ring with S_{Cys} to $C\beta_{Val}$ bond formation by two one-electron steps (**Fig. 13.18**) and concomitant two-electron reduction of the $Fe^{IV}=O$ back to fe^{II}-OH. Analogously, the ring expansion by the DAOCS expandase utilizes the $Fe^{IV}=O$ to break the S-Cβ bond in the thiazolidine and then reclose the sulfur radical onto a CH_2 radical derived from hydrogen atom abstraction from one of the prochiral β-methyl groups. This expands the ring from five to six and generates the endocyclic olefin (**Fig. 13.19**) as the ground state Fe^{II} is regenerated. Presumably the reactivity of the Fe^{IV} oxo iron species is modulated by substrate approach geometrical constraints in each active site and perhaps also by controlled changes in the iron coordination sphere at different points in these complex catalytic cycles.

The carbapenems and oxopenam skeleton of clavulanate are elaborated by a different enzymatic strategy. They do not derive from nonribosomal peptide products. Rather, the simple 5R-carba-2-em-3-carboxylate produced by *Erwinia carotovora* and *Serratia marcescens* is assembled from acetyl-CoA and the amino acid glutamate by a three-enzyme biosynthetic cluster, CarA-C (**Fig. 13.20**) (Li

Figure 13.18 Formation of the second ring of penicillins by IPNS with reduction of the ferryl intermediate.

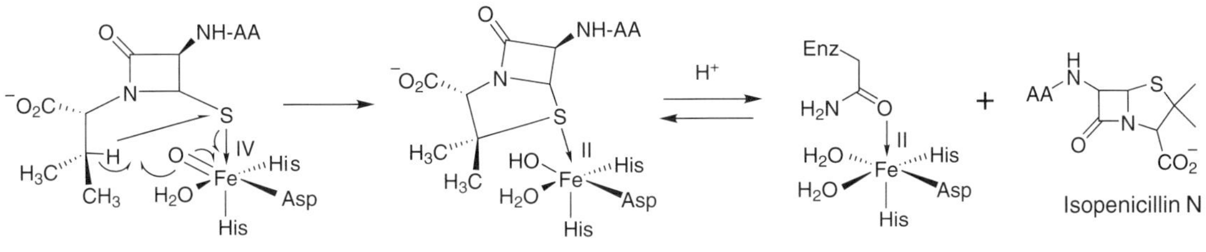

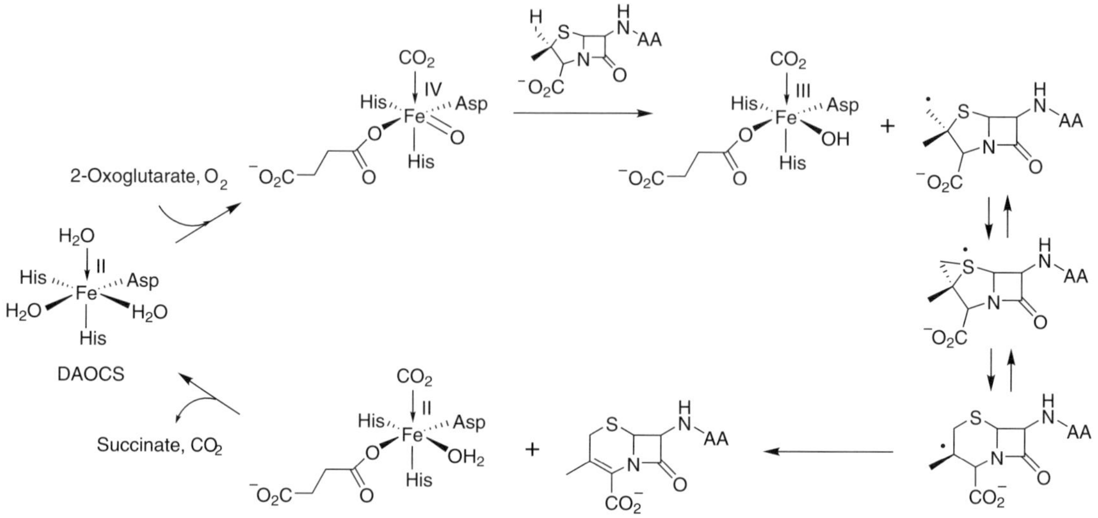

Figure 13.19 Ring expansion by DAOCS with reduction of the ferryl intermediate.

et al., 2000). The five ring is elaborated first, by CarB, to a 2-carboxymethyl proline. The carboxylate is activated by CarA, the β-lactam synthetase, in a reaction that makes the acyl-AMP intermediate on the CH_2-COOH side chain, then uses the amine for intramolecular displacement of AMP as the four-membered lactam forms (Bachmann et al., 1998). This carbapenem intermediate is oxidatively desaturated by CarC and the bridgehead 4/5 configuration epimerized to generate the natural product. CarA and CarB have homologs in the clavulanate biosynthetic pathway (**Fig. 13.21**) where the amino acid arginine and the primary metabolite D-glyceraldehyde 3-phosphate are the precursors. The first step is a thiamine-pyrophosphate-dependent enzymatic generation of carboxyethylarginine, a highly unusual conversion, involving internal redox control and an elimination (of P_i) and addition of the arginine α-NH_2 group. The next step is another ATP-cleaving β-lactam synthase to generate the mono lactam via an architectural variant of an asparagine synthetase (Khaleeli et al., 2001). The X-ray structure of lactam synthetase with bound carboxyethylarginine and an ATP analog suggests preorganized conformer geometry favorable for intramolecular β-lactam formation (Miller et al., 2001).

Then the CAS Fe^{II} dioxygenase acts in three separate steps (Fig. 13.21), first as a hydroxylase to install the OH adjacent to the carboxylate and produce

Figure 13.20 The tandem action of CarA-C to generate the carbapenem nucleus.

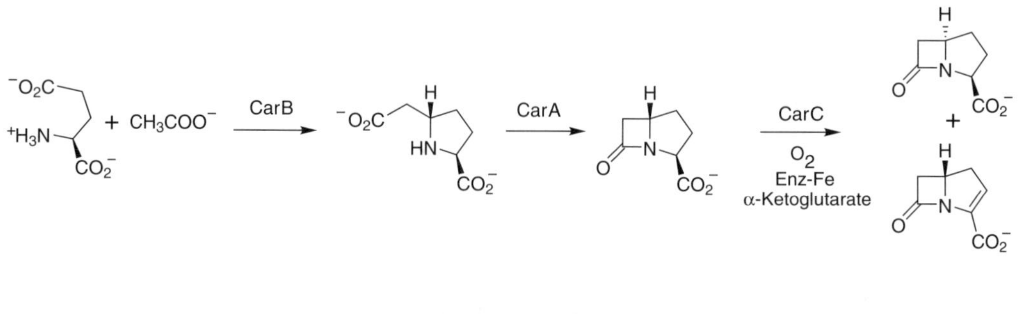

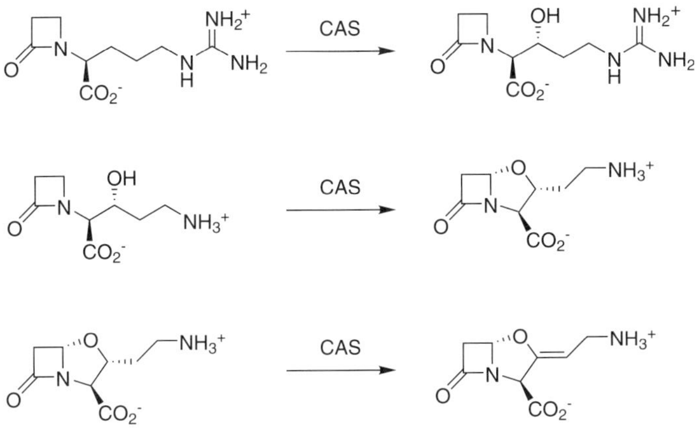

Figure 13.21 Three oxidative transformations by CAS during construction of clavaminate.

proclavaminate. Then CAS acts as an oxidative cyclase adding the alcohol oxygen to C_4 of the β-lactam, generating the 4/5 ring junction in dihydroclavaminate (Zhang et al., 2000). The third consecutive reaction of CAS is an oxidative desaturation, introducing the exocyclic double bond that creates the enol ether in clavaminate. Subsequent enzymes oxidize the amine to an aldehyde and reduce it to the alcohol of clavulanate. The three reactions of CAS show exquisite manipulation of the chemical reactivity of the two-His/Asp platform for the Fe^{II} in the active site.

Post-assembly-line enzymology: oxygenation and glycosylation of the aglycones for vancomycin and teicoplanin and acylation of teicoplanin

Three to four kinds of enzymatic maturation reactions convert the acyclic heptapeptide aglycones of vancomycin and teicoplanin into the active glycopeptide and lipoglycopeptide antibiotics, respectively (see Hubbard and Walsh, 2002). First the free amino group of D-Leu$_1$ of the vancomycin heptapeptide is N-methylated, using S-adenosylmethionine as cosubstrate, carried out by an N-methyltransferase that is ORF 17 in the chloroeremomycin biosynthetic cluster (Fig. 13.9).

Second is the rigidifying cross-linking that occurs in the aryl side chains. In the chloroeremomycin/vancomycin scaffold, the cross-links connect the aryl side chains of residues 2 and 4, 4 and 6, and 5 and 7 (**Fig. 13.22**), while in the teicoplanin scaffold, residues 1-3, 2-4, 4-6, and 5-7 are all cross-linked. The cross-links convert a floppy acyclic peptide into a highly constrained cup-shaped architecture that provides the complementary surface to interact with its target N-acyl-D-Ala-D-Ala in the peptidoglycan terminus of the bacterial cell wall.

The 2-4 and 4-6 cross-links are aryl ether bonds, while the 5-7 cross-link is a direct C-C bond, but both can be formulated as radical couplings of the electron-rich β-OH-chloro-tyrosines (residues 2 and 6), the 4-OH-phenylglycine (residues 4 and 5), and the 3,5-dihydroxy phenylglycine at residue 7 (**Fig. 13.23**). In the chloroeremomycin cluster there are three hemeproteins, ORFs 7 to 9, and there are two homologs in the bahlimycin cluster that are implicated in genetic

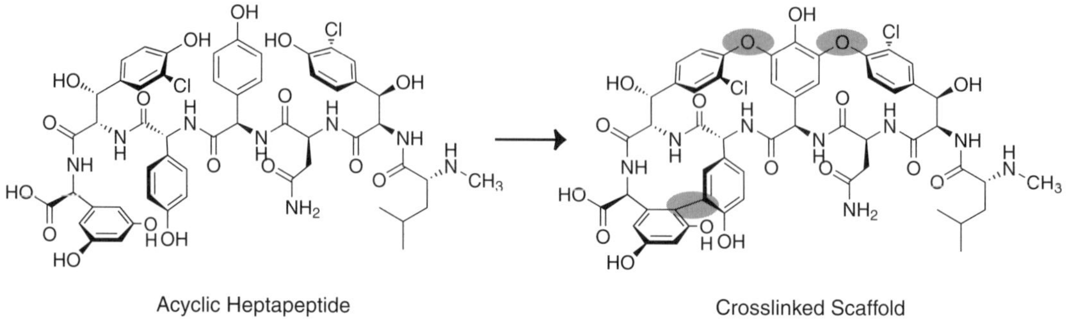

Figure 13.22 Rigidifying cross-links connect the aryl side chains in the vancomycin family of antibiotics.

Figure 13.23 Proposed phenoxy radical cyclization mechanisms for hemeprotein-mediated cross-linking in the vancomycin family.

C-O-C Linkage

C-C Linkage

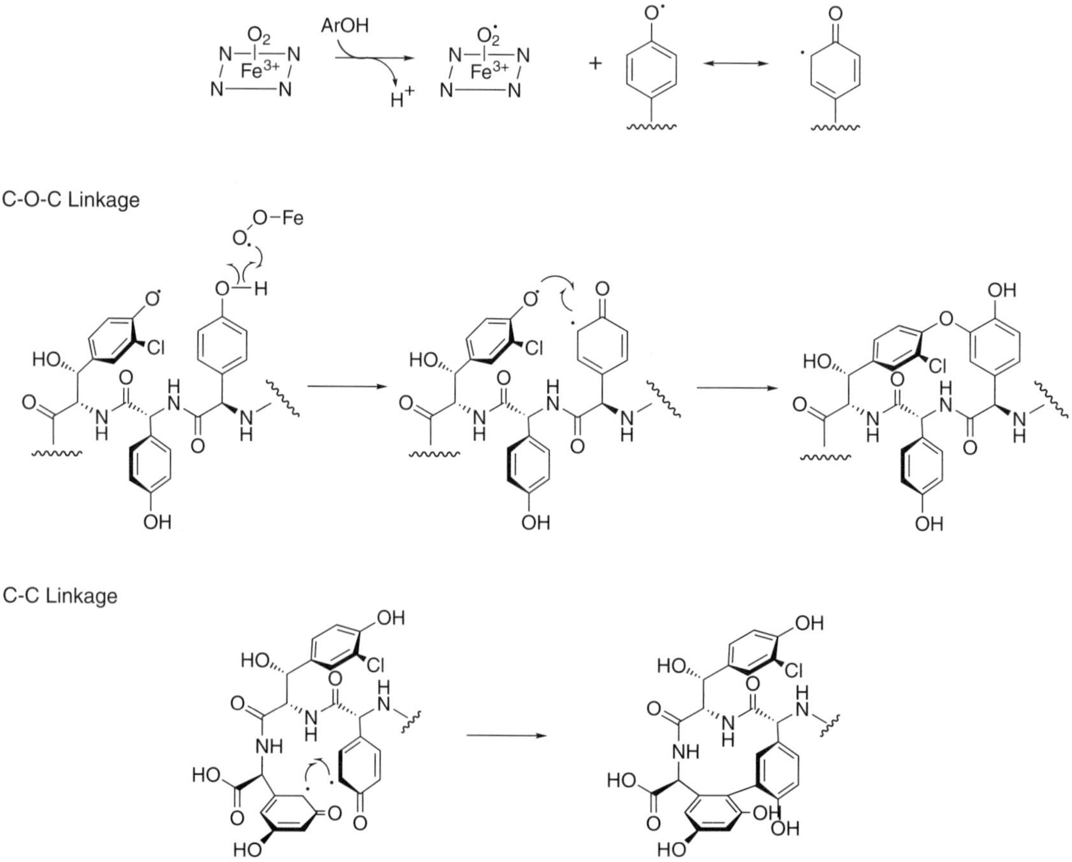

knockouts (Bischoff et al., 2001) as the cross-linking catalysts. These putative cytochrome P450s could generate the phenolic radicals in the side chains of the heptapeptide substrates to initiate the cross-linkings. Whether the individual hemeproteins are regioselective cross-linking catalysts is yet to be determined.

The third set of maturation enzymes are the glycosyltransferases, three (GtfA, GtfB, and GtfC) for the three sugars to be added to chloroeremomycin and two (GtfD, and GtfE) in the vancomycin cluster for the two sugars there (Losey et al., 2001; Solenberg et al., 1997). The first sugar is added to the phenolic-OH of the PheGly$_4$ residue, embedded in the 2-4-6 cross-link (**Fig. 13.24**), and uses TDP-glucose as the donor substrate with GtfB as the catalyst. This glucosyl-cross-linked heptapeptide is now the substrate for the second Gtf (GtfC for chloroeremomycin). The cosubstrate in the chloroeremomycin pathway is TDP-L-β-epivancosamine, while in the vancomycin pathway it is TDP-L-β-vancosamine, differing only in the configuration of the C$_4$-OH in the sugar. The epivancosamine/vancosamine moiety is transferred to the C$_2$-OH of the glucosyl group, creating the 1,2-disaccharide linkage. This completes the biosyn-

Figure 13.24 Three regiospecific glycosyltransferases for tailoring of the aglycone in chloroeremomycin maturation.

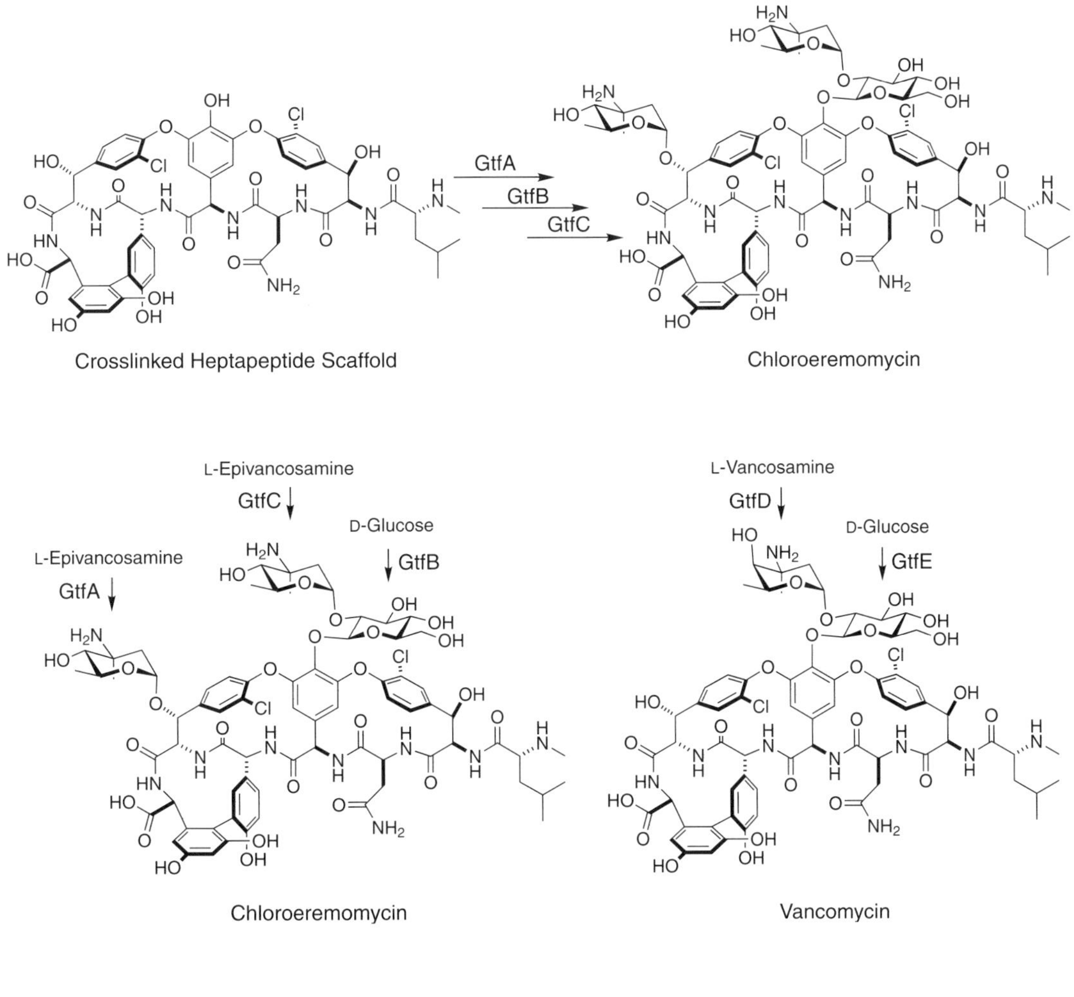

thesis of vancomycin, while the third Gtf (GtfA) in the chloroeremomycin pathway uses another molecule of TDP-L-β-epivancosamine to epivancosaminylate the β-OH of the sixth residue in the peptide scaffold and produce the chloroeremomycin antibiotic.

The fourth type of modification in this family of antibiotics occurs only in the teicoplanin subclass and involves acylation of the amino group of one of the sugars, glucosamine. We will discuss it in the context of other acylations of non-ribosomal peptide antibiotics below. In teicoplanin the identity and placement of the sugars is different, with N-acylaminoglucoses on the phenolic oxygen of PheGly$_4$ and β-OH-Tyr$_6$ and a mannosyl group on residue 7.

Lipopeptide and lipoglycopeptide antibiotics

A number of nonribosomal peptides are lipopeptides by virtue of N-acylation with fatty acyl chains on the amino group of the first amino acid residue. This includes daptomycin, ramoplanin, mycosubtilin, and teicoplanin (**Fig. 13.25**). The acyl chains can be straight chain saturated (mycosubtilin), terminally branched (surfactin), and unsaturated (ramoplanin), reflecting the complement of fatty acids made in those producer organisms. The total synthesis of ramoplanin has been published, opening up structure-activity studies (Jiang et al., 2002). Daptomycin is in phase 3 clinical trials for gram-positive infections (see Bronson and Barrett, 2001a). β-amino fatty acyl substituents appear, as in mycosubtilin, and they are made in situ, as noted below.

In most of the lipopeptide NRPS clusters sequenced to date, the acyltransferase responsible for N-acylation of the N-terminal amino acid does not map with the biosynthetic cluster and little is known about specificity. In the case of mycosubtilin, the first five domains of the MycA subunit (**Fig. 13.26**) are dedicated to construction of the C_{16}-β-NH_2-acyl group (Duitman et al., 1999). The acyl-AMP ligase domain is thought to activate palmitate and install it on domain 2, the immediately downstream ACP$_1$. Domain 3 is a ketosynthase; domain 4 is ACP$_2$, putatively loaded with a malonyl group. Condensation by the ketosynthase would translocate the C_{16} acyl chain and make a β-keto-acyl-C_{18} chain on ACP$_2$. The fifth domain has homologies to aminotransferases and is likely to transaminate the β-keto-acyl-S-ACP to the β-amino at the expense of a cosubstrate amino acid being oxidized to a keto acid.

It is proposed that the next domain, C$_1$, translocates the acyl chain to PCP$_1$, and then C$_2$ condenses it onto the amino group of Asn$_1$ tethered at PCP$_2$ to yield the N-capped Asn-PCP$_2$. Chain elongation proceeds by the normal NRPS assembly line operations from here. The N-acylation of the N terminus of these nonribosomal peptides has analogies to N-formylation of the N-terminal methionine in ribosomal protein synthesis in bacteria, which imposes directionality since formylmethionyl can only act as donor, not acceptor, in a peptide bond-forming step. It is also likely that the nonribosomal peptide N-acylations are providing membrane anchors to localize the products at membrane interfaces. The target for ramoplanin is lipid II in peptidoglycan biosynthesis, which is in such a location. The lipid chain in daptomycin is likely to be crucial for its membrane-perturbing properties. A third use of β-OH and β-NH_2 fatty acyl

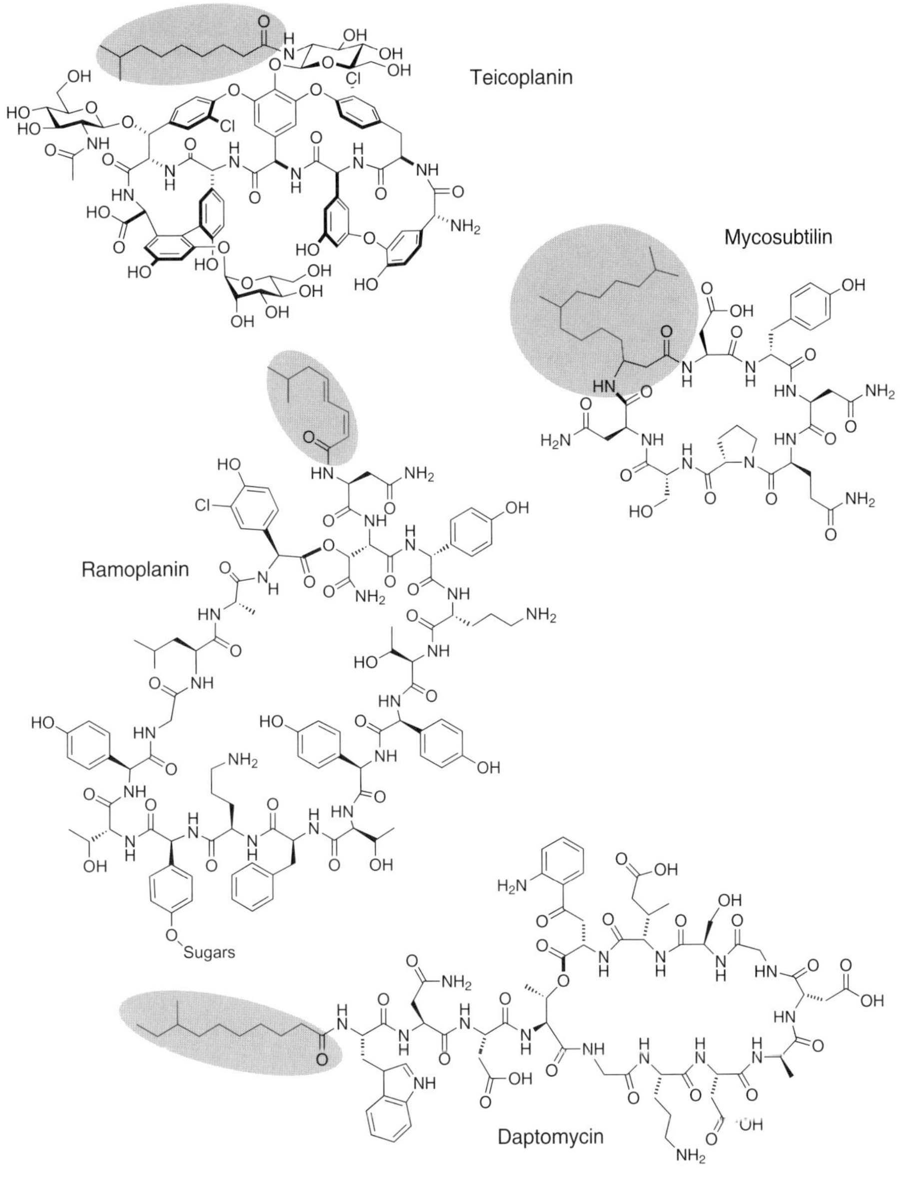

Figure 13.25 Lipopeptides made by nonribosomal peptide synthetase assembly lines.

chains, e.g., in surfactin and in iturin lipopeptide antibiotics, is that these provide intramolecular nucleophiles in TE-mediated cyclizations as termination steps in the NRPS assembly lines. The macrolactone ring of the β-hydroxy acyl heptapeptide surfactin is from the β-O fatty acyl to the carbonyl of Leu_7.

The teicoplanin acylation that completes lipoglycopeptide antibiotic formation is distinct from all the above examples. The acyl chain is not on the N terminus of the peptide scaffold. Instead it is on the amino group of the amino sugar. The acyltransferases are not yet identified, although acyl-CoAs or acyl-S-ACPs are likely cosubstrates. There are analogies in lipid A biosynthesis in gram-

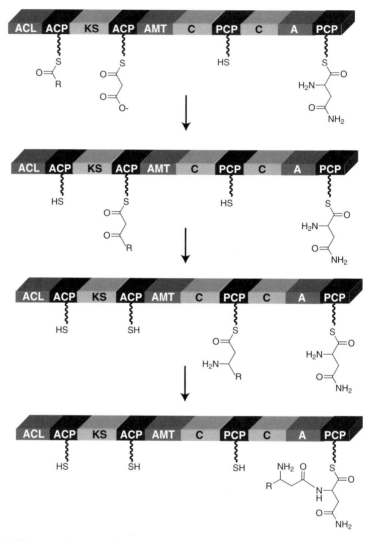

Figure 13.26 *N*-Acylation machinery at the N terminus of the mycosubtilin synthetase assembly line.

negative bacteria, where a GlcNAc residue is first deacetylated enzymatically and then reacylated by a biosynthetic enzyme using a long-chain acyl-*S*-ACP as cosubstrate.

The manipulation of the acyl chains in both forms of lipopeptide antibiotics may be one way to vary structure and improve properties against resistant organisms.

NRPS-PKS hybrid assembly lines: pristinamycins, rifamycin, and bleomycin

Some antibiotics are hybrids of nonribosomal peptides and polyketides (see Du et al., 2001), including pristinamycin IIB, the antitumor antibiotic bleomycin, and rifamycin (**Fig. 13.27**).

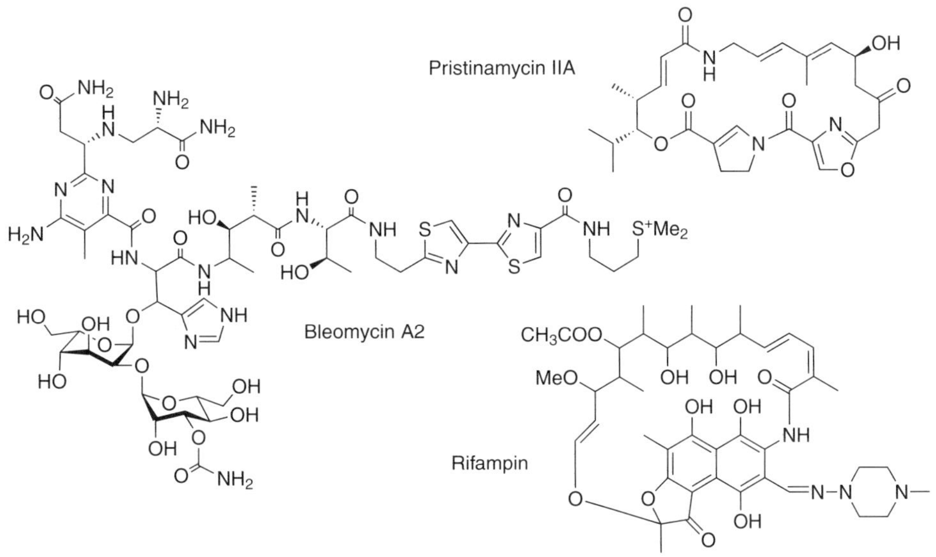

Figure 13.27 NRP-PK hybrids: bleomycin, pristinamycin IIA, and rifampin, a member of the rifamycin family.

The first two compounds clearly show part structures from each kind of assembly line. Pristinamycin IIB has three amino acids, Gly, Ser, and Pro, embedded in between stretches of polyketide. Bleomycin has a short polyketide stretch, encoded by subunit BLM VIII, embedded in a nonribosomal peptide structure. Rifamycin, although apparently a polyketide antibiotic by scanning of its structure, has as starter unit a 3-amino-5-hydroxybenzoate (**Fig. 13.28**) that is activated by a chain-initiating didomain that is an adenylation and aryl carrier protein, reminiscent of the start of nonribosomal peptide siderophore synthetases (Admiraal et al., 2001).

Figure 13.28 NRP and PK modules in the (A) rifamycin and (B) bleomycin assembly lines.

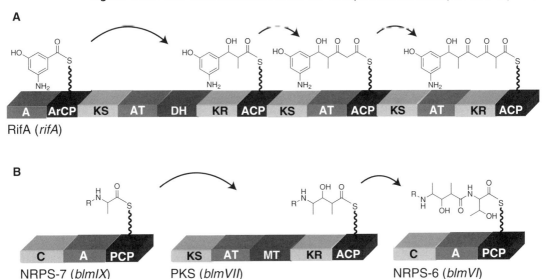

In those instances where the biosynthetic genes have been cloned and sequenced, the assembly lines indeed represent a mosaic of PKS and NRPS modules. The order and placement of the modules predict the polyketide or nonribosomal peptide monomers that get selected and incorporated in the hybrid acyl chains as they grow and translocate as a series of elongating acyl-S-(ACP/PCP) covalent intermediates.

Streptomycin

Novobiocin

Nisin

Diversely synthesized antibiotics.

chapter 14

Biosynthesis of Other Classes of Antibiotics

This chapter discusses the enzymatic logic for the formation of other classes of natural products that have been used in human medicine as antibiotics. The choice of specific topics complements the polyketide and nonribosomal peptide antibiotics of chapters 12 and 13. Other classes of natural products with antibiotic activity are not explicitly discussed, in part because of lack of knowledge of the enzymatic logic of biosynthesis or because of limited use in human therapeutics. For a broader context of natural product classes beyond those described here, the nine-volume series *Comprehensive Natural Products Chemistry* (Barton et al., 1999) can be consulted.

Fosfomycin

The most notable attribute about the antibiotic fosfomycin (**Fig. 14.1**), which inhibits MurA, the first enzyme in peptidoglycan biosynthesis (chapter 3), is the presence of a direct C–P bond in phosphonic acid linkage. Fosfomycin is one of a small group of C-P-containing natural products known, and they all appear to install the C-P bond by the same enzymatic pathway. Aminoethylphosphonate is a component of *Tetrahymena* lipid membranes, while phosphinothricyl-Ala-Ala (Bialaphos) is a C-P tripeptidyl herbicide.

Fosfomycin is produced by an efficient four-step enzymatic pathway, encoded by the genes *fom1-4* in the producer *Streptomyces wedmorensis*, from the primary metabolite phosphoenolpyruvate (PEP) (Seto, 1999) (**Fig. 14.2**). The first enzyme, phosphonopyruvate mutase (Fom1), installs the C-P bond by intramolecular capture by the C_3 enolate anion as the C_2-OPO_3 bond in PEP breaks in the mutase active site. Then the α-keto acid functionality is decarboxylated to the aldehyde (Fom2) and methylated by a methylcobalamin-utilizing enzyme (Fom3). The last step, catalyzed by Fom4, is an unprecedented cyclization of the C_2-OH group onto the C_1-CH_2 to create the epoxide ring and produce fosfomycin.

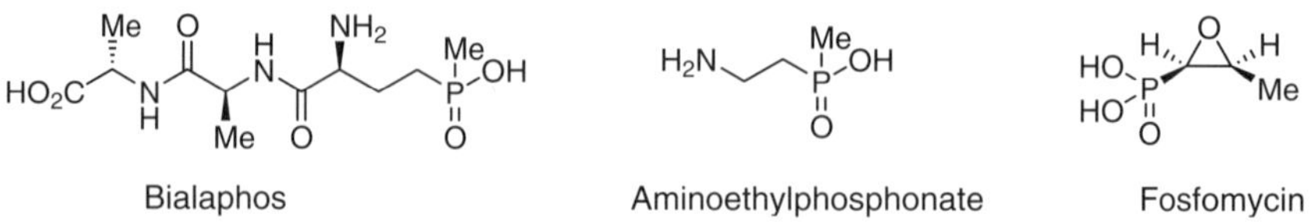

Figure 14.1 Representative C-P-containing natural products: Bialaphos, aminoethylphosphonate, and fosfomycin.

In addition to the four structural genes, several neighboring genes are involved in self-protection of the antibiotic producer. Three genes, *orfI, orfJ,* and *orfK,* appear to be elements of a protein export pump for fosfomycin. Also, OrfA and OrfB confer resistance by phosphorylation of intracellular antibiotic, presumably before its export, to fosfomycin monophosphate and fosfomycin diphosphate, respectively (**Fig. 14.3**). The fosfomycin diphosphate has a side chain analogous to nucleoside triphosphates. Both fosfomycin monophosphate and fosfomycin diphosphate are inactive but can be enzymatically hydrolyzed back to active fosfomycin by phosphatases, such as alkaline phosphatase in the external medium. This reversible self-protection conserves the epoxide chemical warhead, in contrast to the glutathione-mediated epoxide opening in resistant bacteria that are not fosfomycin producers (chapter 10). Phosphorylation of the intracellular form of the antibiotic to deactivate it before export is a strategy also followed by streptomycin producers, as noted in the next section.

Aminoglycoside antibiotic biosynthetic pathways

The aminoglycoside, or aminocyclitol, antibiotics represent products of secondary carbohydrate metabolism and are prevalent among actinomycetes. Starting with the isolation of streptomycin in 1944, various family members were discovered over the following 25 years (Piepersberg, 1997), including tobramycin in 1970. Novel aminocyclitols continued to be reported into the 1990s. Two main categories of these carbohydrate antibiotics are exemplified by the strep-

Figure 14.2 Biosynthetic pathway from PEP to fosfomycin.

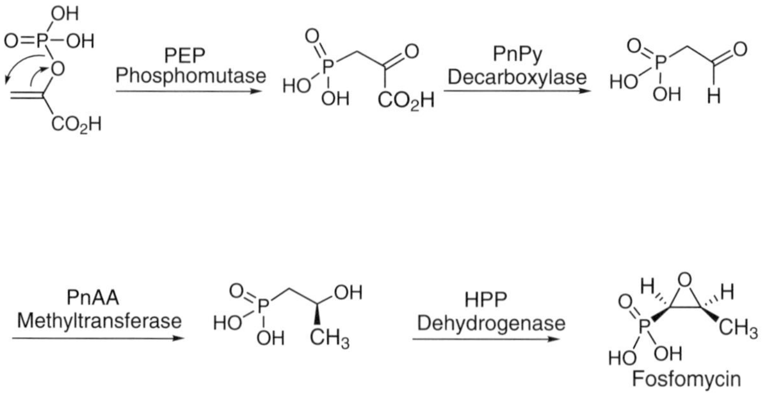

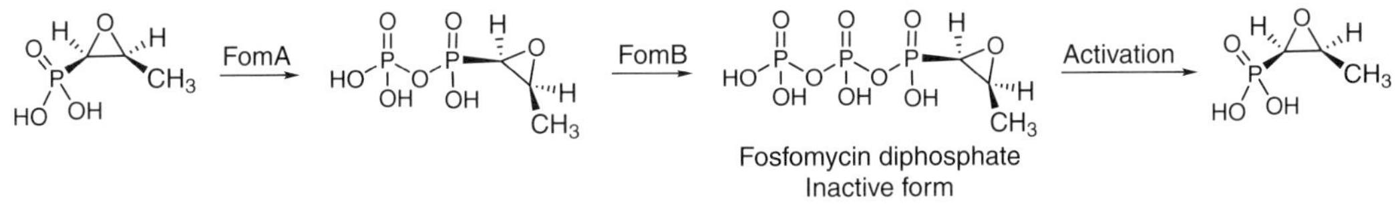

Figure 14.3 Sequential tandem phosphorylation of the phosphonate moiety in fosfomycin as a self-protection mechanism in *S. wedmorensis*.

tomycin class (**Fig. 14.4**) and by the 2-deoxystreptamine-containing antibiotics that include neomycins, kanamycins, and gentamicins (Fig. 14.4). Streptomycin has three sugar constituents: a *scyllo*-inositol-derived aminocyclitol (streptidine) connected to a 6-deoxyhexose component (streptose) connected to an *N*-methyl-L-glucosamine. In antibiotics of the 2-deoxystreptamine class such as kanamycin and gentamicin A, the aminocyclitol is the central ring. Semisynthetic modification of these natural products has been widely practiced. For example, the addition of an α-OH-γ-aminobutyryl side chain to the 1-NH of kanamycin produces the clinically contemporary drug amikacin. The glycoside-to-cyclitol conversion, central to this antibiotic biosynthetic pathway logic, is found in primary metabolism for the generation of inositol-phosphate from glucose-6-phosphate (glucose-6-P) on the way to phosphoinositide membrane lipid biosynthesis (Walsh, 1979).

There are some 30 genes clustered together and regulated simultaneously that are turned on when *Streptomyces griseus* makes streptomycin (see Piepersberg, 1997). These are involved in coding for enzymes of secondary sugar metabolism that make the three sugar monomers, streptidine-6-P, TDP-dihydrostreptose, and nucleoside diphospho-*N*-Me-L-glucosamine, and couple them regio- and stereospecifically. The streptidine-6-P comes from the primary

Figure 14.4 Two major structural classes of aminoglycoside (aminocyclitol) antibiotics: streptomycin and 2′-deoxystreptamine-containing examples kanamycin and gentamicin A.

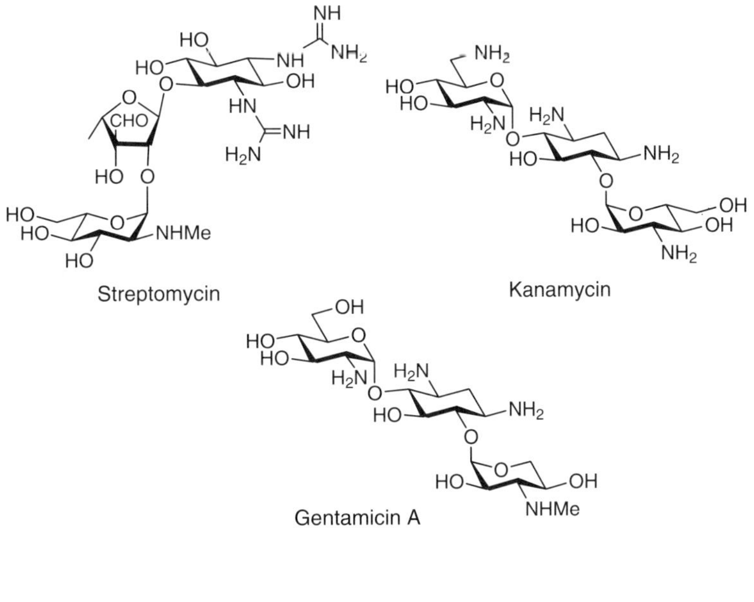

metabolite D-glucose-6-P by an intramolecular aldol enzymatic reaction to make the cyclitol-inositol-3-P, in a well-known reaction (see Walsh, 1979). Then a series of enzymatic generation of keto groups, reductive transaminations, and guanidino transfers produces the bisguanidino-cyclitol-P, streptidine-6-P (**Fig. 14.5A**). The TDP-dihydrostreptose is elaborated from the common intermediate in deoxyhexose biosynthesis, TDP-4-keto-6-deoxyglucose (see chapter 12) by epimerization at C_5 to generate TDP-4-keto-L-rhamnose, followed by conversion to the five-ring furanose structure in TDP-dihydrostreptose, where the dihydro refers to the alcohol oxidation state of the one-carbon CH_2OH unit at C_3 (Fig. 14.5, middle). The NDP-L-glucosamine is similarly fashioned from the NDP-D-glucose via 4-keto,5-epimerization, followed by amination and N-methylation at C_3 (Fig. 14.5, bottom). The 4-OH of streptidine-6-P attacks C_1 of the TDP-dihydrostreptose in the first glycosyltransferase condensation, then the 2'-OH of this disaccharide displaces the NDP of the NDP-N-methyl-L-glucosamine to produce dihydrostreptomycin-6-P. This is the end of the cytoplasmic phase of streptomycin biosynthesis in *S. griseus* and results in an inactive precursor. This is specifically exported via an ATP-dependent pump and oxidized from the dihydro CH_2OH stage to the CHO in streptomycin-6-P during transmembrane passage by an oxidase enzyme. Now the streptomycin-6-P in the extracellular space has the 6-OPO$_3$ group removed hydrolytically by a phosphatase also encoded in the cluster and exported (**Fig. 14.6**). The free streptomycin is the active antibiotic.

The biosynthesis encompasses some 27 enzymatic steps. The producer organisms provide self-resistance by accumulating only the inactive precursor inside the cell, both dihydro and phosphorylated, and execute two chemical steps for activation during and after secretion. This is analogous to the glycosylation of oleandomycin while in the producer cell to keep that macrolide inactive until excreted and specifically deglycosylated (chapter 7). In addition to these self-protective mechanisms, streptomycin producers can rephosphorylate any streptomycin that comes back in, again at C_6 with a phosphotransferase. Analogously, the kanamycin producers elaborate a 6' acetyltransferase. Both of these strategies presage the acquired mechanisms in clinical pathogens that become resistant to these aminoglycoside antibiotics (chapter 10). Finally, in gentamicin producers, an additional layer of self-defense is provided by enzymatic N-methylation of the high-affinity binding site in 16S rRNA (Piepersberg, 1997) to lower affinity for aminoglycosides at the ribosomes.

The streptomycin biosynthetic operons (**Fig. 14.7**) are regulated by quorum-signaling molecules, as described in chapter 11. In *S. griseus* this is the butaneolide A factor (Fig. 11.6), and the hierarchy of global and pathway-specific regulation, through the A factor receptor and then to the strR repressor, applies for the 23 genes in the eight operons of Fig. 14.7.

The logic of the class B aminoglycosides is similar in terms of enzymatic modification of NDP-sugars for deoxygenation and reductive amination and for aminocyclitol generation and glycosyltransferase couplings. The prospects for combinatorial biosynthesis to make new aminocyclitols, e.g., with more rings and new connectivities, may be good, setting up the systems for new rounds of semisynthetic alkylations and acylations, although it remains to be seen if useful new activities will result. The deciphering of the binding sites for class A and B aminocyclitols on 16S rRNA (chapter 4) may aid in design of better aminocyclitol antibiotics.

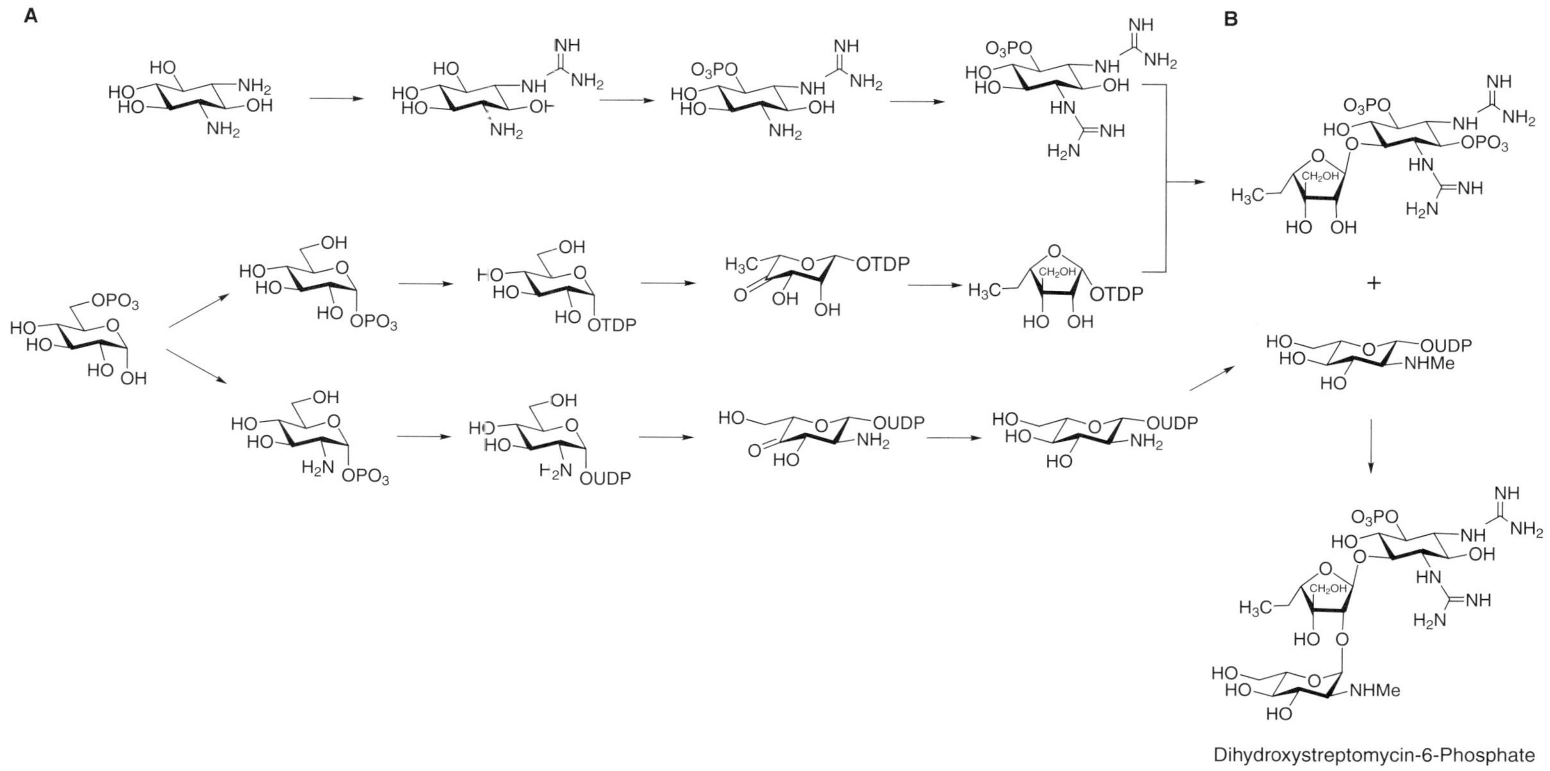

Figure 14.5 Biosynthetic pathway to dihydrostreptomycin-6-P. (A) Upper line: the streptidine-6-P branch; middle line: the TDP-dihydrostreptose branch; bottom line: the NDP-N-methyl-L-glucosamine branch; (B) glycosyltransferase action to produce dihydrostreptomycin-6-P.

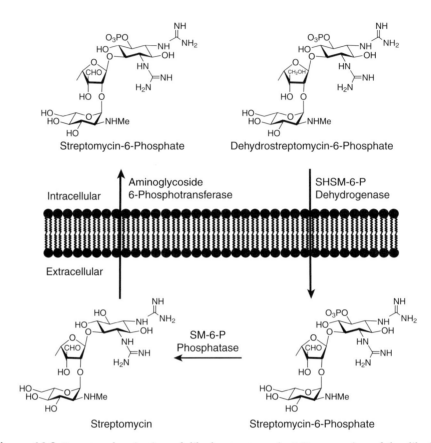

Figure 14.6 Export and activation of dihydrostreptomycin-6-P: conversion of the dihydro CH_2OH to the CHO in streptomycin and extracellular enzymatic dephosphorylation.

Biosynthesis of chorismate-derived antibiotics: the aminocoumarins and chloramphenicol

The DNA gyrase inhibitors chlorobiocin, novobiocin, and the dimeric coumermycin all share an aminocoumarin core and a noviose sugar that are important for binding to the GyrB subunit of DNA gyrase (chapter 5) and blocking DNA

Figure 14.7 A cluster of 22 genes in eight operons for streptomycin biosynthesis.

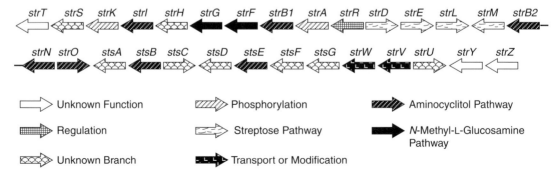

replication. The bicyclic aminocoumarin ring is constructed from tyrosine, in turn derived from chorismate, the key intermediate in aromatic amino acid biosynthesis (**Fig. 14.8A**). The biosynthetic gene cluster for both the novobiocin and the coumermycin cluster from streptomycetes have been sequenced and allow prediction of a pathway in which both halves of the novobiocin derive from tyrosine(**Fig. 14.8B**). The right-hand side arises from prenylation of tyrosine and then oxidative decarboxylation. The left-hand side arises from β-OH-tyrosine, which is then oxidized to the β-keto and cyclized to the coumarin. C-methylation and then glycosylation and condensation with the right-hand prenyl benzoate creates the peptide bond in novobiocic acid. This aglycone is glycosylated by TDP-noviose to complete the novobiocin pathway (**Fig. 14.8C**). Chlorobiocin and coumermycin contain pyrrole substituents in place of the O-carbamoyl group on the noviose sugar and those pyrroles arise from proline. Both the β-hydroxylation of tyrosine and the β-oxidation of proline to pyrrole occur on a sequestered pool of amino acid, activated and tethered on a two-domain aminoacyl-peptidyl carrier protein synthetase with homologies to a loading module of nonribosomal peptide synthetases (chapter 13) (**Fig. 14.9**). The β-hydroxylation of the Tyr-S-PCP (NovH) is carried out by the partner heme-protein hydroxylase (NovI) (Chen and Walsh, 2001), then oxidized to the β-keto-Tyr-S-PCP by NovJ and NovK. This may be set up to cyclize to the coumarin and be released from NovH. A comparable pair of open reading frames (19 and 20) in the chloroeremomycin cluster (Fig. 13.10) make the β-OH-Tyr for positions 2 and 6 in the heptapeptide scaffold of the glycopeptide antibiotics (Hubbard and Walsh, 2002). The Pro-S-PCP is oxidized by a flavo-protein desaturase, akin to a fatty acyl-S-ACP desaturase reaction (Thomas et al., 2002). This logic is also used by *Streptomyces coelicolor* to make undecylpro-digiosin (Thomas et al., 2002). This strategy probably obtains as well for chloramphenicol biosynthesis, noted below.

The antibiotic chloramphenicol was isolated from *Streptomyces venezuelae* in 1948 (see Malik, 1972; Vining and Stuttard, 1995) and was widely used for some decades as a broad-spectrum antibacterial agent, active against both gram-negative and gram-positive bacterial infections by blockade of bacterial protein synthesis as an amino acid antimetabolite. Binding occurs in the peptidyltrans-ferase center of the 50S ribosome subunit (chapter 4) There can be serious hematological side effects, including fatal aplastic anemias, that limit its current use. Chloramphenicol (**Fig. 14.10A**) is a simple molecule with a nitrophenylser-inol skeleton in which the amino group has been acylated with a dichloroacetyl group. The backbone clearly comes via the chorismate pathway, via amination, to produce 4-amino-4-deoxychorismate, that on 3,3-sigmatropic rearrangement and dehydrogenative aromatization gives *para*-aminophenylalanine (**Fig. 14.10B**). The conversion of the β-CH$_2$ to the CHOH of aminophenylserine probably also occurs while the amino acid is installed on an A-PCP reductase three-domain subunit (**Fig. 14.10C**). The aminophenylseryl-S-PCP would then be reductively cleaved by the third domain in the protein to release the amino-phenylserinol. This is two steps away from the antibiotic. One is the dichlo-roacetylation, presumed to occur from dichloroacetyl-CoA (Vining and Stuttard, 1995), and the other is the N-oxidation of the *para*-amino to *para*-nitro sub-stituent (**Fig. 14.10D**). Some of the logic and mechanism of nonribosomal pep-

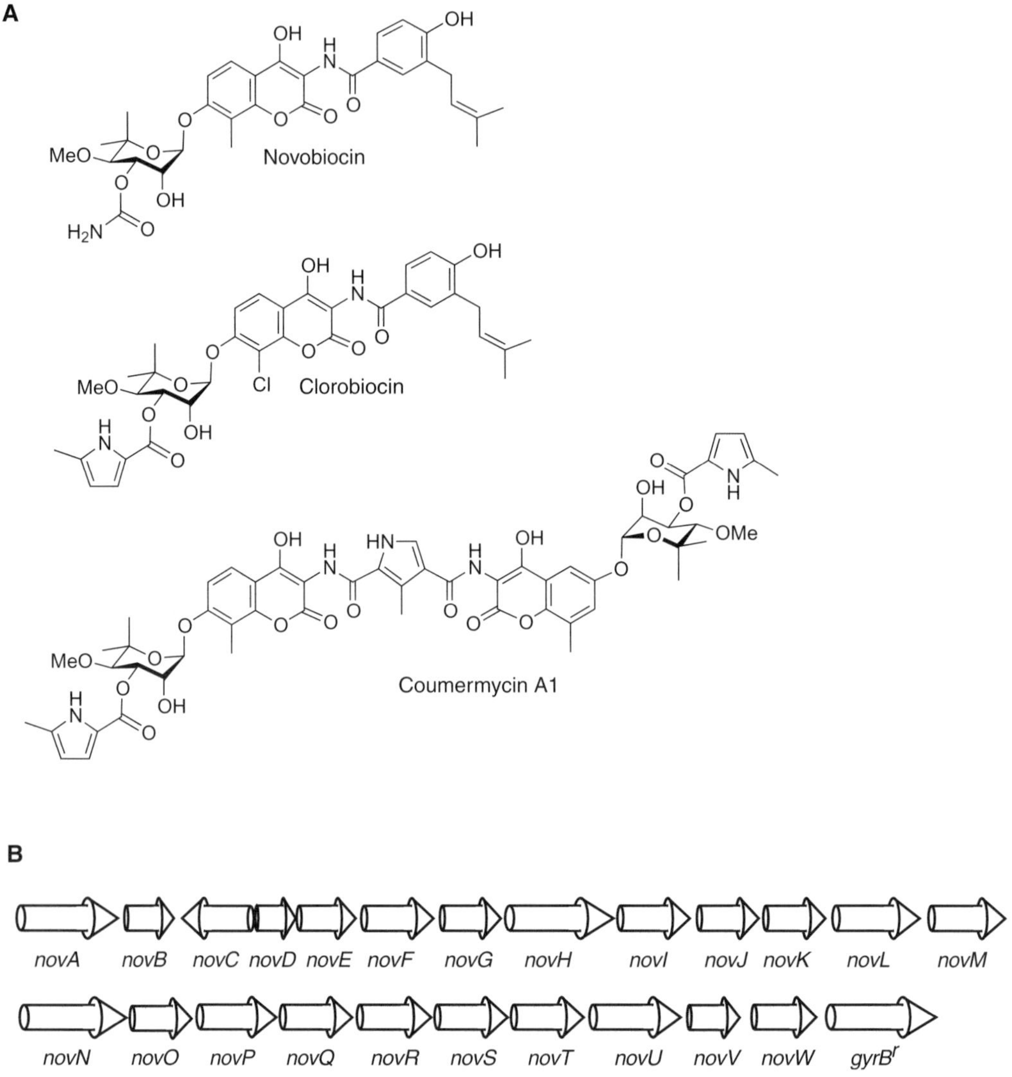

A

Novobiocin

Clorobiocin

Coumermycin A1

B

novA   *novB*   *novC novD novE novF*   *novG*   *novH*   *novI*   *novJ novK*   *novL*   *novM*

novN   *novO*   *novP*   *novQ*   *novR*   *novS*   *novT*   *novU*   *novV novW*   *gyrB^r*

Figure 14.8 Aminocoumarin antibiotics and biosynthetic logic: (A) chlorobiocin, novobiocin, and coumermycin A1 structures; (B) genes for novobiocin pathway; (C) outline of major steps in novobiocin assembly.

tide synthetase selection, activation, and modification of amino acid monomers is utilized in these amino acid-based antibiotics.

Genetics of lantibiotic and microcin B17 biosynthesis

We noted the mechanisms of actions of the class A (e.g., nisin) and class B (e.g., mersacidin) lanthionine-containing antimicrobial peptides, the lantibiotics, in chapter 6. The genes for the ribosomally generated lantibiotic production are clustered (**Fig. 14.11**) and involve the structural gene encoding the precursor

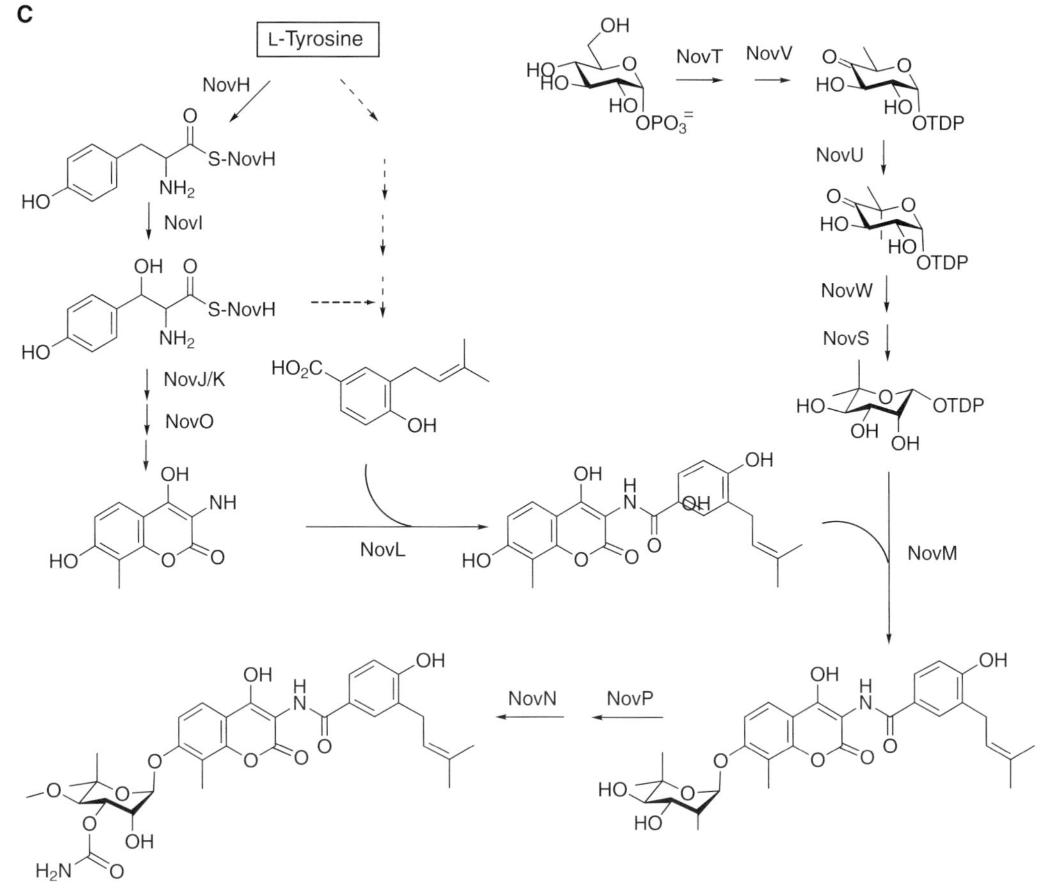

C

Figure 14.8 *Continued.*

peptide, genes for the dehydratases that convert Ser and Thr residues to dehydroalanine and dehydrobutyrine, a leader peptidase gene, and genes for export
pumps for secretion of the mature peptide antibiotic. For example, nisin, an
antimicrobial peptide from *Lactococcus lactis* widely used as a food preservative,
is made from an 11-gene cluster, *nisABTCIPRKFEG*, that spans 14 kbp on a
transposable element and is typical of lantibiotic biosynthetic gene clusters (see
Hansen, 1997, for review). The *nisA* gene encodes a precursor form of the antibiotic peptide: in the case of nisin, this has 57 residues. During enzymatic
maturation, two kinds of modifications occur. First, 13 residues are modified.
Eight β-hydroxy side chains of Ser and Thr residues are dehydrated, probably
by the NisB enzyme, to yield dehydroalanine and dehydrobutyrine residues (**Fig.
14.12A**). Five of these olefinic side chains are captured by five cysteine thiolate
side chains to produce the five thioether linkages, the lanthionine and β-methyl
lanthionine residues (**Fig. 14.12B**), that cross-link the mature nisin and create a
constrained three-dimensional architecture, relevant to the biological activity.
This appears to be the catalytic function of the NisC protein.

At this juncture the second type of modification occurs, proteolytic cleavage
of the N-terminal 23 residues, to yield the 34-residue mature lantibiotic nisin

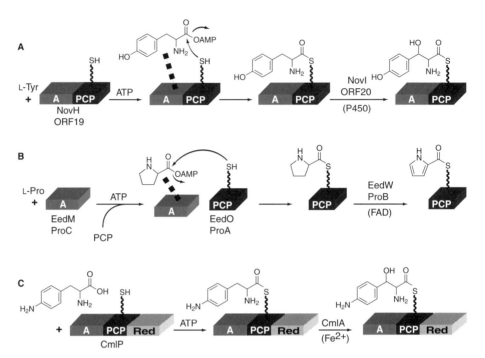

Figure 14.9 β Oxidation of aminoacyl-S-PCPs as a sequestered pool for antibiotic biosynthesis: (A) tyrosine hydroxylation for novobiocin and vancomycin; (B) proline oxidation for coumermycin and undecylprodigiosin; (C) *para*-aminophenylalanine for chloramphenicol.

(**Fig. 14.12C**). The N-terminal 23 residues serve as a propeptide necessary for the dehydration and thioether reactions catalyzed by the NisB and NisC enzymes and may support a fold that allows such recognition. The proteolytic trimming is carried out specifically by the NisP protease encoded in the cluster. Of the other seven genes in the cluster, one, NisI, encodes an immunity function while four (NisT, NisE, NisF, and NisG) are involved in transport or pump functions. NisT is an ATP-hydrolyzing pump of the type discussed in chapter 9 and is thought to be the primary efflux pump for mature nisin and other lantibiotics in related Lan clusters. The NisE, NisF, and NisG proteins are thought to be an additional, fail-safe pump for removing any lantibiotic that makes its way back onto the producing cell and thus constitutes an immunity or self-resistance function. Finally, the *nisR* and *nisK* genes encode two-component regulator (R) and sensor kinase (K) proteins that control transcription of the lantibiotic genes by the two-component pathway logic discussed several times in this book. Analysis of regulation of the related lantibiotic subtilin indicates dual control of biosynthetic gene activation, by a comparable two-component sensor kinase/response regulator and also by derepression of an alternate sigma factor of RNA polymerase that controls transcription of the sensor/response regulator genes (Stein et al., 2002).

Given about two dozen lantibiotic gene clusters currently known, leader peptides and two kinds of side chain modifications, dehydration of β-OH side chains and then capture to make thioether cross-links, the prospects for hybrid peptide engineering is high. It is not yet clear how much the persisting dehy-

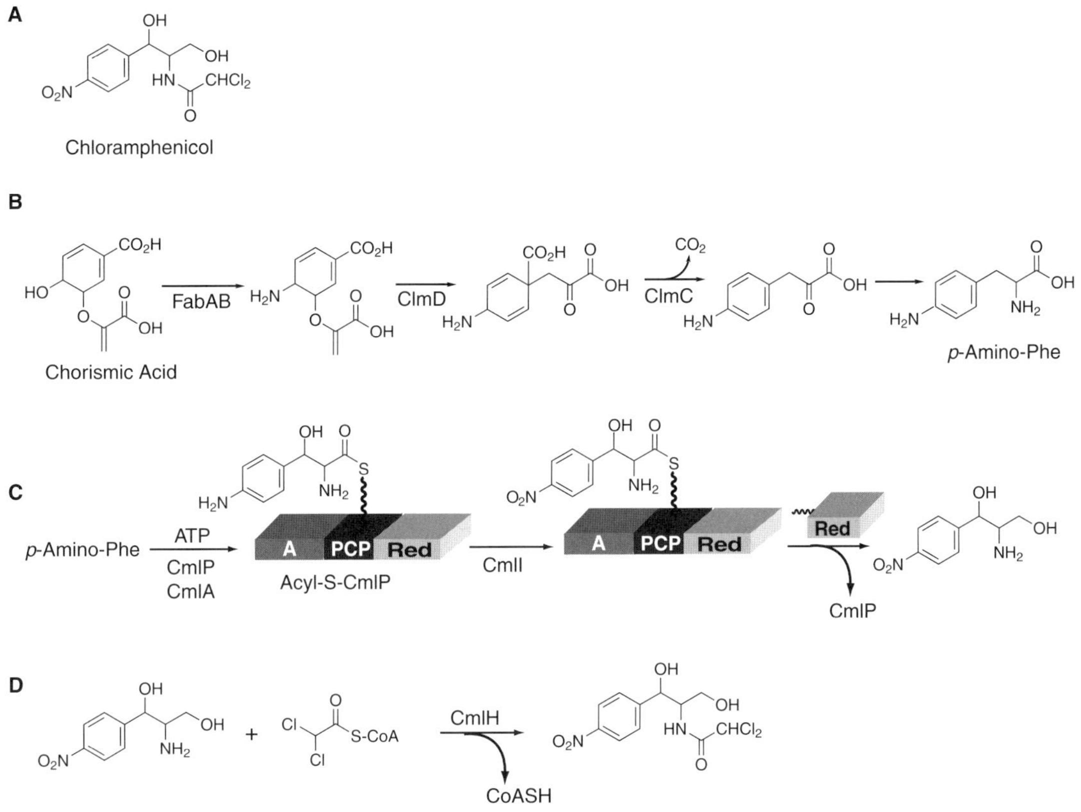

A

Chloramphenicol

B

Chorismic Acid → FabAB → ClmD → ClmC → → *p*-Amino-Phe

C

p-Amino-Phe → ATP / CmlP / CmlA → Acyl-S-CmlP → CmlI → Red / CmlP

D

+ → CmlH / CoASH →

Figure 14.10 Biosynthetic strategy for chloramphenicol: (A) structure of chloramphenicol; (B) chorismate to *p*-aminophenylalanine; (C) β-hydroxylation and carboxyl reduction; (D) dichloroacetylation and N-oxidation.

droalanine and dehydrobutyrine residues (three in nisin), by their rigidifying effects on peptide bonds, set local conformations that contribute to the antibiotic activity. For the class B lantibiotics, which are not primarily membrane pore formers but have specific targets such as lipid II in peptidoglycan biosynthesis, engineering and combinatorial approaches to libraries may optimize activity. Recent structure/function studies suggest the type A and B lantibiotics have different selectivities in interaction with lipid I and lipid II, perhaps indicating distinct recognition of the second GlcNAc residue in lipid II, and suggesting

Figure 14.11 Nisin biosynthetic gene cluster.

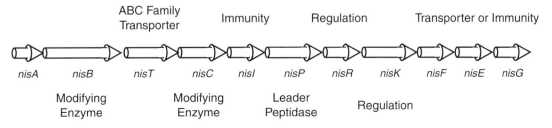

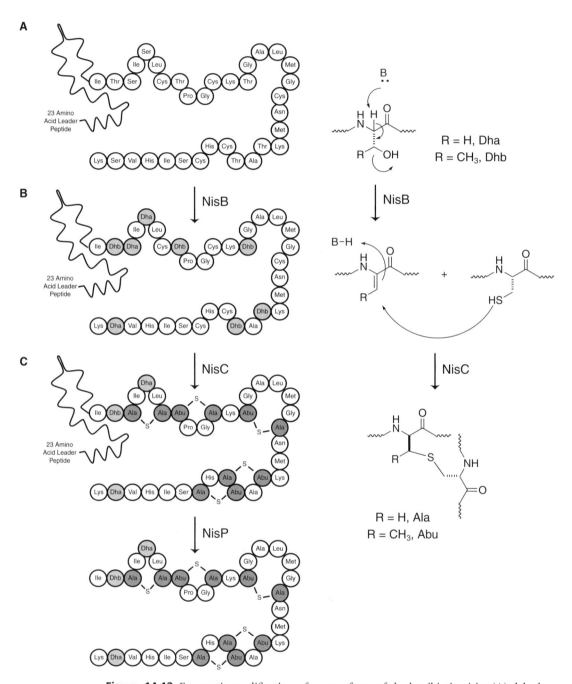

Figure 14.12 Enzymatic modification of prepro form of the lantibiotic nisin: (A) dehydration of Ser and Thr side chains by NisB; (B) thioether formation by attack of Cys side chains catalyzed by NisC; (C) proteolytic cleavage of the N-terminal 23-residue leader sequence by NisP.

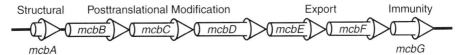

Figure 14.13 Genes for microcin B17 production and enzymatic maturation to the active antibiotic.

Figure 14.14 Enzymatic maturation of prepro microcin B17: (A) thiazole and oxazole ring formation catalyzed by McbB McbC, and McbD; (B) proteolytic removal of the N-terminal 26-residue propeptide.

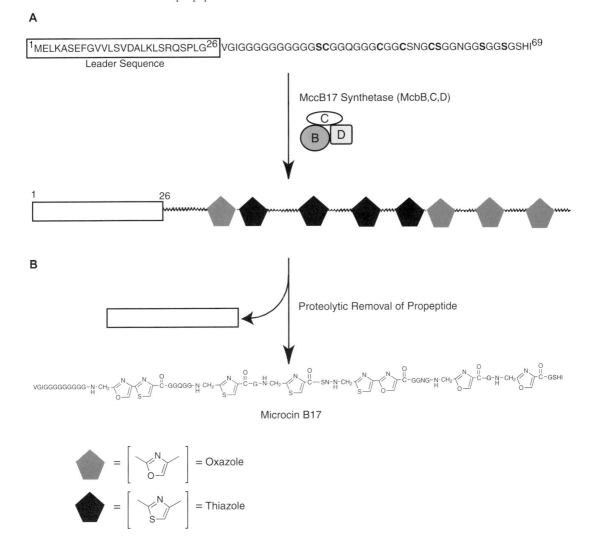

these do not act as nonspecific amphiphilic cationic peptides (Brotz and Sahl, 2000).

A second variant of ribosomal peptide antibiotic maturation with analogous logic to the lantibiotic maturations is found in the operon for the *Escherichia coli* antibiotic microcin B17 (**Fig. 14.13**), a DNA gyrase inhibitor (chapter 15) (see Sinha Roy et al., 1999, for review). Like lantibiotics, microcin B17 is produced from a ribosomally encoded small protein precursor, the 69-residue McbA protein, and enzymatically modified on serine and cysteine side chains, in this case four of each, by the McbB, McbC, and McbD proteins.

The chemical result is not thioether cross-links but instead heterocyclization of Ser to oxazoles and Cys to thiazole rings (**Fig. 14.14A**). These five-membered rings, arising from cyclodehydration enzymology on Gly-Ser, Gly-Cys, or Ser-Cys, Cys-Ser dipeptide moieties in McbA, rigidify the peptide backbone and protect microcin B17 from proteolysis. In particular, the tandem bis heterocycles, generated from adjacent Ser-Cys and Cys-Ser residues, are probably the key determinants for interaction with DNA-DNA gyrase to cleave double-stranded DNA (Heddle et al., 2001).

An additional analogy to lantibiotic maturation is the proteolytic cleavage of the first 26 residues of microcin after the enzymatic heterocycles have been introduced, to remove the propeptide (**Fig. 14.14B**). Again the propeptide is essential for any of the processing by McbB, McbC, and McbD to occur. The mature microcin B17 antibiotic, with 14 of 43 residues modified into the eight heterocycles, is then secreted by the McbE and McbF export pump machinery, in a clear analogy to the NisEFG export protein machinery. The seventh gene in the Mcb operon, *mcbG*, encodes an as yet undetermined immunity function that protects the producer *E. coli* from interdicting its own DNA gyrase.

New Strategies for Finding Novel Antibiotics and Extending Their Lifetimes

S EVERAL STRATEGIES ARE REQUIRED TO come up with new antibiotics, including novel structural and functional classes to deal with the multidrug-resistant bacterial pathogenic populations and to maximize and extend the useful lifetimes of effective antibiotics in human therapeutics. The three chapters of this final section take up several contemporary questions. Where do new antibiotics come from? Can we accelerate the discovery process? Can we slow down emergence of multidrug-resistant clinically pathogenic strains of pathogenic bacteria? The wealth of recent genetic information has provided a clear opportunity to identify and validate new antibacterial targets and screen in high-throughput modes—in vitro, in cell-based assays, and in animals—for genes that are essential to growth or vital to virulence. Some of these approaches are analyzed in chapter 15.

It is clear there is a pressing need for new molecules. One index is to look at the time of introduction of new classes of antibacterial agents since the introduction of the sulfa drugs in 1936. There has been only one new major class introduced in the past 40 years, the synthetic oxazolidinones, in 2000. Several approaches to discovery of new molecules are discussed in chapter 16. Finally, there is the integration of concerns about individual resistance and the public health approach to global problems on the spread of infectious disease and reservoirs of resistance. This highlights the need for a different approach to protect the antibiotic arsenal and to maximize the health of populations against bacterial diseases, taken up in the concluding chapter.

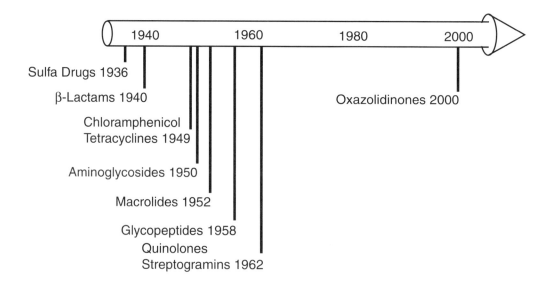

Time line for introduction of new classes of antibiotics into clinical practice.

chapter 15

New Looks at Targets

Defining new targets from bacterial genomics

The goal in contemporary antibacterial target selections to maximize the chance that new drugs can be found and developed begins with bioinformatics to look for open reading frames (ORFs) conserved across the potential bacterial target organisms, from every bacterium in the most general case to all gram-positive or all gram-negative organisms as smaller categories that may still be worth attacking. A second desirable bioinformatics criterion is that the ORF be selectively found in prokaryotes and not eukaryotes, especially higher eukaryotes. The third criterion generally agreed on is an experimental test that the ORF is essential in one or more relevant pathogens by some functional knockout or ablation approach. The genes that pass these filters are the best candidates for going to high-throughput screens to generate initial hits. The screens may involve assay of enzymatic activity if one has been established or ligand binding, e.g., fluorescence change or protection against thermal or chaotrope-induced denaturation. Since compounds in libraries are unoptimized, only modest affinities are expected in initial screens, so concentrations are set for some threshold detection of inhibition or binding, e.g., 10 μM. Positive hits are rescreened, often resynthesized, and tested in secondary assays if available, then serve as starting points for directed chemistry, either small focused library efforts or single-molecule elaborations to increase potency into the nanomolar range.

The complete genomic sequences of most if not all of the major bacterial pathogens reported over the past half-dozen years have turned the infectious disease target area completely around. From a field of research and inquiry that was effectively target poor for the past three decades (peptidoglycan [PG] blockade, ribosome inhibition, DNA gyrase), there is now at least a temporary embarrassment of target riches, with dozens to hundreds of gene products that are candidates as novel targets.

Bioinformatic analysis of the more than three dozen known microbial genomes (as of June 2001, 41 microbial genomes were listed in the The Institute for Genomic Research's microbial database) looks for targets known in one or more organisms to be essential for survival, highly conserved across a broad range of bacterial pathogens, and either absent or distinct in humans (see Rosamond and Allsop, 2000, for review). One limitation to identifying conserved genes of unknown function has been the failure of annotation of putative function by homology, but computational method improvements will continue to drive the unknown genes down to a very small fraction that can be experimentally tested. Even in the absence of a well-described function, various genetic approaches, such as temperature-sensitive mutations or signature-tagged mutagenesis, to name just two (Hensel et al., 1995), can establish the essentiality of a protein and validate it for screening. Rosamond and Allsop (2000) noted an example (**Fig. 15.1**) where the 4,289 genes of *Escherichia coli* were compared against the genomes of seven respiratory disease-causing pathogens (including *Pseudomonas aeruginosa, Haemophilus influenzae,* and *Streptococcus pneumoniae*) to yield 246 genes conserved across all these bacteria, of which 68 genes were absent from humans. Half of these genes (34/68) were of unknown function at the time of the analysis; 16 turned out to be nonessential and 18 were essential, including known targets for quinolones and macrolide antibiotics. In the given example, 3 of these 18 genes were selected as targets for screening to look for new respiratory tract antibacterial drugs.

The identification of 150 genes essential for viability in the important pathogen *Staphylococcus aureus* has been undertaken systematically by expression of antisense RNA to ablate gene function (Ji et al., 2001). The antisense RNA was expressed under control of tetracycline-driven promoters; the presence or absence of tetracycline allowed expression of the conditional phenotype, allowing recovery of the clones that died in the presence of antisense RNA. About 30% of the staphylococcal genes that turned up as critical were of unknown function,

Figure 15.1 Example of a genomics-based approach to new targets for antibacterial drugs in respiratory tract infections. (From Rosamond and Allsop [2000], with permission.)

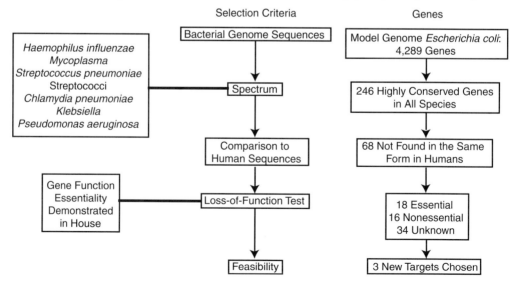

30% were homologs of genes with proposed function, and the remaining 40% were orthologs of bacterial genes known to be essential.

Within *E. coli* strains themselves there will be substantial variation in genes that can contribute to pathogenesis. In *E. coli* O157:H7, 1,387 of the 3,574 genes (Perna et al., 2001) differ from those of the previously sequenced *E. coli* strain MG1655, distributed in hundreds of gene islands where DNA has been shuffled in by horizontal gene transfers, emphasizing recombinational evolution in enterobacterial genomes. More genome sequence data from *E. coli* strains and functional characterization of the several ORFs that encode putative virulence factors (toxins, adhesins, enzymes, type III secretion systems, etc.) will be required to sort out preferred targets in the highly pathogenic strains.

The genomic sequences of methicillin-resistant *S. aureus* (MRSA) strain N315 and vancomycin-resistant *S. aureus* (VRSA) strain Mu50 from clinical isolates in Japan (Kuroda et al., 2001) (see chapter 7) allow a broad view of potential antibiotic targets and reveal up to 70 candidates (out of 2,600 total genes) for new or additional virulence factors that may enable resistant *S. aureus* strains to be such effective human pathogens. For example, two putative PG monofunctional transglycosylases (*sgtA* and *sgtB*) may be targets for assays of new inhibitors (see chapter 16), along with an operon likely to allow *S. aureus* to grow at 3.5 M salt, a molecular correlate of food poisoning by these bacteria. Two large extracellular matrix binding proteins of 722 kDa and 421 kDa may mediate *S. aureus* attachment to the matrix of heart valves in endocarditis. A large set of exotoxin and enterotoxin genes are harbored within pathogenicity islands in the *S. aureus* chromosome, which can now be evaluated for superantigen function in toxic shock syndromes, Kawasaki's disease, and various inflammatory responses caused by these pathogens.

Analogously, the genomic sequence of a virulent strain of *S. pneumoniae* has led to suggestion of novel targets, including surface proteins, both lipoproteins and those anchored via sortase action, that could be candidates for vaccine development (Tettelin et al., 2001). The sortase enzyme in gram-positive bacteria that covalently anchors outer membrane or surface proteins to PG at LPXTG primary sequence motifs will be discussed later in this chapter, but a recent genomics-driven approach to identify such proteins as virulence candidates was conducted in group A streptococci (Reid et al., 2001) and turned up 12 genes encoding such LPXTG motifs. Half of the genes were upregulated in stationary phase and 9 of 12 regulated by virulence gene transcription factors. Finally, on expression of the 12 proteins and immunologic analysis with sera from individuals who had previously had group A streptococcal infections, 10 of the 12 proteins reacted, indicating expression as antigens during the course of infection in humans. These would be candidates for vaccine development and/or antimicrobial targets.

In addition to iterations of computational approaches to connect unknown essential microbial genes to proteins of known function, high-throughput structural genomic efforts (Erlandsen et al., 2000; Mittl and Grutter, 2001) are under way to solve the X-ray structures of hundreds to thousands of proteins and categorize them according to observed architecture and fold rather than just primary sequence and predictions of tertiary structure. In the absence of predicted functions to measure, there are high-throughput assays that do not require a known activity or a known ligand whose binding can be inhibited by potential hits and leads. Rather, one can use fluorescent ligands or thermal cycling or denaturation protection to find tight-binding inhibitors in compound libraries for proteins of unknown function. Candidate ligands can then be tested in whole-cell screening to see if there is a bacteriostatic or bactericidal effect. A sufficiently potent compound can then be used to dissect mechanism (e.g., cell wall, protein, or DNA synthesis inhibition and then zeroing in on specific steps in those pathways). A third approach to identify potential targets is to use bacterial genome microarray chips, or gene expression profiling (see McDevitt and Rosenberg, 2001; Perego and Hoch, 2001), to evaluate the levels of the most abundant mRNAs under various conditions, e.g., exposure to antibiotics of different classes, or a new antibiotic, to catalog the most-affected genes. For example, the effects of addition of the antitubercular drug on *Mycobacterium tuberculosis* gene expression have been assessed (Wilson et al., 1999) on DNA chips covering 97% of the tuberculosis genome and elevations in fatty acid synthase enzymes and trehalose dimycolyltransferase (see Fig. 15.20 and 15.4, respectively) noted.

Figure 15.2 depicts a typical three-stage process for genomics-based approaches to antimicrobial drugs, involving target selection, lead identification, and lead optimization (Rosamond and Allsop, 2000).

Complementary to genetic approaches to defining essential genes are assays for genes required for bacterial pathogens to establish infections in vertebrates. Thus, there are sets of genes dispensable in bacteria growing in petri plates that become essential for them to persist in animal and human infections. One approach to determining genes selectively expressed in vivo and required for bacterial virulence is in vivo expression technology (Mahan et al., 1993; Mahan et al., 1995), which enriches for bacteria that switch on particular genes that enable them to survive and multiply during infections in animals (see Chopra et al., 1997). For example, these include genes that turn on the biosynthesis and directed reuptake of bacterial iron chelators since vertebrate hosts have all the available iron tied up intracellularly or bound to transferrin in extracellular spaces. It remains to be seen if antibiotics that target virulence genes will be

Figure 15.2 Genomics approaches to antimicrobial drugs. (From Rosamond and Allsop [2000], with permission.)

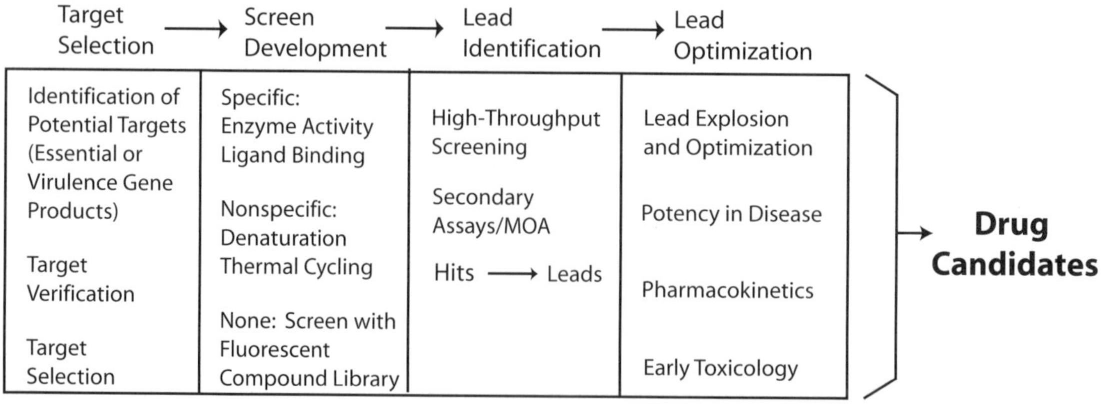

Target Selection →	Screen Development →	Lead Identification →	Lead Optimization	
Identification of Potential Targets (Essential or Virulence Gene Products)	Specific: Enzyme Activity Ligand Binding	High-Throughput Screening	Lead Explosion and Optimization	
	Nonspecific: Denaturation Thermal Cycling	Secondary Assays/MOA	Potency in Disease	**Drug Candidates**
Target Verification		Hits → Leads	Pharmacokinetics	
Target Selection	None: Screen with Fluorescent Compound Library		Early Toxicology	

effective in the clinic and whether there will be reduced frequency of resistance development.

The use of tetracycline promoters to generate conditional phenotypes for antisense RNA inhibition of essential genes to turn up 150 genes in *S. aureus* (Ji et al., 2001) has recently been reported. Bacterial strains have been engineered to regulate the expression levels of target genes (see Trias and Yuan, 1999) to increase the sensitivity of the expressed proteins to candidate inhibitors. DeVito et al. (2002) have reported on arrays of target-specific screening strains engineered to maximize sensitivity of target proteins such as DNA helicases, enoyl-acyl carrier protein (ACP) reductase, DNA gyrase, dihydrofolate reductase, and the MurA gene product (chapter 3) for parallel screening.

New looks at some old targets

While new targets are being turned up by genomics-driven investigations, increases in molecular knowledge about microbial structures and molecular machinery continue to offer new avenues for development of antibacterials with a different focus on aspects of complex targets and improved assays to enhance specificity and throughput.

First we note some prospects in the traditional validated target areas of cell wall biosynthesis, protein biosynthesis, and DNA replication and repair and then point out some less traditional targets that command new attention. Poole (2001), McDevitt and Rosenberg (2001), and Chopra et al. (1997) have reviewed some of these strategies.

Cell wall biosynthesis inhibitors

In the area of the cell wall and cell membrane there are several developments worth investigation.

Staphylococcal sortase and mycobacterial A85

In the biogenesis of the PG layer of the pathogenic staphylococci, the interpeptide cross bridge is not direct between Lys_3 on one chain and $D-Ala_4$ on an adjacent peptide chain, but involves a pentaglycine bridge (**Fig. 15.3A**). These glycines are put in by the *fem* genes, which are auxiliary targets in MRSA (Berger-Bachi and Tschierske, 1998), although no specific inhibitors have been found yet. The main surface antigenic proteins, protein M of *S. pyogenes*, a causative agent of pharyngitis and skin lesions, and protein A of *S. aureus*, are covalently linked to the pentaglycyl bridge through a conserved C-terminal tetrapeptide — LPET moiety (Navarre and Schneewind, 1999). The sequence of the genome of MRSA strain N315 (Kuroda et al., 2001) reveals many new surface proteins that are sortase substrates and likely to have adhesion functions, binding to extracelllular matrix proteins in host tissues and enabling *S. aureus* to cause osteomyelitis and septic arthritis. Blockade of the covalent attachment enzyme, called sortase, may be a promising strategy to reduce virulence in streptococcal infections. The sortase enzyme, whose structure has now been determined and may thereby enable structure-based drug design (Ilangovan et al., 2001), is a trans-

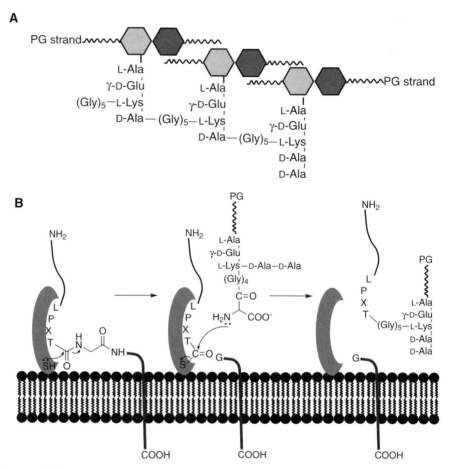

Figure 15.3 Action of sortase to covalently tether outer membrane proteins to the penta-glycine extenders on *S. aureus* peptidoglycan strands: (A) the pentaglycine-containing PG strands; (B) cleavage of LPXTG sequence in precursor protein substrates and transpeptidation by sortase. (From Mazmanian et al. [2001], with permission.)

peptidase, acting in the periplasmic space with specificity for the precursors of cell-surface proteins of gram-positive bacteria that have an LPXTG sequence about 30 to 40 residues from the C terminus of the protein (Mazmanian et al., 1999). The sortase cleaves the precursor (**Fig. 15.3B**) at the T-G peptide bond, releasing the C-terminal fragment and generating a covalent acyl enzyme. This acyl-LPXT intermediate is captured by the amino group of the Gly$_5$ chain of a PG strand, freeing up the enzyme for another catalytic transpeptidase cycle and covalently tethering the protein chain to the PG strand through the pentaglycine bridge. Given that sortase uses the same kind of reaction logic as the penicillin-sensitive transpeptidases, it should be possible to come up with potent and specific inhibitors of this active-site cysteine hydrolase (Ton-That et al., 1999). Bioinformatics analysis (Pallen et al., 2001) has revealed widespread distribution of putative sortases and sortase protein substrates in gram-positive bacteria and multiple sortases within such genomes. The *Streptomyces coelicolor* genome is predicted to have seven sortases, suggesting either partially overlapping cell-surface transpeptidase anchoring of proteins or other functions.

In analogous molecular logic, an acyltransferase in *M. tuberculosis* cell wall biosynthesis of trehalose dimycolate (**Fig. 15.4A**) may be a promising new target for antituberculosis therapy. A complex of three related 30- to 32-kDa mycolyltransferases (Ag85A, B, and C) (Puech et al., 2000) forms a major protein component of the waxy mycobacterial cell wall. They appear to serve as fibronectin binding proteins to assist mycobacteria to enter macrophages. They also transfer the long-chain α-alkyl, β-hydroxy fatty acyl (the mycolyl) chains to the 6-OH of the disaccharide trehalose to produce dimycolyl trehalose, via monomycosyl trehalose intermediates, at the outer surface of the cell walls (**Fig. 15.4B**) (Sathyamoorthy and Takayama, 1987). Blockade of this enzymatic activity might remove the major permeability barrier toward a number of antibiotics. The X-ray structure of Ag85C reveals it is a member of the active-site serine α,β-hydrolase superfamily. This predicts mycolyl-*O*-Ser acyl enzyme intermediates, like the cell wall transpeptidases and the sortase noted above, whose formation and breakdown could be targeted mechanistically. Strategies to screen for blockers of Ag85-fibronectin interactions may also be indicated.

Mycobacteria have arabinogalactan bridges that connect the PG layer with the mycolic acids (Besra et al., 1995), in which the galactose is in the five-ring furanose (Gal$_f$) rather than the common six-ring pyranose form. The connection between the arabinogalactan chains and the PG layer is provided by a 1,3-L-rhamnosyl-GlcNAc disaccharide, and the enzymes that convert dTDP-D-glucose to dTDP-L-rhamnose may be antibacterial targets in *M. tuberculosis* (Ma et al., 2002). The biosynthetic enzyme UDP-galactopyranose mutase is essential for cell

Figure 15.4 Action of the *M. tuberculosis* mycolyltransferase Ag85: (A) trehalose dimycolate; (B) the mycolyl transfer reaction.

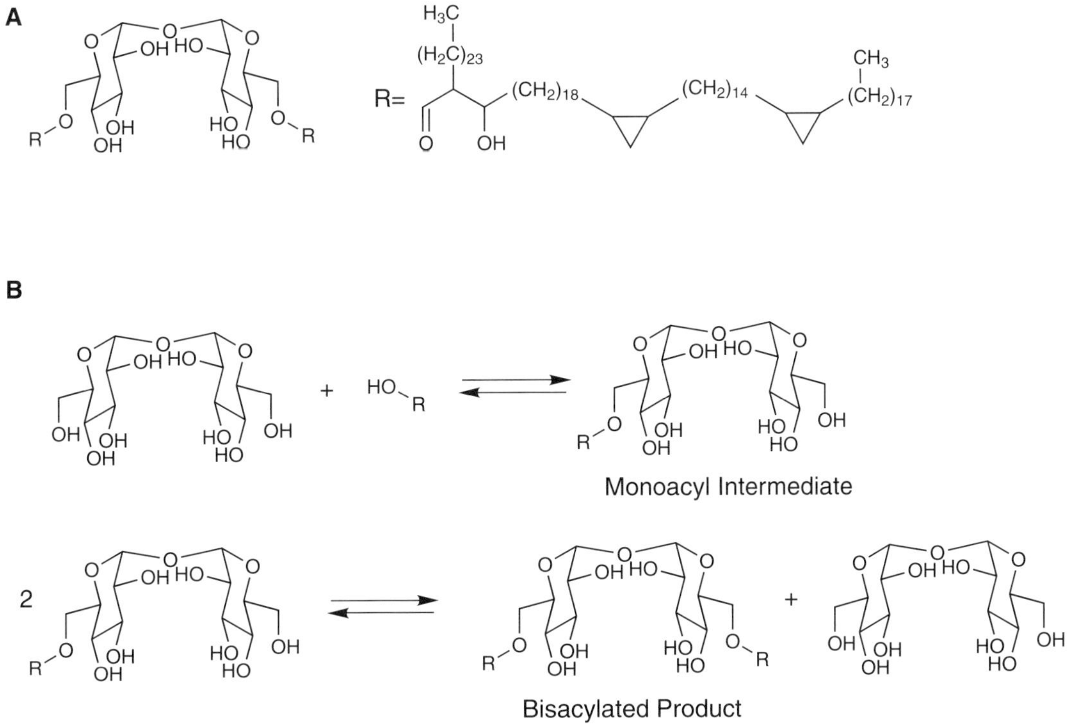

viability in *M. smegmatis*. Gal$_f$ is also found in O-antigens of lipospolysaccharide outer membrane chains of gram-negative bacteria. The X-ray structure of the mutase from *E. coli* has been solved (Sanders et al., 2001), providing insight into mechanism of this flavoprotein catalyst and setting the stage for inhibitor screening and design.

GlmU: a bifunctional enzyme generating UDP-GlcNAc

In chapter 3 we noted that fosfomycin inhibits the first enzyme in the PG biosynthetic pathway, MurA, which catalyzes the enolpyruvylation of the sugar nucleotide UDP-GlcNAc. UDP-GlcNAc is produced in a two-step sequence (GlmU) from glucosamine-1-P, in turn generated from the primary metabolite fructose-6-P (by amination from cosubstrate glutamine [GlmS] and then conversion of glucosamine-6-P to glucosamine-1-P by the GlmM mutase) (see van Heijenoort, 2001b, for review). The enzyme GlmU is bifunctional in many bacteria, with two independent domains, catalyzing first the N-acetylation, via acetyl-CoA, and then transfer of the UMP moiety of UTP onto the 1-phosphate to produce UDP-GlcNAc (Gehring et al., 1996). Because UDP-GlcNAc is a key metabolite, *glmU* is an essential gene, and in gram-negative bacteria UDP-GlcNAc is a branch point metabolite, serving as precursor for both PG biosynthesis and outer membrane components: lipid A and O-antigen chains. To date no potent specific inhibitors of either the acetyltransferase domain activity or the uridylyl transfer domain activity of GlmU have been reported. The crystal structure of the *S. pneumoniae* GlmU trimer has been reported (Kostrewa et al., 2001), allowing structure/function as well as screening approaches.

Transglycosylases

While it has been known for years that transglycosylases were crucial components of late-stage polymerization of disaccharyl pentapeptide units into existing PG strands, they have been understudied as a class due to unavailability of substrates for assay and their membrane-associated nature, which has made purification and characterization difficult (see van Heijenoort, 2001a, for review). Genome sequencing has now indicated four transglycosylases in *E. coli* and comparable numbers in primary pathogens, some as bifunctional transglycosylases/transpeptidases and some as monofunctional transglycosylases. Some recent reports are worth note, highlighting two areas of development.

First, the combined chemoenzymatic approaches of S. Walker and colleagues, using lipid I analogs (chapter 3) and the MurG glycosyltransferase, have allowed access to a variety of lipid-disaccharyl-pentapeptide lipid II analogs (**Fig. 15.5**) that could be used to assay membrane-associated transglycosylases (Ye et al., 2001). In particular, a C$_{35}$ lipid chain with 4-*cis*-olefinic links was active, was less prone to aggregation than the natural C$_{55}$ isoprenoid chain, and suggested that a useful assay protocol could be established to test for substrates and inhibitors. Additional syntheses of lipid II analogs (Cudic and Otvos, 2002) and lipid II itself (VanNieuwenhze et al., 2002) along with design of improved assays (Schwartz et al., 2001) promise to move the field. The second facet is that the natural product moenomycin (chapter 3) inhibits transglycosylases, and displacement assays could be readily established for screening (Vollmer and Holtje, 2000). We noted in chapter 13 that teicoplanin is a natural lipoglycopeptide,

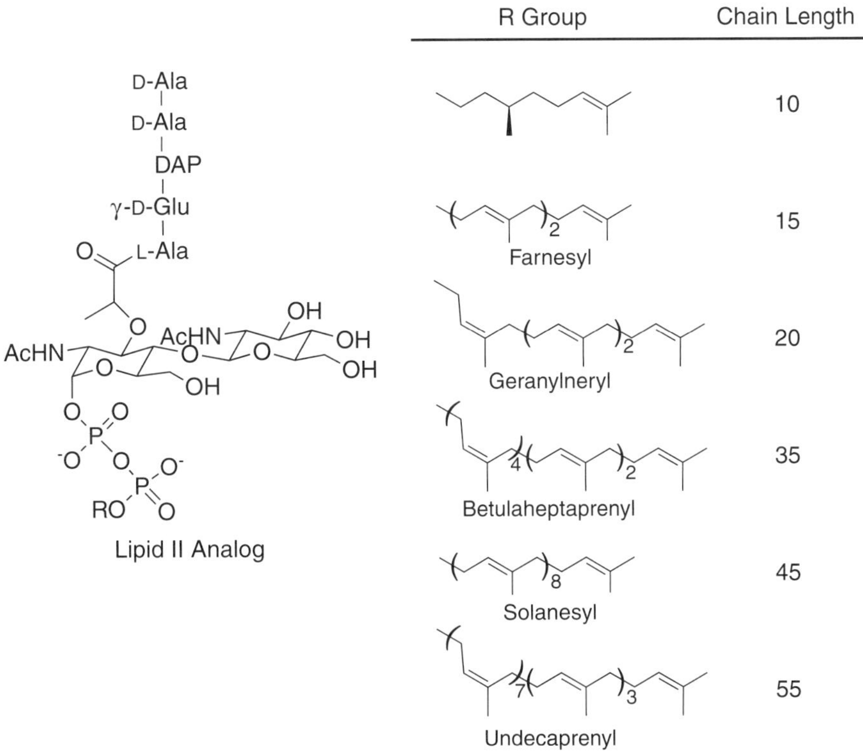

R Group	Chain Length
	10
Farnesyl	15
Geranylneryl	20
Betulaheptaprenyl	35
Solanesyl	45
Undecaprenyl	55

Lipid II Analog

Figure 15.5 Defined lipid II substrate analogs for membrane transglycosylase assay.

acylated on the glucosamine amino group at the top of the glycopeptide dome (Fig. 13.26). Semisynthetic *N*-aryl derivatives, such as the chlorobiphenyl vancomycins and chloroeremomycins (**Fig. 15.6A**), are about 80-fold more active against vancomycin-resistant enterococci (VRE) than the parent glycopeptides. Since these *N*-aryl glycopeptides do not bind *N*-acyl-D-Ala-D-Lac any more tightly than vancomycin or chloroeremomycin, it has been hypothesized that they seek out a second target (Ge et al., 1999; Sun et al., 2001). Indeed, destruction of the *N*-acyl-D-Ala-D-Ala/D-Ala-D-Lac binding site by removal of *N*-MeLeu$_1$ (**Fig. 15.6B**) maintains activity against VRE. Kahne and coworkers have suggested the transglycosylases could be the additional target (Ge et al., 1999), a hypothesis that would open new avenues to VRE reversal. A gene responsible for the susceptibility of *E. coli* cells to glycolipid derivatives of vancomycin but not vancomycin itself has recently been reported (Eggert et al., 2001), validating a molecular basis for distinction. Also, hydrophobic *N*-aryl derivatives of vancomycin that are active against VRE and that inhibit transglycosylase activity in vitro (Sinha Roy et al., 2001) have been used in affinity chromatography to isolate a subset of *E. coli* membrane proteins, including penicillin-binding protein 1B (PBP1B), PBP2, PBP3, PBP5, and PBP6, consistent with transglycosylases as targets.

The ability to produce large carbohydrate libraries by synthesis (Baizman et al., 2000) may lead to ligands with specificity and potency for transglycosylase inhibition. The structure of the lytic transglycosylase from *E. coli*, SLT$_{35}$, which

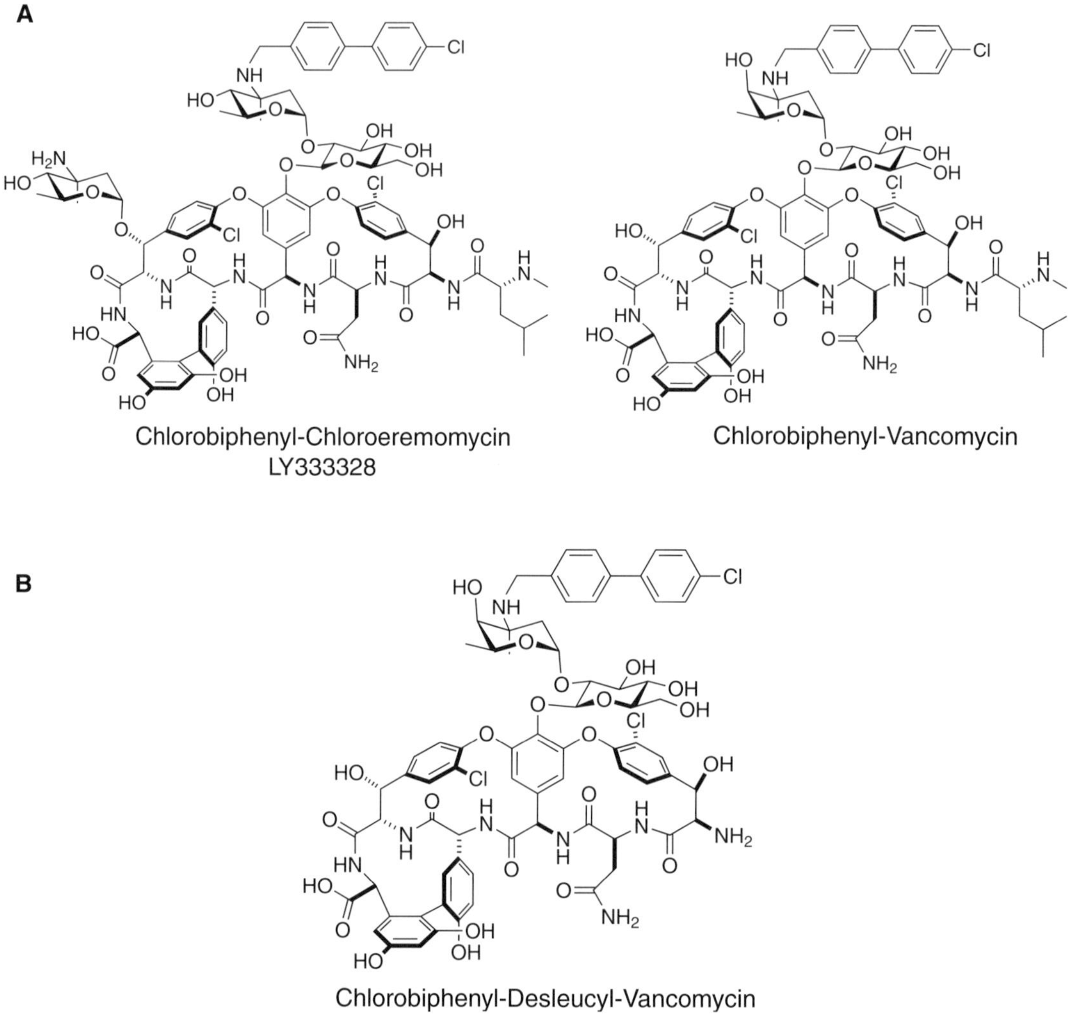

A

Chlorobiphenyl-Chloroeremomycin
LY333328

Chlorobiphenyl-Vancomycin

B

Chlorobiphenyl-Desleucyl-Vancomycin

Figure 15.6 Chlorobiphenyl analogs of chloroeremomycin and vancomycin active against VRE: (A) specific compounds; (B) aryl glycopeptides active against VRE with the D-Ala-D-Ala binding site destroyed.

participates in release of anhydromuramyl peptides by intramolecular attack of the C_6-CH_2OH on the C_1 glycoside link during β-lactamase-induced signaling (van Asselt et al., 2000), has been solved and may be a prototype for design and evaluation of glycosylase inhibitors.

Protein biosynthesis inhibitors

In the second classical target area for antibacterial drugs, protein synthesis inhibition, there are also several opportunities for further investigation of new antibiotic targets.

Antibiotics targeted against the ribosome

The X-ray structures of the 30S and 50S ribosomal subunits and the full 70S complexes (chapter 4) are sure to aid in assay development and evaluation of new antibiotics that bind both at the classical sites and nonclassical sites in either the 16S or 23S rRNA molecules, which together make up two-thirds of the mass of the ribosome.

The region of domain V of the 23S rRNA includes the peptidyltransferase center from the peptidyltransferase site to the beginning of the exit tunnel for the nascent polypeptide chain (Ban et al., 2000; Nissen et al., 2000) and encompasses the binding site for both the 14-membered macrolide erythromycin and the 16-membered ring macrolide tylosin (Douthwaite et al., 2000; Poulsen et al., 2000). It also overlaps partially with other antibiotics such as the streptogramins and lincosamides, e.g., clindamycin. Structure-based design of novel antibiotics that fill one or more of these RNA subsites should be a productive enterprise. The peptide exit channel is about 100 Å long (see Nissen et al., 2000), lined mostly with RNA from domains I to V of the 23S rRNA but also with some contacts from proteins L4, L22, and L39. Whether inhibitors can be found that fill the tunnel is unclear, but it is worth noting that the nonsteroidal anti-inflammatory drug flurbiprofen blocks a tunnel into the active site of the prostaglandin cyclooxygenases (Selinsky et al., 2001).

The macrolide carbomycin apparently binds slightly differently than erythromycin since, unlike erythromycin, it inhibits the actual peptidyltransferase reaction in aminoacyl transfer assays to puromycin (Poulsen et al., 2001). The extended sugar chain on the C_5-OH of the carbomycin macrolide scaffold reaches back towards the peptidyl transferase RNA center (Hansen et al., 2002). Two antibiotics used in veterinary medicine, tiamulin and valnemulin, semisynthetic derivatives of the natural product pleuromutilin (**Fig. 15.7**), may be starting points for defining these targets further. Tiamulin and valnemulin show footprints that affect the nucleotides in domain V of 23S rRNA that have been implicated as part of the dynamically mobile peptidyltransferase center (Poulsen et al., 2001), and they completely block peptide bond formation. These compete with carbomycin but not erythromycin, suggesting that both the pleuromutilins and erythromycin can bind at the same time in adjacent, but non-overlapping, regions. The pleuromutilins may overlap with pristinamycin IIA binding (Poulsen et al., 2001), suggesting there will be fruitful analysis in fine-structure mapping of antibiotics in and around the peptidyltransferase center of the 50S subunit, with design of new composite antibiotic structures likely.

One example for the existence of nonclassical ribosome sites for antibiotic binding is provided by recent studies on the natural product everninomycin (**Fig. 15.8**), a member of the oligosaccharide orthosomycins (Belova et al., 2001).

Figure 15.7 Structures of pleuromutilin family members that block the peptidyltransferase center on the ribosome.

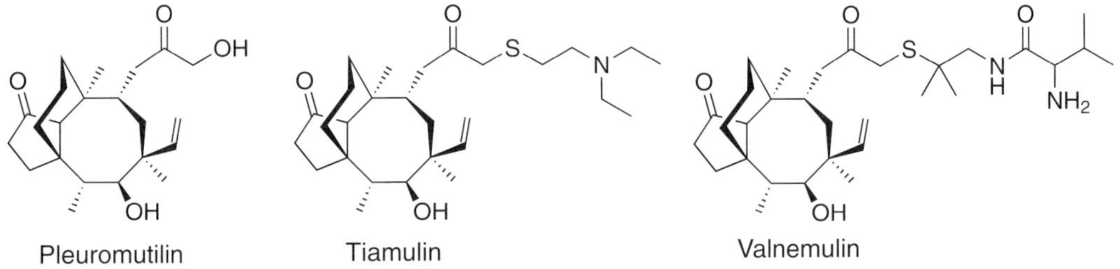

Pleuromutilin   Tiamulin   Valnemulin

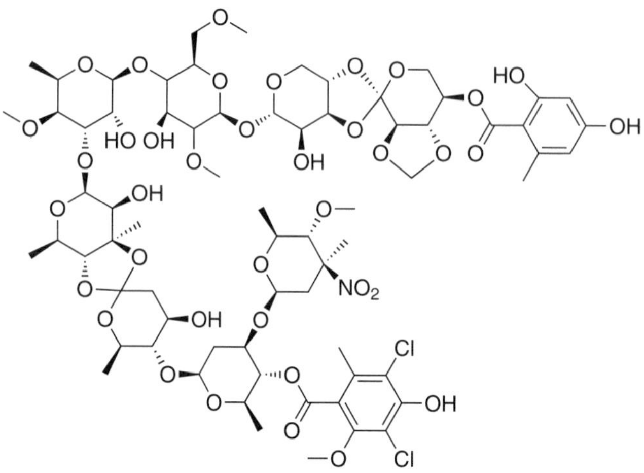

Everninomycin

Figure 15.8 Everninomycin structure.

Everninomycin is an octasaccharide capped at both ends with phenolic aryl carboxylic esters. It binds to the 23S rRNA far from the peptidyltransferase center that is the target for macrolides and streptogramins. Resistance mutations were used to determine that everninomycin binds at loops 89 and 91 (**Fig. 15.9**) and may block the binding of the initiation factor protein IF2, which brings in the initiator formylmethionyl (fMet) tRNA. Belova et al. (2001) note that this is a distinct site from the known ribosome-binding antibiotics that target the peptidyltransferase centers and the exit site for nascent peptide chains. This site may be a good target for other small molecules, which could be assayed by displacement of everninomycin. Everninomycin is used as an animal growth promoter because toxicity has limited its development in humans, but nontoxic variants based on such structural information may be possible.

A second class of natural products that act as antibiotics by interdicting one of the proteins that acts as a partner for the ribosome during protein biosynthesis is the thiopeptide class, represented by GE2270A, thiostrepton, and nosiheptide (**Fig. 15.10**) (see Sinha Roy et al., 1999, for review). These nonribosomal peptides contain Ser and Cys residues which have been cyclodehydrated and dehydrogenated to create thiazole, thiazoline, and oxazoline ring systems that introduce rigidity. Thiostrepton and nosiheptide target 23S rRNA in the region of A_{1087}, as well as blocking the binding of the elongation factor EF-G to the ribosome at the peptidyltransferase site. The thiazole peptide GE2270A blocks ribosome-mediated peptidyl transfer by targeting the GTPase EF-Tu, a chaperone protein that delivers aminoacyl-tRNAs to the mRNA codons at the peptidyltransferase site (see chapter 4). The antibiotic binds to the EF-Tu complex, tightening GTP binding, slowing GTPase action, and preventing formation of the releasable EF-Tu-GDP complex, stalling the ribosome peptide elongation process (**Fig. 15.11**). The X-ray structure of the EF-Tu–GE2270A complex has been determined (Anborgh and Parmeggiani, 1991), and, more generally, EF-Tu offers several sites for interaction with other antibiotics, including pulvomycin and kirromycin (see Sinha Roy et al., 1999). These findings suggest a structure-based optimization program against EF-Tu might be worthwhile. Following on the theme of anti-

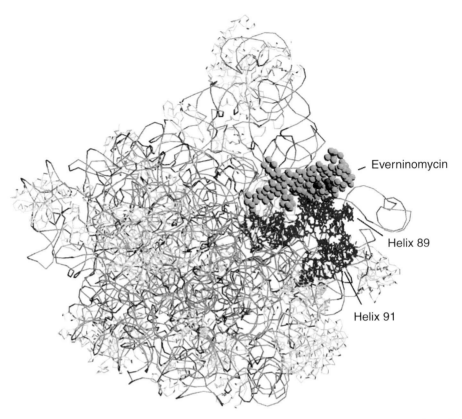

Figure 15.9 Binding site of everninomycin on 23S rRNA. (From Mazmanian et al. [2001], with permission.)

biotics that target RNA sequences, Sucheck and Wong (2000) have reviewed recent approaches to design and testing of small molecules that interact with specific sequences in mRNA and rRNA.

The interaction of aminoglycosides with 16S rRNA both from X-ray and nuclear magnetic resonance imaging studies offers a structure-based paradigm for the design of new molecules. In a complementary approach, Wong and colleagues (Sucheck et al., 2000) have used the neamine tetra-amino disaccharide (**Fig. 15.12**) as a core element to probe binding determinants for 16S rRNA. Dimers of neamine were linked to produce a bivalent synthetic aminoglycoside with the properties of retained high affinity for the rRNA and reduced recognition by aminoglycoside-modification enzymes. Simple N,N'-methyl diamine linkers (Fig. 15.12) provided binding activity yet were poor substrates for modifying acetyltransferases and phosphotransferases that deactivate aminoglycosides. This is a promising starting point for new approaches to aminoglycoside mimetics.

Peptide deformylase and methionine aminopeptidase
Bacterial protein biosynthesis starts with fMet tRNA as the initiator aminoacyl-tRNA, escorted to the peptidyltransferase center on the ribosome by the IF2

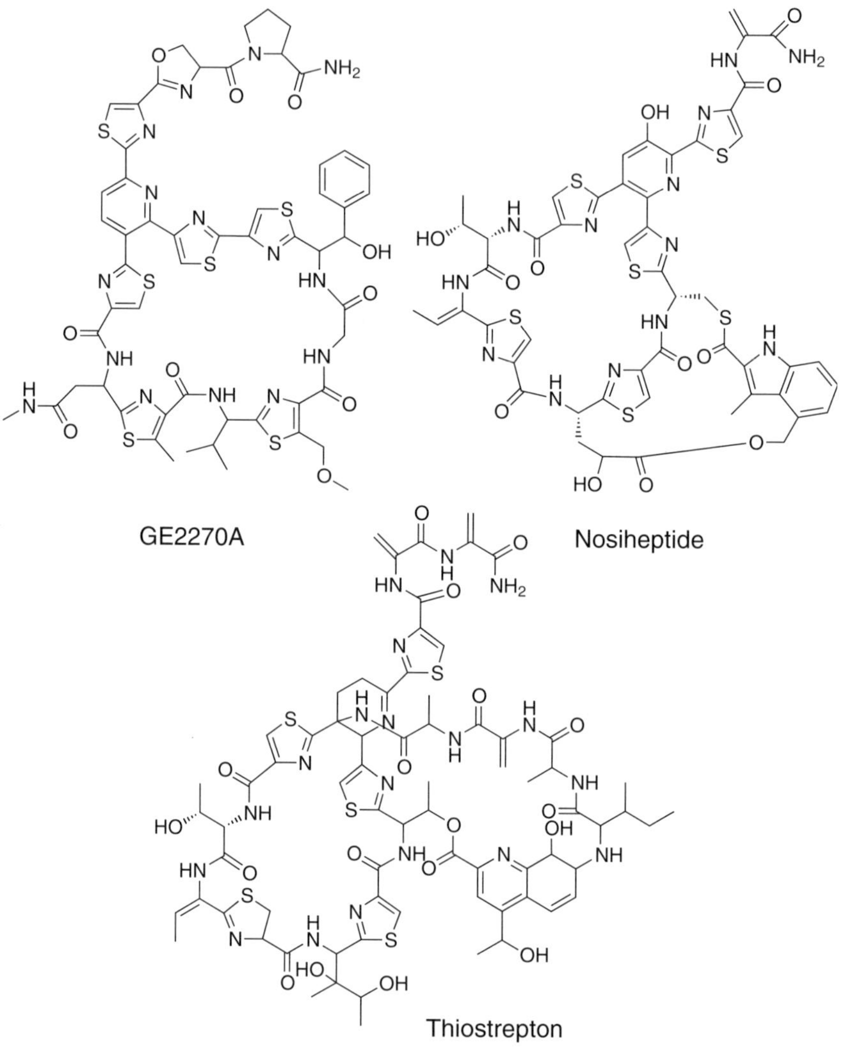

Figure 15.10 Examples of the thiopeptide class of antibiotics containing thiazole and oxazole rings.

protein chaperone noted above. The *N*-formylation of the methionyl amino group ensures that fMet can act only as a donor and not as an acceptor in peptide bond formation, imposing a directionality to the start process. As the elongating peptide chain emerges from the ribosome, the *N*-formyl group is removed enzymatically by the enzyme known as peptide deformylase (Huntington et al., 2000; Rajagopalan et al., 1997) (**Fig. 15.13**). The N-terminal methionine is then removed hydrolytically by methionine aminopeptidase. Both the deformylase and the aminopeptidase are essential by gene deletion analysis in *E. coli*, raising the prospect that these two enzymes are valid targets for antibacterials. The deformylase is a metallopeptidase, inhibited by metal-chelating ligands (Apfel et al., 2001; Chen et al., 2000) such as the hydroxamate found in the natural dipeptidyl hydroxamate actinonin (**Fig. 15.14**) (Trias, 2001) and many analogs. These compounds are bacteriostatic rather than bactericidal and

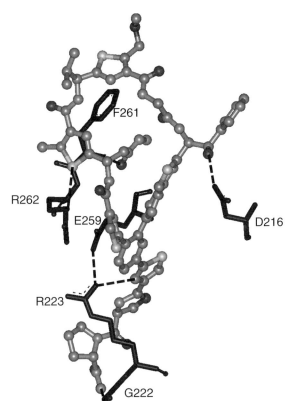

Figure 15.11 Binding site for thiopeptide GE2270A on the elongation factor EF-Tu. (From Heffron and Jurnak [2000], with permission.)

mutations arise at a high frequency, although these tend to reduce the fitness of the mutants. It remains to be seen how broadly effective peptide deformylase inhibitors will be.

Mupirocin and other inhibitors of aminoacyl-tRNA synthetases

Mupirocin is a natural product (**Fig. 15.15**) that prevents isoleucine incorporation into proteins by blocking the Ile-tRNA synthetase. It is marketed as the topical antibacterial agent Bactroban. The structure of the complex of mupirocin with the *S. aureus* Ile-tRNA synthetase has been determined (Silvian et al., 1999), validating its ligation at the active site, competing against Ile-AMP binding. Screening programs against other tRNA synthetases, both bacterial and eukaryotic for control purposes, have been conducted, but no analogs have been advanced to clinical evaluation. This is not for lack of activity against the isolated tRNA synthetases. For example, carbocyclic analogs of tyrosine inhibit tyrosyl-tRNA synthetase with nanomolar potency (Jarvest et al., 2001), including the natural product SB-219383, with a 50% inhibitory concentration of 1 nM (Qiu et al., 2001), some 12,000-fold lower than the 12 μM K_m for L-Tyr. The X-ray structure of the inhibitor-enzyme complex has been solved to give insights into subsequent inhibitor design (Qiu et al., 2001). Ester analogs of aminoacyl-AMP intermediates have been prepared, including Ile-esters of hydroxamates with the adenine ring replaced by isovanillin to yield an Ile-AMP analog with low-micromolar 50% inhibitory concentrations against Ile-tRNA synthetase (Lee et al., 2001). Glutamyl-γ-boronates inhibit the Glu-tRNA^{Gln} amidotransferase with

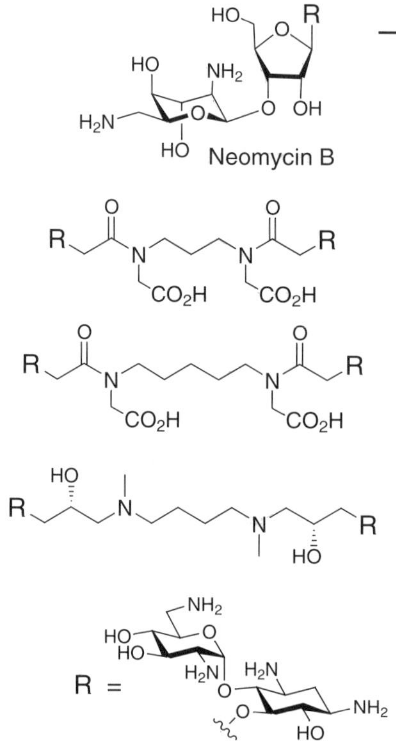

	16S RNA A-Site K_d (μM)	E. coli MIC (μM)	AAC-(6') K_m (μM)	APH-(2") K (μM)
Neomycin B	0.2	3.1	3.64×10^5	1.9 (K_m)
	1.1	31	1.6×10^4	0.78 (K_i)
	0.8	125	2.26×10^4	0.15 (K_i)
	0.04	6.25	9.26×10^3	0.94 (K_i)

R = Neamine

Figure 15.12 Synthetic dimers of neamine derivatives as RNA-targeting aminoglycoside mimetics.

low-micromolar potencies (Decicco et al., 2001). However, both of these types of inhibitors fail to show any antibacterial activity for lack of uptake into bacterial cells. The problem of delivery of such hydrophilic inhibitors continues to be unsolved.

DNA replication and repair inhibitors

DNA gyrase: novel quinolone and nonquinolone inhibitors

DNA gyrase is the classical target of quinolone antibacterials, as noted in chapter 5, and new quinolones continue to be developed (see Bush and Macielag, 2000), including levofloxacin for penicillin-resistant *S. pneumoniae* in community-acquired pneumonias. Trovafloxacin was approved in 1998 but restricted in use

Figure 15.13 Action of peptide deformylase and methionine aminopeptidase to trim away fMet residues at the N termini of bacterial proteins.

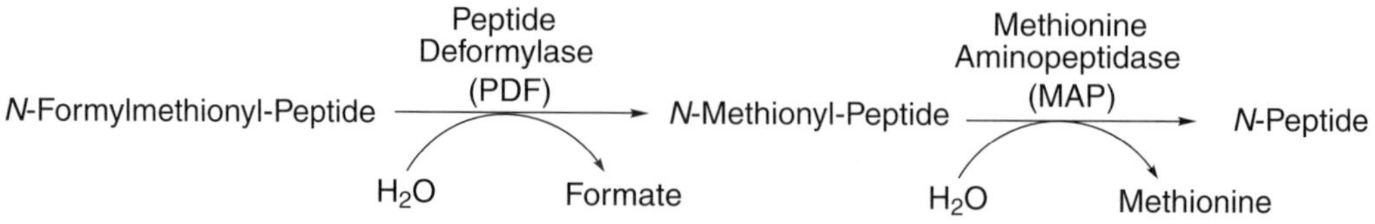

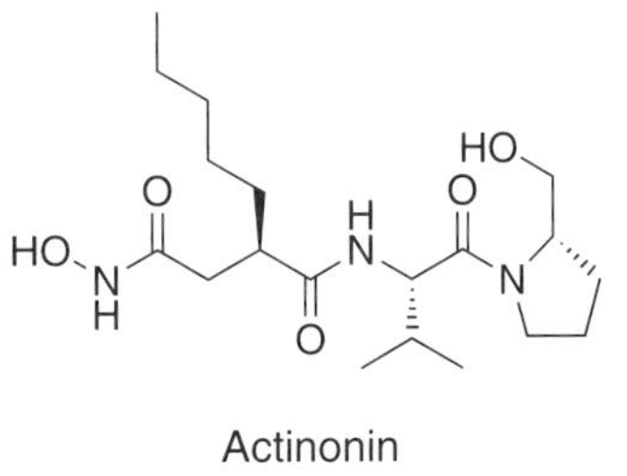

Figure 15.14 The natural product actinonin is a metal-chelating inhibitor of peptide deformylase.

Actinonin

in 1999 due to liver toxicity. The 8-methoxyquinolones moxifloxacin and gatifloxacin were approved in 1999, intended to provide enhanced activity against staphylococci and to treat community-acquired pneumonia, bronchitis, and sinusitis (Bronson and Barrett, 2001b; Cubbon and Masterton, 2000). Variants of quinolones contain a bridgehead nitrogen, producing 2-pyridone ring systems that maintain potency against some of the more common gyrase mutants with quinolone resistance (Chu, 1999). Clinafloxacin and sitafloxacin have been reported to be active against both GyrA (gyrase subunit) and ParC (topoisomerase IV subunit) mutants (Onodera et al., 1999; Schmitz et al., 2000). There are other kinds of molecules that offer leads for inhibitory ligands for DNA gyrase and/or the cognate type II topoisomerase, topoisomerase IV.

The coumarin natural products (chapter 14) elaborated by streptomycetes—novobiocin, chlorobiocin, and the dimeric coumermycin (**Fig. 15.16**)—actually bind one to three orders of magnitude more tightly ($K_i = 10^{-7}$ to 10^{-9} M) to gyrase than do typical quinolones (10^{-6} M), with coumermycin perhaps spanning the two GyrB subunits in the A_2B_2 tetramer to give the most potent inhibition.

Novobiocin and chlorobiocin have been cocrystallized with a 24-kDa N-terminal fragment of the *E. coli* GyrB subunit (**Fig. 15.17**) that overlaps with the adenine ring site of ATP, consistent with the observed competitive inhibition of ATP binding (see Holdgate et al., 1997; Lewis et al., 1996; Tsai et al., 1997).

While the coumarins have been of great value in sorting out gyrase domain functions, they have not succeeded clinically, perhaps because of the combination of poor solubility, weak activity against gram-negative bacteria (poor penetration through the outer membrane barrier), and vertebrate toxicity. It may be that these natural product pathways (see chapter 14) will be amenable to combinatorial biosynthetic manipulations to increase structural diversity and separate out desired antibacterial activities from unwanted side effects.

Another natural product, again from the ever-productive streptomycetes, that shows potent activity against pure DNA gyrase in vitro is the nonribosomal pentapeptide cyclothialidine (**Fig. 15.18A**). The side chains CH_2OH of Ser_3 and CH_2SH of Cys_4 have been captured in ester linkage and thioether linkage, re-

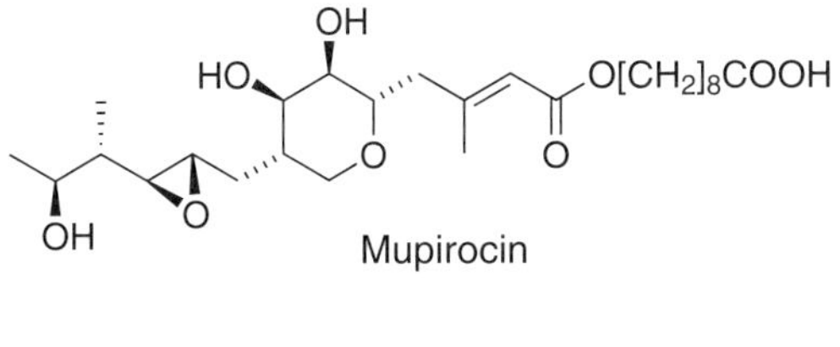

Figure 15.15 Mupirocin: an inhibitor of Ile-tRNA synthetase.

Mupirocin

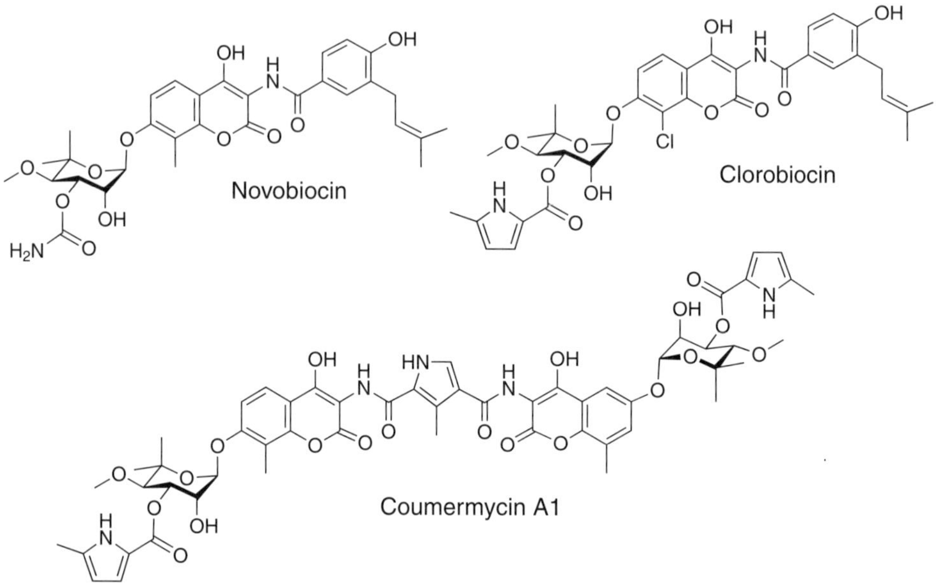

Figure 15.16 Naturally occurring aminocoumarin inhibitors of DNA gyrase.

spectively, by a 2,6-dimethyl-3,5-dihydroxybenzoyl moiety, to create a 12-membered macrolactone that provides the steric organizing constraint to populate the gyrase-inhibitory conformer of cyclothialidine (**Fig. 15.18B**).

Somewhat surprisingly, the cocrystal of cyclothialidine with the N-terminal fragment of GyrB also reveals overlap in the ATP site, revealing that coumarins and the cyclic depsipeptide demonstrate equivalent ways to occupy that binding space along with the purine ring of ATP (Lewis et al., 1996). Cyclothialidine is not active against intact bacteria because of poor penetration, probably due to

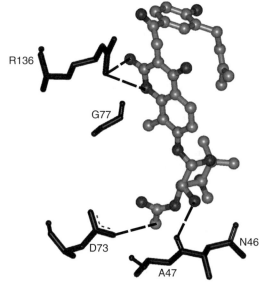

Figure 15.17 Binding of novobiocin to the ATP site on the GyrB subunit with selected key interactions displayed. (From Lewis et al. [1996], with permission.)

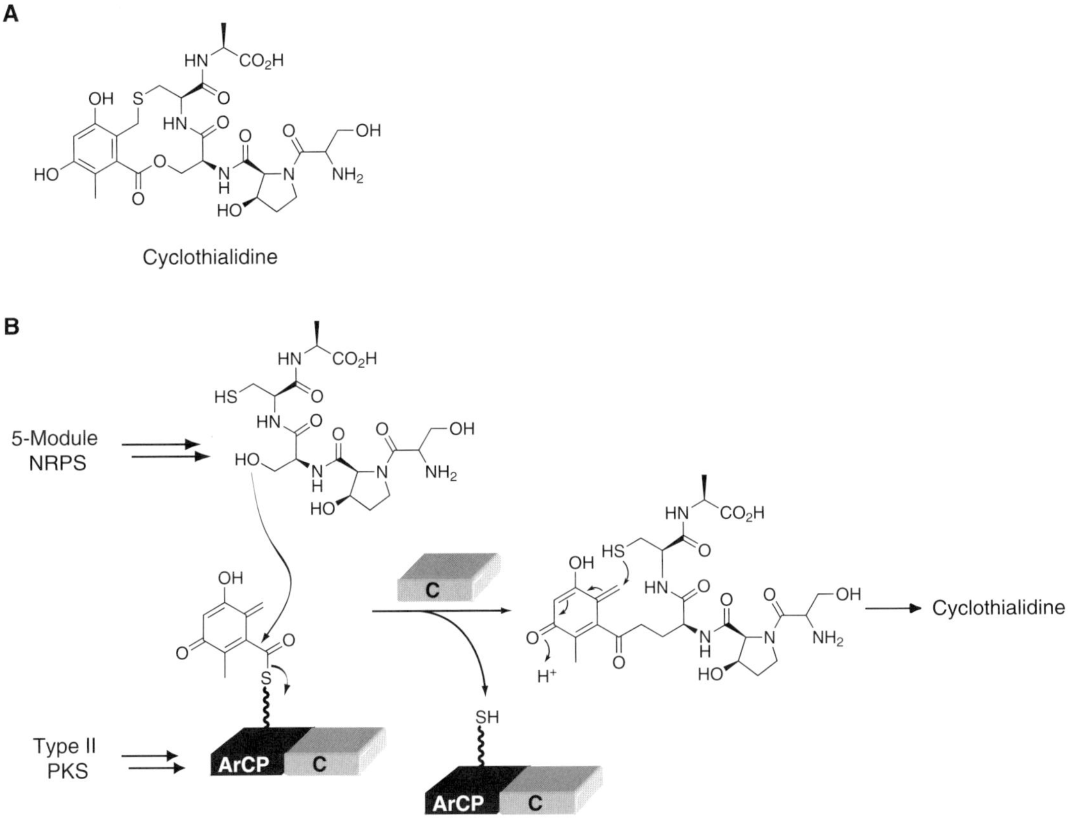

A

Cyclothialidine

B

5-Module
NRPS

Type II
PKS

Cyclothialidine

Figure 15.18 (A) The peptide macrolactone cyclothialidine is a DNA gyrase inhibitor; (B) proposed route for cyclization of a linear nonribosomal pentapeptide precursor.

its polar peptide constituents. As delineated in chapter 16, this nonribosomal peptide thioether macrolactone might be an interesting pathway for combinatorial biosynthetic manipulation.

A third natural product that inhibits DNA gyrase and, like the quinolone drugs, leads to irreversible accumulation of the doubly cleaved DNA-gyrase covalent intermediate is the 43-residue peptide microcin B17 (Fig. 5.5C and 14.14) produced by certain strains of *E. coli* as a peptide antibiotic. As noted in chapter 14, microcin B17 is encoded ribosomally as a 69-amino-acid precursor from which the N-terminal 26 residues are cleaved after 14 of the 43 (six Gly, four Ser, four Cys) have been posttranslationally modified to four oxazole and four thiazole rings. There are two 4,2-tandem bis heterocycles constructed in this maturation process and these appear to be important determinants of antibacterial activity (Sinha Roy et al., 1999). Microcin-resistant *E. coli* present with a mutation at the C terminus of GyrB, and gyrase has recently been shown to be the killing target (Heddle et al., 2001). There are mechanistic similarities to the action of quinolones on gyrase, but microcin shows an absolute dependence on ATP or a noncleavable ATP analog to induce accumulation of the cleaved DNA-enzyme intermediate. Inspection of the microcin B17 sequence suggests the presence of a polyglycine random coil interspersed by heterocycles, likely to be DNA and protein binding moieties. It is not known what the minimal fragment of microcin is that confers the gyrase inactivation or whether small bis heterocyclic fragments would be pharmacologically and medicinally tractable.

A small bacterial protein toxin, CcdB, also traps DNA gyrase in a complex with DNA double-strand breaks. CcdB (11.7 kDa) and CcdA (8.7 kDa), its partner protein antidote, are encoded in the *E. coli* F plasmid. The F plasmid encodes a cell death program that turns on in bacterial daughter cells that did not inherit a copy of the F plasmid during cell division (see Couturier et al., 1998, for review). If the F plasmid is lost, CcdA degrades first, by action of the Lon protease, and then the released CcdB subunit can attack gyrase and lead to cell death. Analysis of the mechanism of CcdB inhibition of gyrase, compared to quinolones, coumarins, and microcin B17, may yield new design insights into novel gyrase inhibitors.

Recent structural biology advances have indicated that the ATP binding region of the GyrB subunit has folding homology to a superfamily of other ATP binding proteins termed the GHL family (from gyrase B, chaperone Hsp90, and DNA repair enzyme MutL [Ban and Yang, 1998]). A variety of both natural products and synthetic ligands (see McMahon et al., 1998, for review) have been found that are potent and selective inhibitors of ATP binding to proteins (in particular protein kinases), and such libraries may be sources of potent ligands that could be optimized for specificity and potency against bacterial type II topoisomerases.

Proteins that interact with RNA

In the dynamics of RNA metabolism, transient complexes form between RNA and DNA, RNA and RNA, and RNA and proteins (see Tanner and Linder, 2001, for review) and must do so with specificity and kinetic efficiency. RNA molecules need to be folded, unfolded, and refolded in some or all of their length for biological function. Enzymes that unwind RNA molecules (and probably rewind them) are RNA helicases (Tanner and Linder, 2001), using the energy of NTP hydrolysis to drive the unwinding, e.g., of double-stranded RNA. RNA helicases are identified by seven to eight conserved sequence motifs, and structures of RNA and DNA helicases show close three-dimensional resemblance. Some RNA helicase functions occur in prokaryotes, including transcription, ribosome biogenesis, translation initiation, and RNA degradation. Other functions occur in eukaryotes, including mRNA editing, splicing, and RNA transit to the cytoplasm. Given that RNA helicases are translocation motors for RNA, they have been considered as "RNA chaperones, maturases and unwindases . . . temporary 'clamps' that permit the rearrangement of RNA interactions in a controlled manner" (Tanner and Linder, 2001). These analyses lead to the suggestion that since RNA helicases are required for bacterial function, they could be appropriate antibacterial enzyme targets for inhibition provided selectivity versus eukaryotic congeners can be achieved.

New looks at some new targets

In addition to the traditional validated targets, there are indications that many other aspects of bacterial metabolism and physiology should be vulnerable to new antibiotics (Allen, 1985; Sutcliffe, 1988). In addition to the targets that are and will be emerging from the genomics approaches noted at the beginning of this chapter, there are some other enzymes and processes for which there is already reasonable to strong justification for study as novel antibacterial targets.

Bacterial fatty acid synthesis

Fatty acid biosynthesis is essential for bacterial growth and survival. We have noted in chapter 12 the similarity of the assembly-line enzymatic logic for both fatty acids and for polyketide natural products, in both type I and type II configurations of modular catalysts or separate subunits, respectively. In eukaryotes the fatty acid synthases (FASs) are organized in multimodular subunits, as discussed for type I systems, whereas in most bacteria the FASs are organized as type II systems with separate subunits, raising the prospect of selective inhibition. Natural products are known that have antibiotic action by inhibition of fatty acid biosynthesis, such as cerulenin (**Fig. 15.19**), which alkylates and inactivates the active-site nucleophilic cysteine of the ketosynthase enzyme in FASs by epoxide ring opening. A more selective inhibitor of bacterial ketosynthase catalysts could be effective.

Recently, antibacterial antiseptics of the triclosan class (**Fig. 15.20**) have been found to block the olefin saturation step in fatty acid biosynthesis catalyzed by the enoyl-ACP reductase enzyme FabI in *E. coli* (McMurry et al., 1998), confirming that these are good targets. Triclosan-resistant mutants in *P. aeruginosa* pump out this widely used antiseptic agent through the MexC-MexD-OprJ efflux pump (Chuanchuen et al., 2001). Synthetic 1,4-disubstituted imidazoles are also reported to be low-micromolar inhibitors of FabI (Heerding et al., 2001). The *M. tuberculosis* homolog of the *E. coli* enoyl-ACP reductase gene (*fabI* in *E. coli*) is *inhA*, with 36% identity. The InhA enzyme is much less susceptible to triclosan but is particularly sensitive to isoniazid, one of the staples of antituberculosis combination chemotherapy. Isoniazid (Fig. 15.20B) requires oxidative activation by the mycobacterial KatG catalase and then acylates NAD bound in the active site of InhA to inhibit the enzyme (Rozwarski et al., 1998). Structure-function studies of both FabI and InhA starting from triclosan- and isoniazid-based libraries may lead to new antibiotics and antiseptics.

To function in catalysis the FASs of both type I and type II require posttranslational priming of the apo forms of the ACPs by phosphopantetheinyltransferases (PPTases), which install the phosphopantetheine (Ppant) tether, derived from the cosubstrate CoASH (Lambalot et al., 1996), in the holo ACP (**Fig. 15.21**). The holo forms of the ACPs now have the —SH group of the Ppant prosthetic group, which is the site of acyl chain growth. The structures of both the apo and holo forms of the *Bacillus subtilis* ACP have been determined (Xu et al., 2001), as have those for *E. coli* ACP and the ACP subunit for the actinorhodin type II polyketide synthase (Crump et al., 1997).

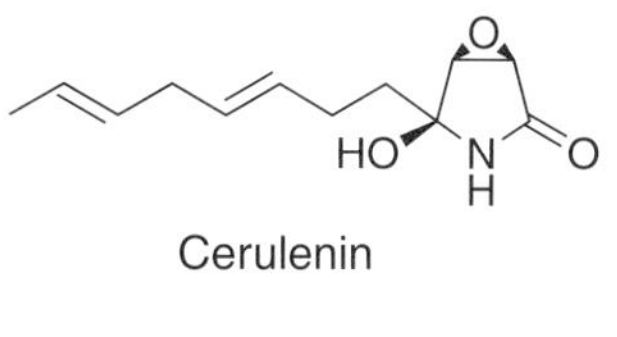

Figure 15.19 Structure of the natural product cerulenin: an alkylating inactivator of fatty acid synthases.

Cerulenin

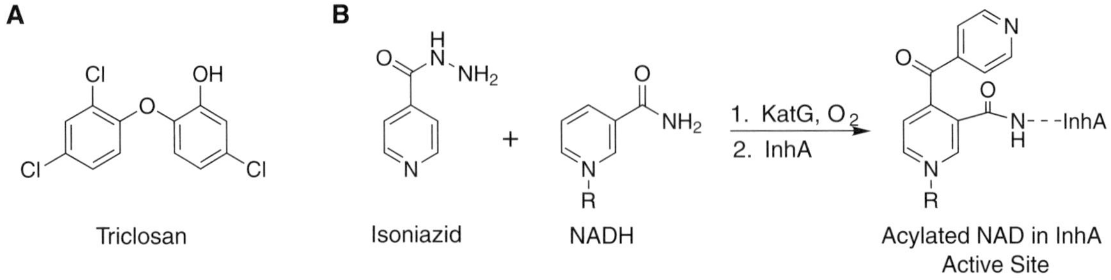

A

Triclosan

B

Isoniazid

+

NADH

1. KatG, O$_2$
2. InhA

→

Acylated NAD in InhA
Active Site

Figure 15.20 (A) Triclosan, an antibacterial antiseptic, inhibits enoyl-ACP reductase. (B) The antitubercular drug isoniazid requires metabolic oxidation to generate an acylated NAD in the active site of the target enoylreductase.

Animal cell FASs also use similar Ppant priming of FAS, so it is unclear if specific inhibition of the prokaryotic PPTases can be achieved. However, structures have been determined for bacterial PPTases, including an ACP-PPTase complex (Chirgadze et al., 2000; Parris et al., 2000; Reuter et al., 1999), allowing a structure-based approach to inhibitor design in order to test this premise. Both the ACPs and the PPTases that modify them are potential targets for antibiotics.

Bacterial isoprenoid biosynthesis

Nonclassical pathway enzymes

For 50 years the mevalonate pathway to isoprenoid natural products has been known and well studied. The essence of this pathway (**Fig. 15.22**) is construction of the six-carbon branched-chain mevalonate skeleton from three molecules of acetyl-CoA, condensed sequentially by thiolase and hydroxymethylglutaryl-CoA synthase enzymes. The thioester then undergoes four-electron reduction to convert the thioester carbonyl to the primary alcohol of mevalonate. Pyrophosphorylation at the primary alcohol and phosphorylation at the tertiary alcohol by two kinases set up the olefin-forming decarboxylation/P$_i$ elimination reaction to yield the allylic isomer dimethyallyl-pyrophosphate (dimethylallyl-PP) (Δ^3). Finally, the isopentenyl-PP isomerase moves the double bond to the Δ^2 isomer, isopentenyl-PP, so both isomers are available for elongation reactions (Walsh, 1979).

In recent years it has become apparent, initially from labeling studies and more recently from work with purified enzymes (see Rohdich et al., 2001, for

Figure 15.21 Reaction catalyzed by phosphopantetheinyltransferase in priming of apo ACP domains.

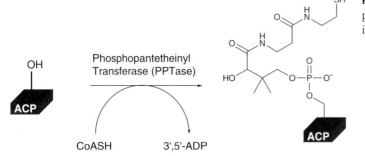

CoASH   3',5'-ADP

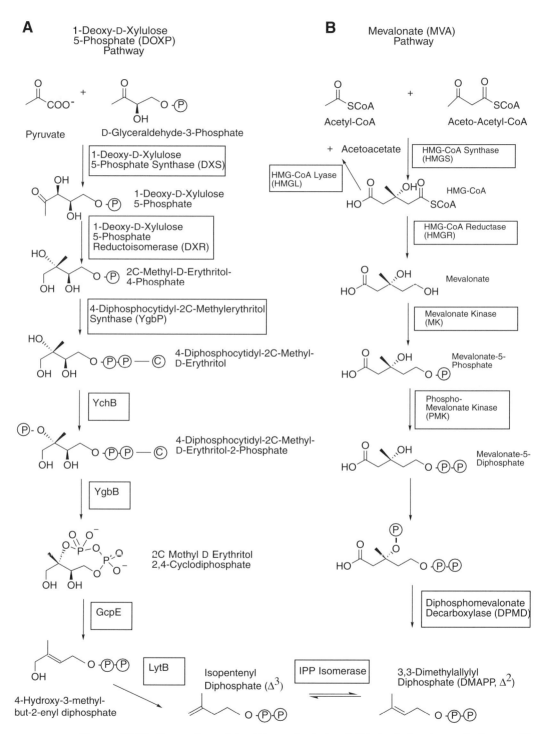

Figure 15.22 Comparison of the (A) nonclassical and (B) classical pathways for isoprenoid biosynthesis in bacteria: new enzyme targets.

review), that acetyl-CoA was not the source of either the Δ^2 or Δ^3 isoprenyl-PP isomers, required for biogenesis of the essential bacterial isoprenoid quinones (coenzyme Q) and the C_{55} undecaprenyl phosphates that act as carriers in PG assembly in gram-negative bacteria. Instead, the bacterial pathway is nonclassical (Fig. 15.22), condensing pyruvate and glyceraldehyde-3-P to make deoxyxylulose-5-P (DX-5-P), also an intermediate in thiamine and pyridoxal biosynthesis. Clearly an inhibitor of this first DX-5-P synthase enzyme would be a promising antibacterial, blocking a key step for three essential metabolites. DX-5-P is then converted from the straight-chain to the branched-chain skeleton by an NADPH-dependent reductoisomerase, yielding the 2-C-methyl-D-erythritol-4P (ME) intermediate. This enzymatic process is inhibited by the natural product phosphonate fosmidomycin (K_i = 10 nM) (Koppisch et al., 2002), presumably acting as an analog to the aldehyde intermediate and a reasonable starting point for practical inhibitor design. The next two enzymes are a CMP-nucleotidyltransferase, to generate ME-CDP, and then a kinase, to release CMP and produce the ME cyclic PP. The structure of the ME cyclic PP synthase has recently been reported (Kemp et al., 2002). The subsequent enzymatic steps for breaking the C-OPP bond (carbon-oxygen bond of the alcohol-PP linkage) and the loss of both —OH groups to yield Δ^2 isopentenyl-PP are still obscure, although mechanisms have been proposed (Hecht et al., 2001).

It is likely that any of the several enzymes in the nonmevalonate pathway will be good antibacterial targets since it is the mevalonate pathway that is used in plants and animals. Hedl et al. (2002) have noted that bacterial bioinformatics suggests genes encoding the mevalonate pathway are essential in *S. aureus* and other gram-positive cocci. For example, *Enterococcus faecalis* and *E. faecium* use the classical pathway, where the thiolase and hydroxy methyl glutaryl-CoA reductases are fused into a single protein, so classical pathway inhibitors should work against these gram-positive pathogens.

C_{55} undecaprenyl-PP synthase

The C_{55} isoprenoid lipid carrier in the membrane phase of PG biosynthesis, undecaprenyl-PP, is assembled by a *cis*-prenyltransferase, undecaprenyl-PP synthase (Fujihashi et al., 2001). This enzyme differs from the *trans*-prenyltransferases that elongate C_5 to C_{15} isoprenyl units and maintain the *trans* double bonds in the 1,5-arrays characteristic of natural isoprenoids. The transferases that elongate isoprenoids by C_5 increments to make *trans* (E) double bonds remove the prochiral ProR C_1 hydrogen from the C_5 allylic monomer, while the transferases that elongate to *cis* (Z) double bonds abstract the ProS C_1-H of the Δ^3 allylic monomer. The C_{30-40} ubiquinone isoprenoid side chains are all E isomers.

Undecaprenyl-PP synthase instead uses a farnesyl-PP (C_{15} with three *trans* double bonds) unit as a primer and carries out eight successive *cis* elongations with isopentenyl-PP (C_5 unit) as donor substrate to build up the C_{55} undecaprenyl chain (**Fig. 15.23**), generating eight *cis*-prenyl (Z) units and the three *trans*-prenyl (E) units at the distal end of the C_{55} chain. It is not known how the E_3/Z_8 isomer composition of the 11 double bonds constrains function of the C_{55} lipid as a PG carrier in cell wall synthesis.

The same type of *cis*-prenyltransferase is involved in eukaryotes to produce the long-chain isoprenoid dolichol-PP involved in oligosaccharide chain assem-

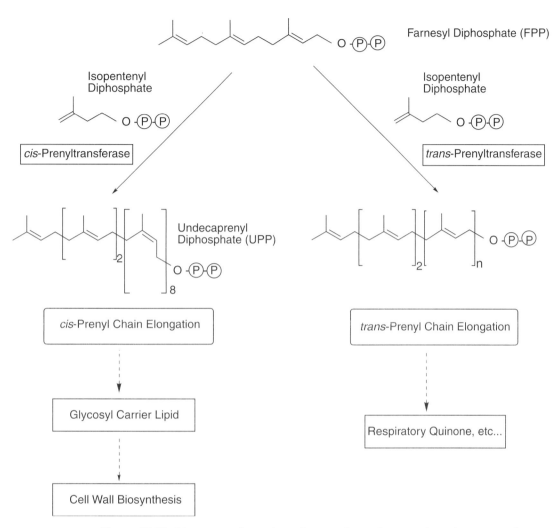

Figure 15.23 Divergence of prenyltransferase pathways between *cis*- and *trans*-prenyl transfers.

bly for protein glycosylation (Bugg and Brandish, 1994). Therefore, it is not known if one could obtain selective inhibition of the prokaryotic *cis*-prenyltransferase, but if achievable that would block the formation of lipid I and lipid II in PG biosynthesis. The X-ray structure of the *Micrococcus luteus* undecaprenyl-PP synthase (Fujihashi et al., 2001) suggests a binding orientation for the farnesyl-PP acceptor/template and the isopentenyl-PP donor in the first (of eight) C-C bond-forming step and suggests the growing chain, elongating five carbons at a time, can fill a hydrophobic cleft. Perhaps the cleft could be targeted by inhibitors.

Isocitrate lyase

A variant of fatty acid metabolism that appears to be a novel target in *M. tuberculosis* is the conversion of carbons from fatty acids through the glyoxylate shunt to glucose. Although the glyoxylate shunt enzymes, such as isocitrate lyase

(**Fig. 15.24**), are not essential for survival of *M. tuberculosis* in culture plates, they are essential for virulence in animals (McKinney et al., 2000), indicating that the pathogenic bacteria depend on fatty acids for energy during in vivo infections. This is an example where a virulence screen rather than a bactericidal screen reveals a potential novel target. No selective inhibitors of isocitrate lyase have yet been reported. The glyoxylate cycle has likewise been implicated as a requirement for fungal virulence (Lorenz and Fink, 2001).

Lipid A biosynthesis in gram-negative bacteria

A strategy that could target gram-negative bacterial infections, but not gram-positive ones, is to block the biosynthesis of the lipid A core of the lipopolysaccharide component of the bacterial outer membrane (**Fig. 15.25A**). The lipid A core of lipopolysaccharide causes many of the toxic side effects associated with gram-negative infections (Raetz, 1987). The lipid A core is a glucosamine disaccharide, hexa-acylated and containing phosphate esters at 1 and 4′. The precursor of the glucosamine moieties is the common precursor nucleoside diphosphosugar UDP-GlcNAc that is esterified at the 3-OH with a 3-R-3-OH-myristoyl group donated by the corresponding 3-R-3-OH-myristoyl-*S*-ACP. This metabolite is then deacetylated on the N-acetyl moiety (**Fig. 15.25B**) by the enzyme LpxC, before N-3-OH-myristoylation (LpxD). The LpxC deacetylase is a zinc metalloenzyme that has been inhibited by metal-chelating phenyl-oxazolyl hydroxamates (**Fig. 15.25C**) (Jackman et al., 1999; Onishi et al., 1996). These inhibitors have not progressed because of poor penetration into intact bacteria, but they validate that LpxC is a killing target in gram-negative bacteria. Screening of a metalloenzyme inhibitor library has also turned up leads that target LpxC (Clements et al., 2002).

Two-component regulatory systems

The general mechanisms bacteria use for sensing some chemical change in their immediate external microenvironment most often utilize two-component signal

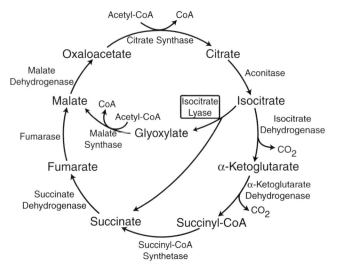

Figure 15.24 The glyoxylate shunt and the role of isocitrate lyase.

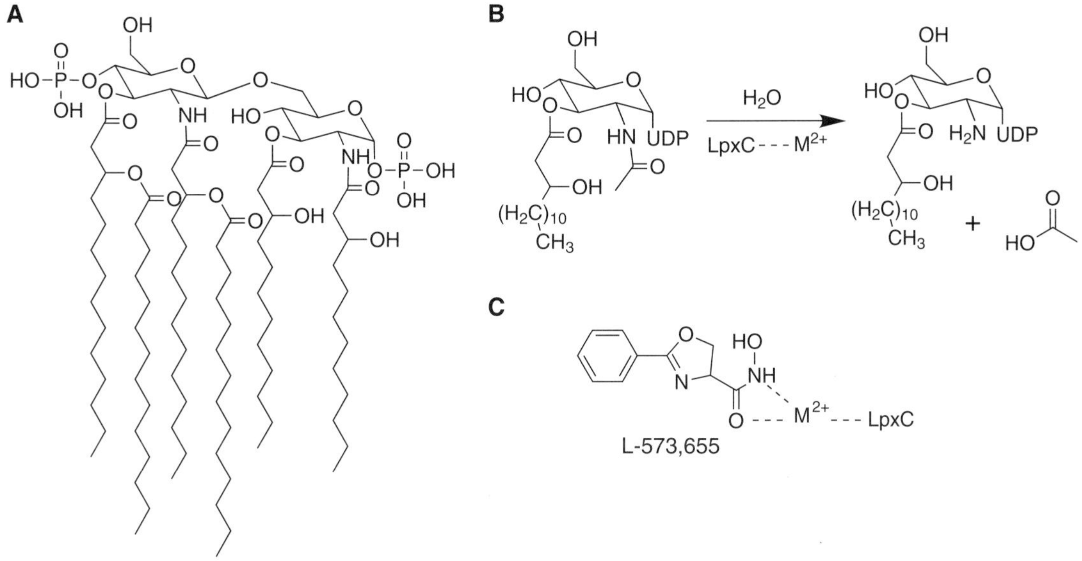

Figure 15.25 (A) Structure of the lipid A core; (B) deacetylation of UDP-GlcNAc by LpxC; (C) phenyl-oxazolyl hydroxamate inhibitors of the zinc enzyme LpxC. M^{2+} is the enzyme-bound metal cation required for catalysis.

transduction systems, with sensors and response regulators as the two protein components (Barrett and Hoch, 1998). The sensor is typically a transmembrane histidine kinase and the response regulator a DNA transcriptional activator (**Fig. 15.26**) (see Matsushita and Janda, 2002). Ligand sensing by the periplasmic loops and transmembrane domain of the sensor leads to autophosphorylation of an active-site histidine in the cytoplasmic histidine kinase domain of the sensor and subsequent phosphoryl group transfer from the P-His to a conserved Asp-β-carboxylate in the amino half of the response regulator. The P-Asp form of the response regulator induces an allosteric change in the conformation of the DNA binding domain, and the activator can derepress transcription of target genes (if it has been a repressor in its basal state) and start the programmed response.

We have noted that the VanS-VanR two-component system is a crucial sensor/transducer element for the VanA and VanB phenotypes in clinically important VRE (chapter 10). There have been other indications that two-component systems are determinants of bacterial virulence. A genomics-driven approach has been used to characterize the two-component regulatory systems in *S. pneumoniae* (Throup et al., 2000), in which 14 two-component gene pairs were detected. Although the physiologic functions of the 14 pairs could not readily be determined from sequence, each pair could be knocked out and the pathogenicity of the *S. pneumoniae* mutants evaluated in a murine respiratory tract infection model. One response regulator, in the OmpR subfamily, was essential for growth, and this had essential homologs in *S. aureus* and *B. subtilis.* Seven other two-component gene pairs, when mutated, showed some attenuation of *S. pneumoniae* growth in the mouse respiratory tract infection model.

In *S. aureus,* disruption of the *srhS-srhR* two-component pair led to a 3-log attenuation of growth of this *S. aureus* strain in a kidney pyelonephritis model

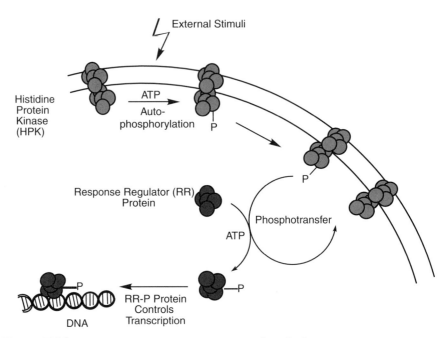

Figure 15.26 Two-component sensor/response regulator logic.

in mice (Throup et al., 2001). mRNA array analysis indicated that this two-component pair is important for the ability of the pathogen to grow at low oxygen tension when it switches to anaerobic routes of energy generation. The facultative anaerobiosis of *S. aureus* is one of the key attributes that allows it to produce deep-tissue, persistent infections. These results set the stage for analysis of the particular role of these eight two-component sensor/transducer pairs in pathogenesis, including such processes as adhesion and autolysis, and may help prioritize which two-component pairs are preferred antibacterial targets. Analysis of the *P. aeruginosa* genome reveals 63 or 64 two-component systems, suggesting sophisticated and complex control strategies for integration of external signals by this versatile pathogen (Rodrigue et al., 2000). One of these *P. aeruginosa* response regulators, PvrR, has been identified as a modulator of phenotypic switching from antibiotic-resistant to antibiotic-susceptible forms and also participates in biofilm formation (Drenkard and Ausubel, 2002).

Two-component systems have also been linked to virulence. In *S. aureus* strains the two-component *agr* signaling circuit is an essential element in genetic control of expression of virulence determinants, including the secretion of exoenzymes, protein toxins, and adhesins (Lyon et al., 2000). The *agr* two-component pair, AgrC and AgrA, is under quorum-sensing control (see below). In the gram-negative pathogen *Salmonella enterica* serovar Typhimurium, the PhoP-PhoQ sensor/transducer pair is turned on by Mg^{2+} or Ca^{2+} limitation after the bacteria are engulfed by macrophages or epithelial cells. PhoP-PhoQ activates transcription of genes that remodel the outer membrane, including alterations to lipid A (Guo et al., 1998). These include addition of aminoarabinose to the lipid A phosphate groups and addition of a seventh acyl group, a palmitoyl chain, to lipid A, catalyzed by PagP. Among the effects are alterations in the surface charge of the outer membrane that produce resistance to cationic antimicrobial peptides, including those from the macrophages and also the cationic polymyxin B antibiotic (chapter 6) (Guo et al., 1997). Compounds that would block both the Agr sensor/transducer pair in *S. aureus* or the PhoP-PhoQ pair in *Salmonella* serovar Typhimurium would have promise as new antibacterial agents, as would inhibitors of *Salmonella* PagP acyltransferase.

Screening approaches to the KinA protein histidine kinase from *B. subtilis* turned up several inhibitors, including closantel tetrachlorosalicylanilide and atrityl amidine (RWJ-49815), but all of these are probably nonspecific denaturants, structure perturbants, and protein aggregants rather than specific leads (Hilliard et al., 1999; Stephenson et al., 2000). Microarray analysis has been applied to the *B. subtilis* two-component systems (Kobayashi et al., 2001).

The X-ray structure of several response regulators and catalytic domains of sensor kinases have been determined (Robinson and Stock, 1999), leading to their inclusion in the GHL subfamily of ATP-hydrolyzing proteins noted above for DNA gyrase. Again, the large collection of ATP-site inhibitors from protein kinase research should be good starting points for detection of leads that would be selective for binding to the adenine pocket of the ATP sites of histidine sensor kinases.

Quorum sensor biosynthesis: inhibition to attenuate virulence

We noted in chapter 11 the use of quorum-sensing systems by which bacteria sense population density and make genetically mediated responses to produce virulence factors, including antibiotics. As noted above, the Agr locus in *S. aureus* is part of the global virulence response. As shown in **Fig. 15.27**, the AgrC and AgrA proteins of the five-gene *agr* operon are the transmembrane sensor kinase and response regulator (Lyon et al., 2000). AgrB is a peptide efflux pump that is dedicated to proteolytic processing and secretion of the AgrD gene product, a propeptide form of the mature autoinducing peptide (AIP).

The AIP, once proteolytically processed and secreted, is the external ligand for AgrC, turning on the further transcription of the Agr locus in the producing cell and in neighboring cells. The density-dependent quorum sensing is provided by the concentration of the secreted, diffusible AIP and its specific reception by AgrC. The AIP structure is intriguing. It is a thiolactone of eight to nine residues, arising from capture of the C-terminal phenylalanine residue by the side chain of Cys_5. The corresponding cyclic lactams or cyclic lactones, replacing N or O for the S of the thiolactone, are inhibitors, binding to the extracellular domain of AgrC but not transducing the signal (Lyon et al., 2000). This suggests approaches to antagonize the Agr signaling pathway and generate global inhibitors of this virulence response pathway. Four AIP variants have been seen, leading to the classification of four *S. aureus* AIP pheromone groups (McDowell et al., 2001). Quorum-sensing systems in other gram-positive bacteria also seem to be mediated by small peptides acting as pheromones (see Kleerebezem et al., 1997, for review). These include the development of genetic competence in *B. subtilis* and *S. pneumoniae* and the regulation of the operons for the production of the lantibiotic class of antimicrobial peptides (chapter 14).

Quorum-sensing systems also appear to be important determinants of morphology and communication when bacteria grow in aggregates in biofilms, which

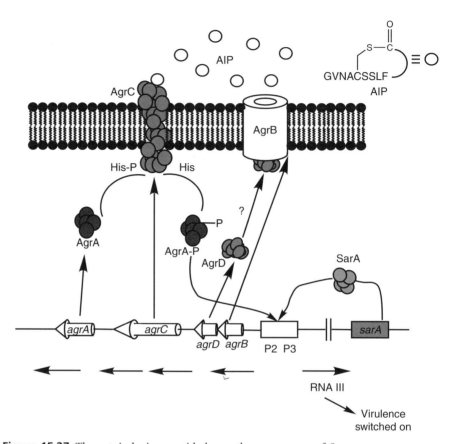

Figure 15.27 The autoinducing peptide locus, the *agr* operon, of *S. aureus*.

occur, for example, on indwelling catheters in hospitalized patients. Under these conditions the bacteria are often refractory to antibiotics because of poor penetration through the polysaccharide coats elaborated in these phenotypes (Miller and Bassler, 2001). A more direct approach to inhibition would be to block biosynthesis of the quorum signalers that initiate biofilm development. In the specific Agr context above, where a peptide is the signal molecule, this would be either the AgrD enzyme making the propeptide form of the inducer peptide or the protease activity of the AgrB export pump.

In the general case for gram-negative organisms in which acylhomoserine lactones are the intercellular signaling quorum molecules, the LuxI family of synthases would be the target. The acylhomoserines are produced from *S*-adenosylmethionine (SAM) and an acyl-*S*-ACP cosubstrate (Hanzelka et al., 1999). Although little is known about the detailed mechanism, the LuxI enzyme superfamily is thought to act first as amide synthases (**Fig. 15.28**) to generate the *N*-acyl-SAM and free ACP, followed by cyclization of the carboxylate oxygen on the β-carbon of the SAM-methionyl moiety, with cleavage of the C_β-S bond. This is the lactone-forming step and releases coproduct thiomethyladenosine. It should be possible to find or make specific and potent inhibitors of this enzyme superfamily and block production of the quorum signals. The X-ray structure of the lactone synthase EsaI from *Pseudomonas stewartii* has recently been solved

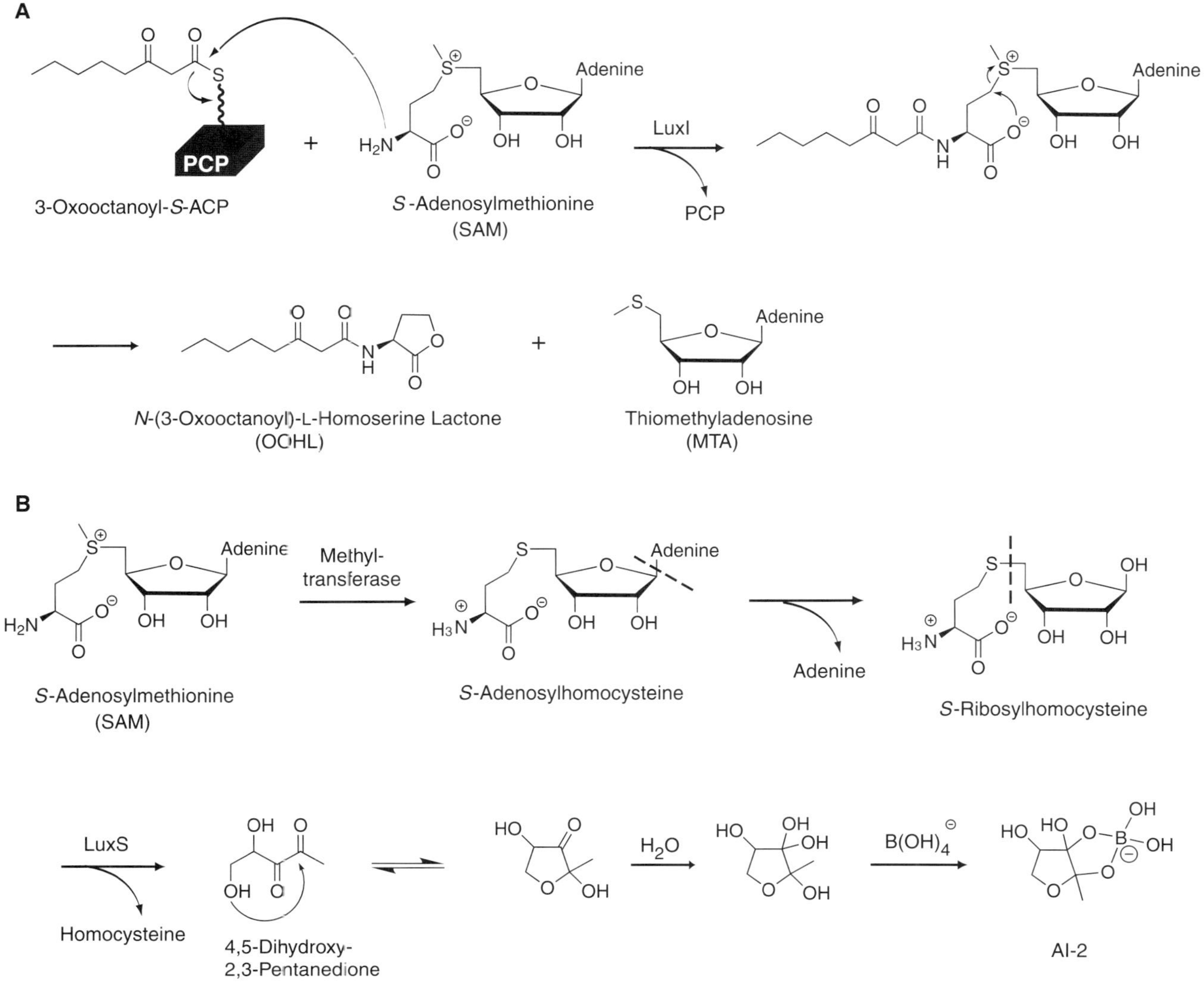

Figure 15.28 (A) The proposed reaction mechanism for acylhomoserine lactone (AHL) synthases. (B) Enzymatic generation of the AHL quorum signals.

and will be a starting point for structure-based design of drugs (Watson et al., 2002).

Recently a second family of quorum autoinducers, AI-2, to go along with the AI-1 homoserine lactones, has been detected in gram-negative bacteria, including enterohemorrhagic *E. coli* O157:H7, and the hypothesis advanced that AI-1 is involved in intraspecies communication while AI-2 is for interspecies sensing. Both the acylhomoserine lactones and the AI-2 quorum signaling derive from SAM. While LuxI cleaves SAM to methiothioadenosine and uses the homoserine chain as part of the AI-1 signal molecule, in the AI-2 pathway SAM is converted to *S*-adenosylhomocysteine by various methyltransferases. The *S*-adenosylhomocysteine skeleton is then acted on by two enzymes, Pfs to release adenine and produce *S*-ribosylhomocysteine, followed by LuxS, which produces 4,5-dihydroxy-2,3-pentanedione (DPD). DPD in the form of its cyclic hydrate (1,2-diol) complexes with $B(OH)_3$ in the medium to produce the active bicyclic borate ester form, AI-2, which is bound specifically and stoichiometrically to its target protein, LuxP, a soluble periplasmic protein related to ribose binding proteins (Chen et al., 2002) (Fig. 15.28B). This signaling role is a novel biological function for a boron-containing metabolite. The AI-2–LuxP complex is the ligand for the autophosphorylating two-component sensor kinase LuxQ (Schauder and Bassler, 2001; Schauder et al., 2001). The zinc-containing enzyme LuxS (Lewis et al., 2001) could be a target for agents that would reduce virulence.

Other targets to attenuate virulence

A variety of successful bacterial pathogens, such as *Yersinia, Listeria*, and *Salmonella*, have gained the ability to modulate intracellular activities of vertebrate hosts to blunt destruction. This is particularly relevant to these pathogens, as they induce internalization into host cells, such as macrophages, and then neutralize the killing machinery of the phagocytic host cells (Groisman, 2001). Stebbins and Galan (2000), Galan and Collmer (1999), and Lee and Schneewind (2001) have noted examples of structural mimicry by bacterial proteins of host cell homologs that control host cell responses. Both *Yersinia* and *Salmonella* species secrete proteins across host cell membranes by type III secretion machinery (Galan and Collmer, 1999; Lee and Schneewind, 2001), as noted in chapter 9. Among the bacterial proteins injected are tyrosine phosphatases, YopH from *Yersinia* spp. and SptP from *Salmonella* spp. (Guan and Dixon, 1990; Stebbins and Galan, 2000), which dephosphorylate macrophage proteins including the tyrosine kinase FAK (focal adhesion kinase), resulting in paralysis of the macrophage attack on the bacterium (Persson et al., 1997). When *Salmonella* injects the SopE protein into host cells, it acts as a guanine nucleotide exchange factor (GEF) to accelerate exchange of GDP by GTP at the active site of Rac1 and cdc42 GTPases (see Galan and Collmer, 1999; Lee and Schneewind, 2001; and references therein). In turn, these rearrange the actin cytoskeleton and promote uptake of the *Salmonella* into the host cell, wherein it can restore the normal functioning of the host cell cytoskeleton by delivery of the bacterial SptP protein, which acts as a GAP (GTPase accelerating protein), to promote accumulation of Rac1 and cdc42 in the original, resting, inactive GDP states. This limits the perturbation of the host GTPases and the cytoskeleton and internalization machinery, allowing the infected host cell to survive and the *Salmonella* to "hide out" in a sequestered microenvironment. Either the SopE GEF or the SptP GAP proteins of *Salmonella* would be potential targets for reducing the virulence and pathogenicity of such *Salmonella* colonizations. So would agents that block the assembly or functioning of the type III secretion machinery via both inner membrane and outer membrane components (chapter 9).

Efflux blockers

Screens for efflux pump blockers have been undertaken against the MexA-MexB-OprM, MexC-MExD-OprJ, and MexE-MexF-OprN systems of *P. aeruginosa*, as well as the AcrA-AcrB-TolC three-component pumps of *E. coli*, in an effort to reduce fluoroquinolone efflux. Lead compounds inhibited the pumps, lowered both intrinsic resistance and acquired resistance, and lowered the frequency of emergence of gyrase-resistant mutants (Lomovskaya et al., 2001).

The plant natural product 5′-methoxyhydnocarpin D (**Fig. 15.29**) is one such active pump blocker of fluoroquinolone efflux (Stermitz et al., 2000), suggesting structure-activity work will be possible. Analogously, modification of tetracycline structures have produced chloropropylthio derivatives that block Tet efflux proteins. (Chopra and Roberts, 2001). As noted in chapter 4, the new glycylcyclines (Fig. 4.5) are also Tet efflux pump blockers as well as being active in strains with the ribosomal protection factors TetM and TetO (Lee and Hecker, 1999; Mitscher et al., 1999).

The intrinsic resistance of *P. aeruginosa* to antibiotics was alluded to in chapter 9, reflecting both barriers to antibiotic entry by porins and antibiotic efflux by the pump systems noted above. The sequencing of the *P. aeruginosa* genome (Stover et al., 2000) sets the stage for genomics-based approaches. At first glance, the bacterium's ability to encode outer membrane proteins (150 genes) appears disproportionately large, with 19 genes of the OprD porin family, 34 members of the TonB gated porin family, and 18 genes of the OprM efflux pump family. This suggests multiple routes for *P. aeruginosa* to balance and regulate the flux of molecules through the outer membrane both inward and outward. Knockout approaches could delineate an essential subset in each category, allowing design of assays targeted against such subsets both for antibiotic uptake, e.g., to yield "fifth-generation" cephalosporins, and for antibiotic efflux blockers.

Figure 15.29 Inhibitors reported for efflux pumps.

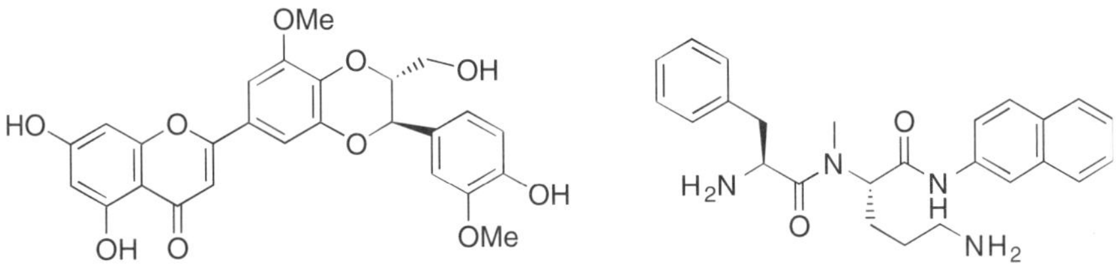

5′-Methoxyhydnocarpin D

Naphthyl Dipeptide

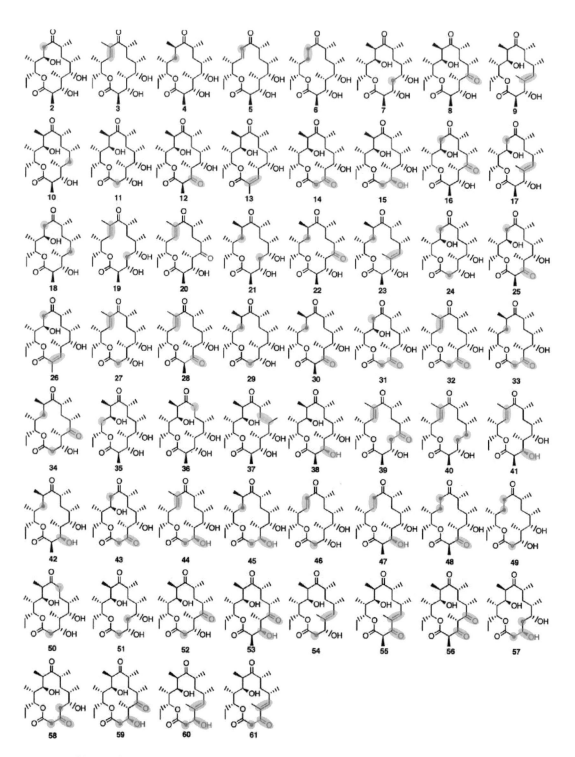

A library of erythronolide macrolide variants by reprogramming the DEBS synthase domains. (From McDaniel et al. [1999], with permission.)

chapter 16

New Molecules

With the new targets that will be identified and validated by bacterial genomics, the sets of screens that allow for high throughput and automation, and the increasing sophistication of analysis of classes of gene products such as those which are essential for virulence and persistence in animals but not for growth on culture plates, there is evidence that dozens to hundreds of new targets, many of currently unknown function, will be available in the near future. Automated high-throughput screens can deliver the capacity to assay as many as 100,000 compounds per week, such that a typical inventory of a million compounds could be run in less than three months.

The limiting resource for antibacterial drug discovery and development in this context may be the sources of new molecules that can serve as initial hits as ligands and/or inhibitors of new target proteins or RNA sequences. Historically, natural products have been a rich source of bioactive compounds, in particular antibiotics, and they remain one starting point, although there is the question of whether valuable new classes of natural products, e.g., new antibiotics, are still undiscovered after 50 years of exhaustive natural product isolation efforts. The second main approach over the past decade has been to make libraries of synthetic compounds. We will briefly take up the subject of synthetic compound libraries, then turn to new approaches with natural products as antibiotic candidates.

Chemical libraries and the chemical genetic approach

We have noted in earlier chapters that synthetic compounds have been the source of three classes of antibiotics in contemporary therapeutic use: the sulfa drugs, the quinolones, and the oxazolidinones. There is reason to believe that new molecules can be crafted that will be useful against novel targets, where the probability of preexisting gene-based resistance is low, especially if the new synthetic structures have not been seen in nature. For example, the inhibition of class B metallo-β-lactamases by biphenyltetrazoles fits this paradigm.

One approach to synthetic compound discovery and development is to use mechanistic and structural knowledge, e.g., from structural genomics programs, to build architectures that are designed to dock onto a predicted or known binding site on a target protein. A variant is to pursue this strategy in a library format, in which a few hundred molecules are made in a focused library. For example, this approach has been followed with heterocyclic libraries (see Chang et al., 1999) intended to bind to the adenine sites in ATP-utilizing enzymes, notably against protein kinases, but translatable to any ATP-hydrolyzing enzyme such as DNA gyrase or bacterial Hsp90 (discussed in chapters 6 and 15).

A more ambitious goal would be to assume that chemists can produce enough architectural and functional group diversity in large libraries of synthetic compounds that there is reasonable probability that a ligand can be found for any protein. If such a ligand could be optimized for specificity and potency such that one could approach the limit that only the single target protein would be inhibited in a cellular context, then one would have arrived at the actualization of chemical genetics. Schreiber has used the term chemical genetics to describe such a context, where a chemical inhibitor would have the specificity and power to interrogate a complex biological system to evaluate the function of the target protein with power equivalent to classical genetic knockout of the encoding gene. Schreiber (2000) has also noted that this kind of objective stands synthetic chemistry precepts upside down, refocusing the goal from target-oriented synthesis, where one particular synthetic product was made in a series of steps designed to control yield and stereo- and regiochemistry, to diversity-oriented synthesis, where the goals of synthetic schema are to produce as many compounds as possible with maximal diversification.

Combinatorial chemistry represents this approach and has revolutionized the practices in medicinal chemistry, including antibiotic synthetic chemistry, with high-throughput parallel or "mix and split" technologies to increase dramatically the number of organic compounds accessible in short periods of time. The quality of combinatorial chemical libraries depends on several features, including numbers of molecules, purity, and diversity. A central parameter for medicinal chemistry applications has been to achieve natural product-like complexity in the library molecules. This includes both control of architecture, in three dimensions, and the density of functional groups, especially those which mimic natural product ligands for protein and nucleic acid target interactions. In some contexts one may want rigidly controlled, three-dimensional structures, while for blocking protein-protein interactions one may want flat molecules with distributed functionality. In all cases the larger the number of diverse molecules in the library the more likely a positive hit will be garnered in any assay.

Recent reviews by Arya et al. (2001, 2002) summarize some of the approaches used to build diverse libraries around different templates that fix architecture. For example, the Schreiber group produced a tetracyclic template for library synthesis, starting from the natural product shikimic acid and ending with a library estimated at two million members (Tan et al., 1998; Tan et al., 1999) (Fig. 16.1A). A second approach, also from the Schreiber group (Lee et al., 1999), used ring-closing metathesis strategies to create macrocyclic templates

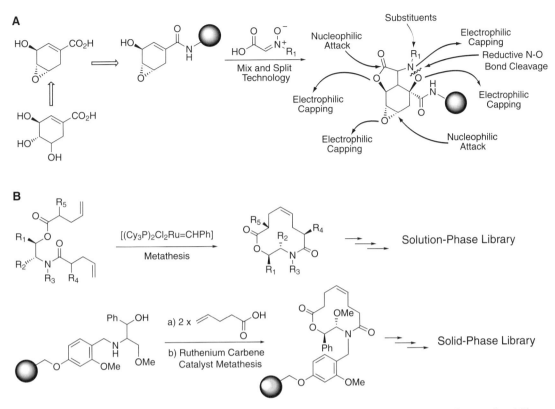

Figure 16.1 Examples of approaches to templated libraries: (A) tetracyclic templated libraries; (B) macrocyclic templated libraries. (From Arya et al. [2001], with permission.)

with controlled complexity and diversity (**Fig. 16.1B**). In each of these approaches, high functional group diversity was introduced in scaffolds of distinct architectures and complexities. These presage the kinds of approaches that are likely to create natural product-like properties in synthetic combinatorial libraries. These approaches can use biomimetic reactions to approximate final products that are analogs of natural products but with a great diversity of substituents not found in nature. For example, Shair and colleagues (Lindsley et al., 2000) have described approaches to benzoxanthenone scaffolds such as those found in the natural product carpanone, and Nicolaou et al. (2000a, 2000b, 2000c) have assembled natural product-like combinatorial libraries derived from benzopyrans.

Lists of libraries built from particular scaffolds, e.g., those known to inhibit proteases, kinases, phosphatases, and other enzymes, are available (e.g., Dolle, 2000), and these can be tested against new bacterial examples. Also, Dolle notes libraries of special relevance to antibacterial efforts, including some designed against the Erm rRNA methyltransferases (chapter 10) and against multidrug resistance pumps (chapter 9). Hall et al. (2001) have summarized the literature on chemical libraries recently built to mimic natural product templates and scaffolds, including cycloserine, chalcones, epothilone, and vancomycin. All indications are that focused combinational chemistry libraries will continue to be prepared. Trias (Trias, 2001) has described combinatorial chemistry approaches for optimization of activity in expanded-spectrum oxazolidinone antibiotic candidates and also for converting screening hits to leads for inhibition of peptide deformylase (chapter 15).

Wess et al. (2001) have noted that generation of leads is only a starting point for medicinal chemistry and delineate several of the tasks and bottlenecks in medicinal chemistry efforts in drug development that would apply to development of new antibacterial agents. Thus, the discovery of new targets and initial screening hits against these targets, described in this and the preceding chapter, will not in and of themselves result in new drugs or shorten time to approval unless the lead optimization and preclinical and clinical development cycles can also be accelerated in time and in efficiency.

Libraries of natural products by combinatorial biosynthetic strategies

The availability of genome sequences from many microbes that produce natural products has begun to allow prediction of and testing for the genes encoding the enzymes of secondary natural product metabolic pathways, especially those of therapeutic interest. In chapters 12 and 13 we outlined the general principles for the biosynthetic assembly lines of polyketides (PKs) and nonribosomal peptides (NRPs); these are ones where combinatorial biosynthesis has been widely practiced already in nature. We will summarize below some recent efforts on reprogramming of these assembly lines and of the post-assembly-line enzymatic tailoring reactions to create new variants of natural products, "unnatural natural products." Carrying out combinatorial reprogramming on a large scale will require large numbers of polyketide synthase (PKS) and nonribosomal peptide synthetase (NRPS) gene clusters, an understanding of the rules for cutting and pasting to maximize autonomously folding modules, and rapid methods for gene shuffling. Progress is being made on all three of these fronts. Strohl (2001) reported that 115 natural product biosynthetic gene clusters are known, with about half representing type I and type II PKS clusters. Of the 115 clusters, 70 were from streptomycetes. Efforts have been made to find oligonucleotide probe sequences that have high utility for cloning both bacterial and fungal (Nicholson et al., 2001) PKS gene clusters to increase the number of starting clusters. It has been estimated that as few as 1% of the microbes in soil and aquatic environments may be culturable in the laboratory. To avoid missing the 99% of microbial diversity for antibiotic biosynthetic genes, the cloning of 50- to 150-kb inserts from nonculturable organism samples has progressed. DNA-shuffling techniques to accelerate combinatorial evolution between clusters have been reduced to practice, for example, by the scientific team at Maxygen (Zhang et al., 2002).

Combinatorial biosynthesis in polyketides

With the availability of the erythromycin biosynthetic cluster over the past decade, this system has been the workhorse for developing and refining genetic reprogramming of the enzymatic machinery, with initial focus on the three-subunit deoxyerythronolide B synthase (DEBS) assembly line (Fig. 12.16) for production of the 14-membered macrolide 6-DEB. Mutations in almost every catalytic module (ketosynthase [KS], acyltransferase, ketoreductase, dehydratase, enoylreductase) of the DEBS1, 2, and 3 subunits have been engineered and the altered product profiles analyzed. **Figure 16.2** summarizes the changes implemented at positions 2-13 of the macrolactone scaffold of 6-DEB (Katz, 1997; Strohl, 2001).

The redox state of any β-carbon in any of the six elongation cycles can be controlled, as can the use of malonyl or methylmalonyl at any extender site. The loading module has been bypassed through a mutation to inactivate the KS domain in the loading module and exogenous feeding acyl diketide thioesters. One can also fuse different loading modules to alter the starter units that get incorporated.

To make a start toward combinatorial reprogramming, the group at Kosan Biosciences has used a three-plasmid system to mix one mutation on each of the three DEBS subunits and reported a library of some 50 macrolactone variants (McDaniel et al., 1999).

While the normal erythronolide ring size is 14 atoms, the tylosin assembly line has one more module and produces a 16-membered lactone. Sixteen-membered versions of the erythronolide skeleton have been detected in a stuttering mutant of *Saccharapolyspora erythraea* (Wilkinson et al., 2000) and also by feeding a triketide in place of a diketide to the inactivated loading module of the DEBS assembly line (**Fig. 16.3**) (Kinoshita et al., 2001), suggesting altered macro ring size is achievable by thioesterase domain cyclization at the C terminus of the DEBS3 subunit. While the technologies have been intensively implemented only in the DEBS system to date, there is reason to believe these approaches will be generalizable to reengineering of other PKS assembly lines, in combinatorial fashions.

The subsequent tailoring reactions on the erythronolide macrolactone involve two cytochrome P450-type hydroxylases, EryF and EryK, introducing hydroxyls at C_6 and C_{12}, and bis glycosylation at C_3 (with TDP-L-mycarose) and

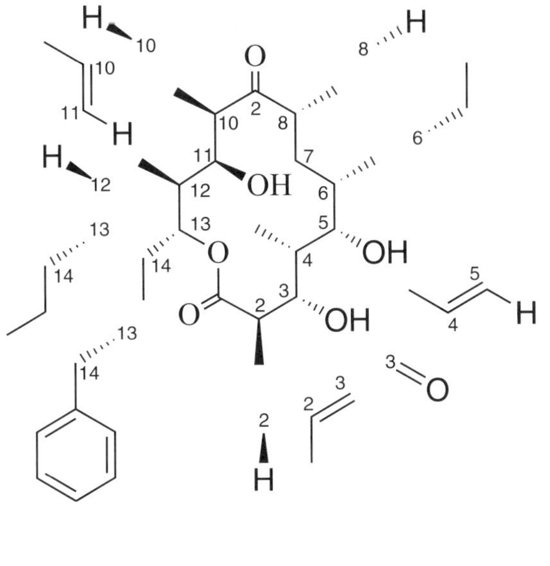

Figure 16.2 Changes that have been engineered in the 6-DEB macrolide scaffold. (From Strohl [2001], with permission.)

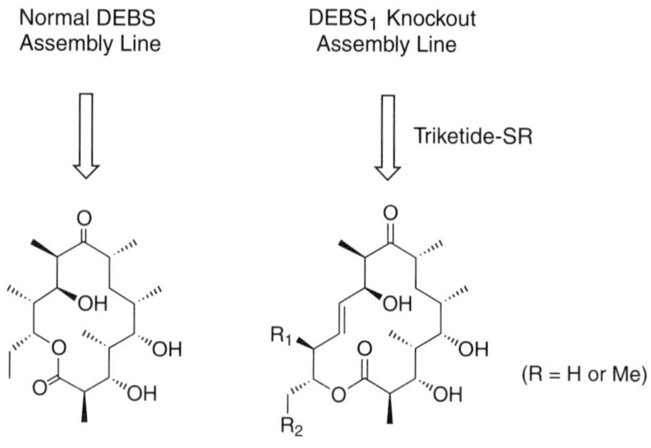

Normal DEBS
Assembly Line

DEBS₁ Knockout
Assembly Line

Figure 16.3 Routes to altered macrolactone ring size in the DEBS assembly line.

C_5 (with TDP-D-desosamine) (see Fig. 12.19). Many cytochrome P450 hydroxylases exist, and it may be that some will hydroxylate the 14-membered lactone with altered regiospecificity. The combinatorial possibilities for glycosylation can operate at two levels: TDP-deoxysugar biosynthesis and then action of the glycosyltransferases (Gtfs). The pathways from the common nucleotide diphosphosugar TDP-glucose to TDP-D-desosamine and to TDP-L-mycarose are known and individual enzymes performing the net deoxygenations at C_6, C_4, and C_2 are identified, as are those epimerizing C_5 and reductively aminating C_3 (see Fig. 12.20).

It is possible to knock out one or more of these genes and to replace them with other enzymes to manipulate the TDP-deoxyhexose pathways in vitro and in vivo. For example, in the *Streptomyces venezuelae* biosynthetic pathway to pikromycin, a 3-keto macrolide lacking the 3-α-mycarosyl substituent (**Fig. 16.4A**) (see Xue and Sherman, 2001, for review), the desosamine biosynthetic genes are in the PKS cluster.

To establish that the TDP-desosamine pathway could be reprogrammed, the *desI* gene was knocked out and replaced with the *calH* gene from the calicheamycin biosynthetic pathway, to produce a 4-amino-6-deoxy TDP-hexose novel intermediate (**Fig. 16.4B**). This was recognized by the downstream enzymes, the new amino group N-acetylated (for self-protection?), and the novel sugar transferred either to the C_3 of the 12-ring macrolide or to the C_5 of the 3-keto-14-membered macrolide to produce two new antibiotics (Zhao et al., 1999). If CalH is omitted, then the D-quinovose sugar is installed at C_5 (Borisova et al., 1999). These results set the stage for combinatorial manipulation of TDP-deoxysugar intermediate structures. They also indicate that DesVII, the pikromycin glycosyltransferase, shows enough promiscuity that it will transfer deoxysugar analogs of the normal TDP-hexose substrates. McDaniel and colleagues (Tang and McDaniel, 2001; Rodriguez and McDaniel, 2001) have reconstructed the TDP-desosamine biosynthetic pathway in a heterologous host and established that several of the compounds in the library shown in Fig. 16.12 can thereby be glycosylated to gain antibiotic activity. Many Gtfs from PKS clusters could be cloned and tested for promiscuity and permissivity both toward altered aglycone macrolide structures, such as the library of Fig. 16.3, and toward variant TDP-deoxyhexoses and -aminohexoses.

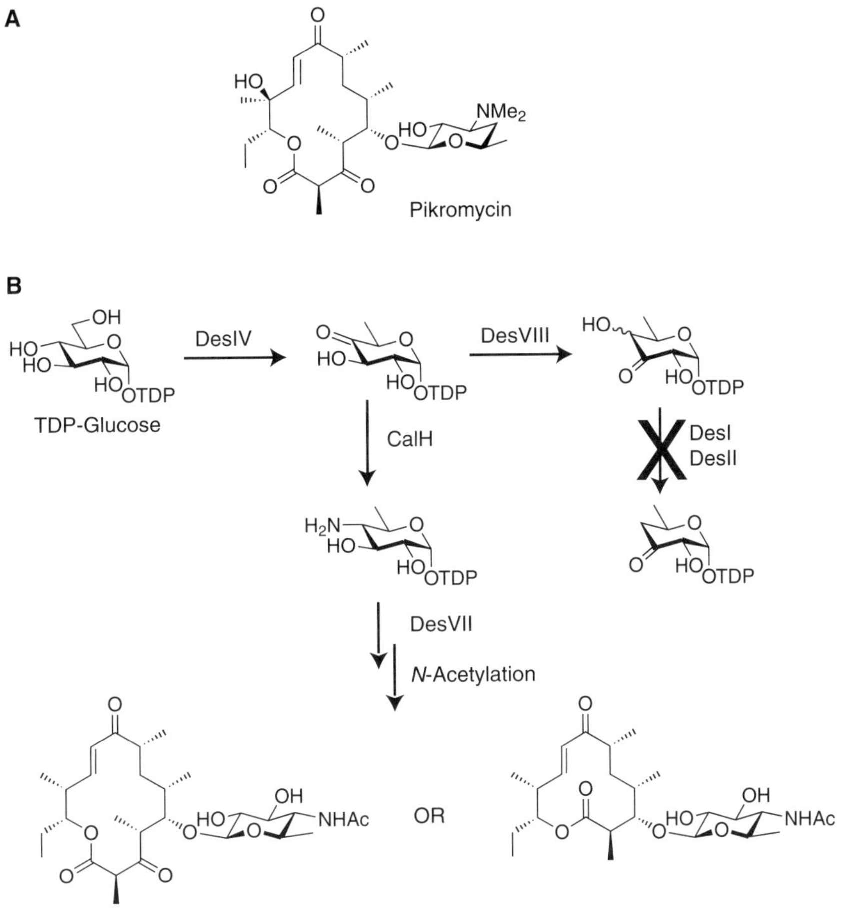

Figure 16.4 Manipulation of the TDP-deoxyhexose pathways in *S. venezuelae*: (A) lack of desosamine moiety when the 3-position remains as a ketone in pikromycin; (B) replacement of *desI* by *calH* to alter the sugars on the macrolide scaffold.

In sum, one can presently vary macrolide ring size, macrolide starter units, substituent identity and redox state at almost every carbon site on the macrolide, deoxy- aminohexose identity, and site of glycosylation. By such combinatorial strategies it should be feasible to generate biosynthetic libraries of a few tens of thousands of novel macrolides at a time.

One of the practical limitations is the linear length of large PKS assembly lines. They get distributed into multiple subunits (e.g., DEBS1, 2, and 3). Then the subunits have to find each other and orient for directed transfer of the growing chain directionally between subunits. This can be of value in combinatorial reprogramming, provided one can decipher the logic by which subunits find each other and line up. Khosla and colleagues (Gokhale et al., 1999) have made a start by discovering the existence of C-terminal and N-terminal linker regions in the DEBS subunits and demonstrating their portability. If this strategy is generalizable, libraries of PKS modules could be constructed with appropriate linkers to direct module-module interaction and increase the probability of efficient chain transfer and growth across module and subunit interfaces in libraries of engineered modules.

Combinatorial biosynthesis in NRPs and in NRP-PK hybrids

NRPS gene clusters are found in both bacteria and fungi. Dozens of cluster sequences have been reported and hundreds of clusters are likely to be sequenced within the near future, producing the parts lists for swapping of modules and testing of combinatorial biosynthetic approaches to new peptide antibiotics. One of the attractive features of NRPS natural product peptides is the great diversity of amino acid (and hydroxy acid) monomers that are incorporated, >100, compared to the limit of 20 proteinogenic amino acids in ribosomal peptides.

Biosynthetic genes for nonproteinogenic amino acid monomers have been found embedded in NRPS clusters, such as four enzymes for 4-OH-phenyl-glycine and another four open reading frames for $3,5-(OH)_2$-phenylglycine biosynthesis (**Fig. 16.5**) in the vancomycin and teicoplanin class of glycopeptide producers (Hubbard et al., 2000; Hubbard and Walsh, 2002; van Wageningen et al., 1998). These genes appear to be moved as a cassette to other organisms that make these unusual amino acids, suggesting a strategy to import this biosynthetic capacity into any cluster. If cassettes of tandem genes are the rule for nonproteinogenic amino acid construction, the ability to move such cassettes will aid in reprogramming efforts for NRPS assembly lines.

Marahiel and colleagues (for reviews, see Doekel and Marahiel, 2001; Konz and Marahiel, 1999) have begun to work through practical rules for combination of NRPS catalytic domains and modules and have reconstituted hybrid di- and trimodular systems, with chain-cleaving thioesterase domains placed at the ends of these reconstructed assembly lines. These successes raise the prospect for combinatorial approaches to module swaps, insertions, and deletions to increase or decrease the number of amino acids incorporated into the growing chain and change their identity at specific sites. The coding logic for amino acid recognition by the adenylation (A) domains of NRPS assembly lines has been deciphered (Stachelhaus et al., 1999), allowing in situ reprogramming to be undertaken. For assembly lines that generate D-amino acid residues via epimerization domains, such as the D,D,L,D,D,L,L-configuration for the vancomycin heptapeptide aglycone, epimerase domains could be inactivated to combinatorialize the L- or D-configuration at any site. Presumably the condensation (C) domains in such assembly lines that are downstream of E domains are D-specific (see Hubbard and Walsh, 2002). These could be used in modular reassembly as general reagents for making D,L-, L,D-, and D,D- peptide bonds in chain elongations.

As in PKS assembly lines, there are tailoring enzymes in NRPS assembly lines, some embedded in *cis* and some acting in *trans*. For example, the *N*-methyltransferases (MT domains) that produce the seven *N*-methyl amino acids in the cyclic undecapeptide cyclosporin A are found in four-domain (C-A-MT-PCP [peptidyl carrier protein]) elongation modules (**Fig. 16.6A**), suggesting the portability of peptide bond formation and *N*-methylation activity at any NRPS site. Some of the most intriguing natural products have five-ring sulfur and oxygen heterocycles, thiazoles, and oxazoles, which arise from cyclization of cysteinyl-SH and seryl-OH side chains on the preceding peptide bond carbonyl (**Fig. 16.6B**), catalyzed by cyclization (Cy) domains that are variants of the peptide bond-forming condensation domains (Cy-A-PCP modules). These may be

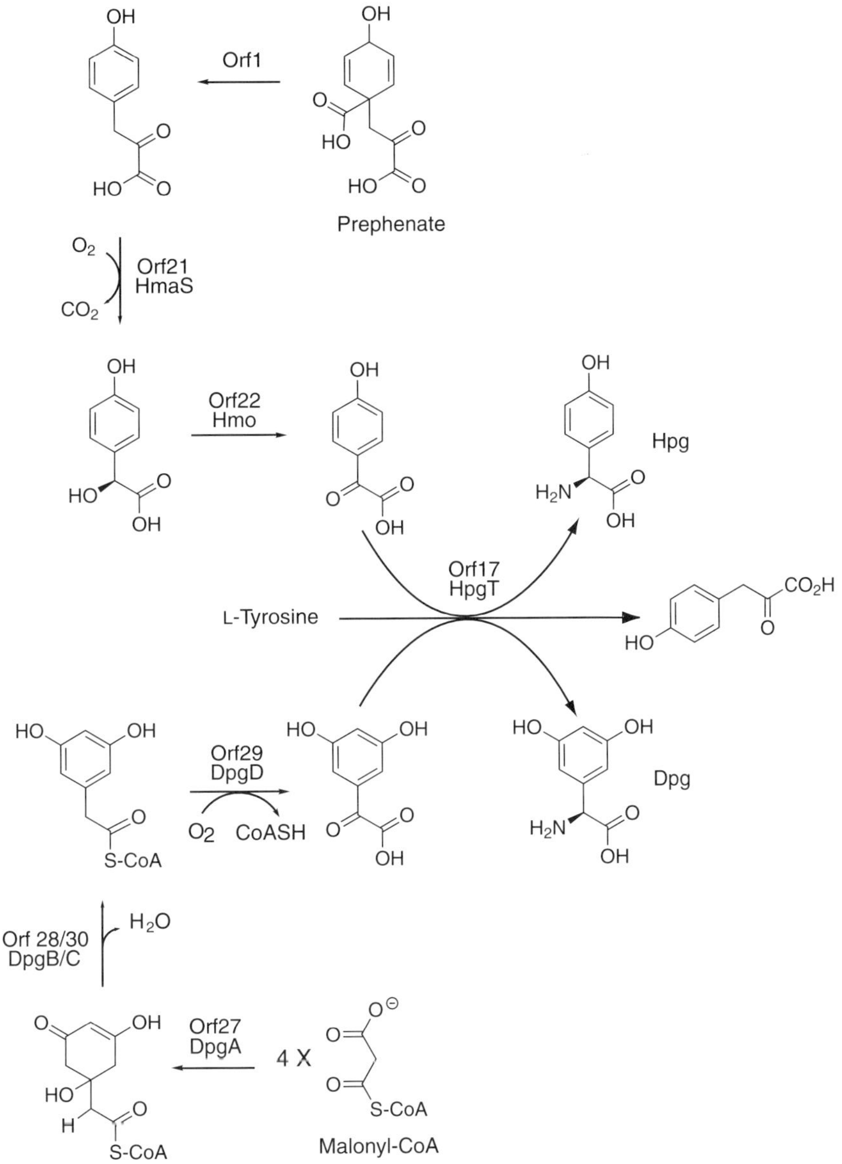

Figure 16.5 Four-enzyme cassettes for de novo generation of the 4-OH-PheGly and 3,5-(OH)$_2$-PheGly monomers for vancomycin and teicoplanin biosynthesis.

portable elements in combinatorial approaches to NRPS assembly lines. The tailoring enzymes for NRP molecules can be oxidoreductases, hydroxylases, and glycosyltransferases.

Among the most useful natural products are hybrids of PKs and NRPs, including bleomycin, epothilone, and pristinamycin II (**Fig. 16.7**). About a dozen hybrid PKS-NRPS assembly lines have now been sequenced (see Doekel and Marahiel, 2001; Du et al., 2001; Hubbard and Walsh, 2002), revealing the logic of how these modules and domains are intermingled.

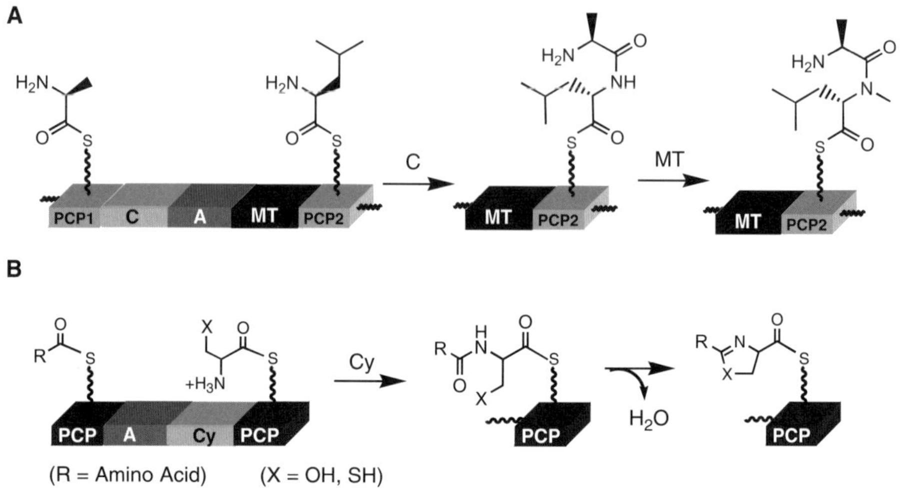

Figure 16.6 Tailoring enzymes embedded in *cis* in NRPS Assembly Lines: (A) *N*-methyltransferases; (B) cyclization domains to make oxazoline and thiazoline rings.

Reconstitution of PKS-NRPS and NRPS-PKS interfaces has been achieved with purified components in vitro to establish the recognition patterns of the the KS, C, and Cy catalytic, chain-elongation domains (Miller et al., 2002; Patel and Walsh, 2001), as a prelude to combinatorial strategies that would make novel hybrid PK-NRP-PK structures. For example, the pristinamycin II component (Fig. 16.8) of the antibiotic Synercid is an NRP-PK-NRP-PK hybrid. The assembly line is proposed to have 10 modules for selecting the four amino acid (Gly, Ser, Pro, Val) and six (methyl)malonyl-CoA monomers (**Fig. 16.8**). In the putative module arrangement, Gly will be activated by module 4 and the Ser-Pro-Val tripeptide fashioned by modules 9, 10, and 1. The first PK segment would

Figure 16.7 NRP-PK hybrid molecules: bleomycin A2, epothilone D, and pristinamycin IIA.

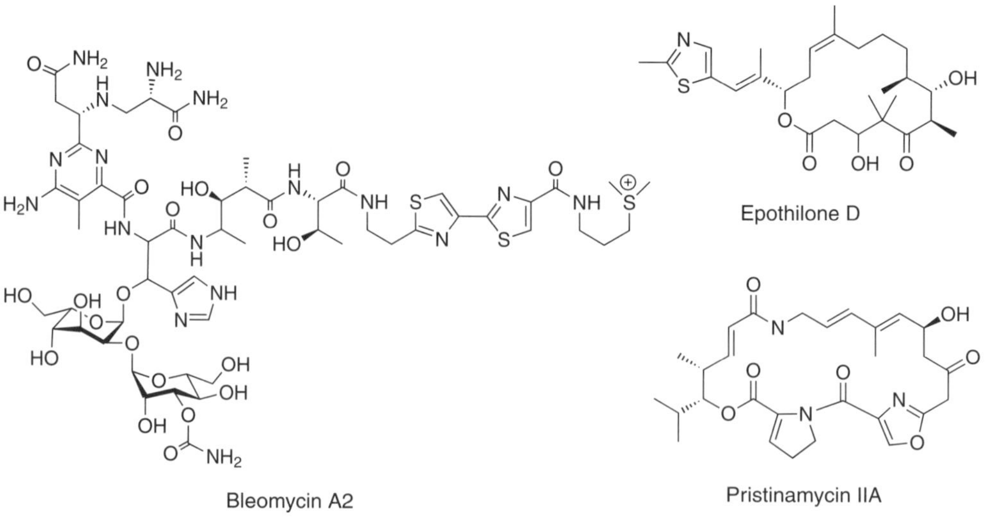

Bleomycin A2

Epothilone D

Pristinamycin IIA

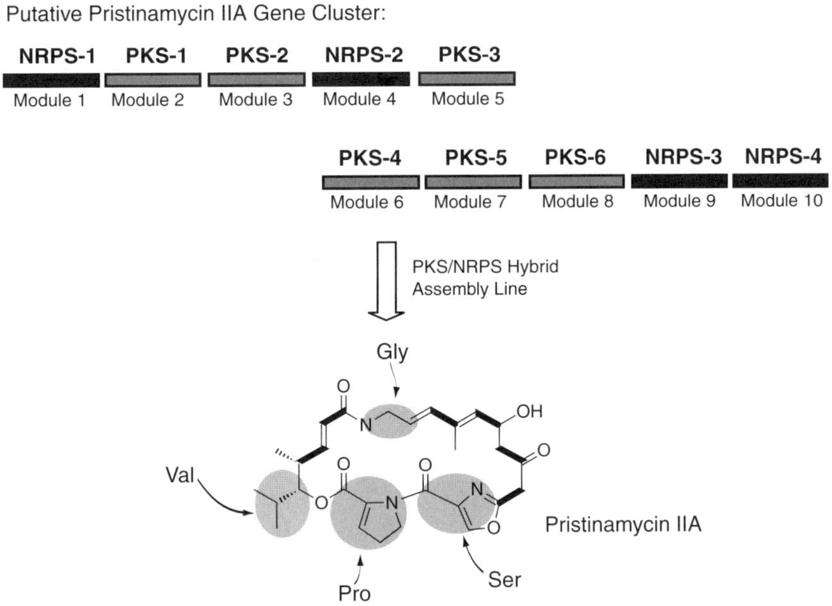

Putative Pristinamycin IIA Gene Cluster:

Figure 16.8 Pristinamycin IIA is a product of a putative hybrid assembly line of NRPS-PKS-NRPS-PKS modules.

arise from modules 2 and 3. After glycine insertion, a stretch of four PKS modules, modules 5 to 8, would assemble the nine-carbon PK chain portion preceding the Ser-Pro-Val tripeptide unit. All four PK-NRP-PK-NRP modules could in principle be manipulated separately and combinatorially.

In analogy to the macrolactone antibiotics noted above, some of the NRPs are also hydroxylated and glycosylated in post-assembly-line enzymatic maturation steps. The same approaches to test altered specificity of cytochrome P450 hydroxylases and the two stages of glycosyl group variation, TDP-deoxyhexose pathway manipulation and glycosyltransferase replacement and/or specificity relaxation, can also be undertaken. For example, the enzymes in the pathway converting TDP-glucose to TDP-L-epivancosamine have all been characterized (Chen et al., 2000), and replacement or deletion strategies as described above in the pikromycin system can be attempted to alter sugar identity. It is likely that one could use a library of TDP-deoxyhexoses and -aminohexoses and a battery of glycosyltransferases (Losey et al., 2001; Solenberg et al., 1997) to decorate a library of peptide aglycones and create new combinations. As an example, the aglycone of vancomycin has been glycosylated with TDP-glucose and then TDP-L-epivancosamine by two Gtfs, one from the vancomycin cluster (GtfB) and one from the chloroeremomycin cluster (GtfC) (**Fig. 16.9**) to produce the unnatural glycopeptide epivancosamycin. The same two Gtfs working on the aglycone of teicoplanin produce a novel teicoplanin analog.

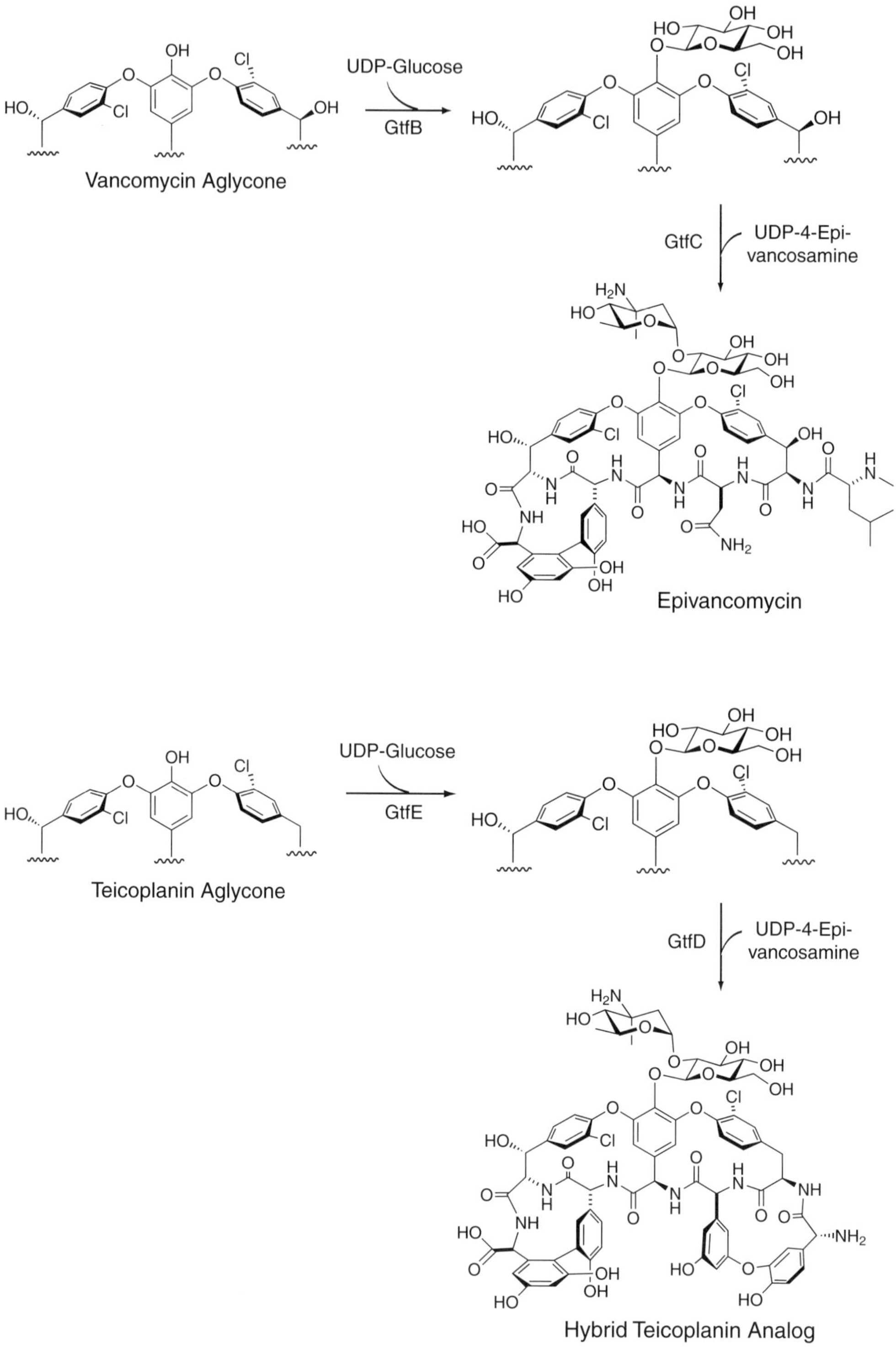

Figure 16.9 Enzymatic biosynthesis of hybrid glycopeptides in the teicoplanin and vancomycin class by combinations of TDP-sugars and glycosyltransferase swaps.

Problem pathogens

- Methicillin-resistant *Staphyloccus aureus* (MRSA)
- Vancomycin-resistant *Staphylococcus aureus* (VRSA)
- Vancomycin-resistant enterococci (VRE)
- Multidrug-resistant *Streptococcus pneunomiae*
- Multidrug-resistant *Mycobacterium tuberculosis*
- Multidrug-resistant *Salmonella* (e.g., *Salmonella* sp. strain DT104 resistant to ampicillin, chloramphenicol, streptomycin, sulfonamides, trimethoprim, tetracycline, kanamycin, ciprofloxacin)

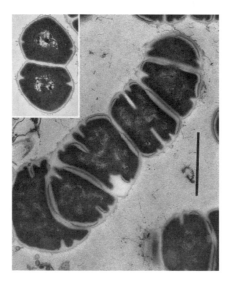

Problem pathogens. Electron micrograph of vancomycin-resistant enterococci exposed to vancomycin, with inset of a control cell grown in trypticase soy broth alone. Bar = 1 μm. (From Lorian and Fernandes [1997], with permission.)

Contexts and Challenges for the Use of New Antibiotics

The efforts described in chapters 15 and 16, to identify and evaluate new molecular and cellular targets for antibiotics and create molecular structures in novel classes of antibacterial drugs, will be played out in the context of existing drug-resistant pathogenic bacteria as well as newly emerging infections. The useful lifetimes of current and future antibiotics will depend on the pace of resistance development and therefore on the use patterns of the antibiotics, not only as human therapeutics but also in animal husbandry, agriculture, and horticulture. Unless public health infrastructures are strengthened and global monitoring and pathogen surveillance systems are implemented to guide the choice of antibiotics, we will squander the opportunities to maximize the efficacy of antibiotics.

In the preantibiotic era, some 100 years ago, the three main causes of death in the United States were bacterial infections: tuberculosis, pneumonia, and gastrointestinal (GI) tract infections (Wenzel and Edmond, 2000) accounted for 30% of deaths, and the life expectancy was 47 years (Cohen, 2000). At the end of the 20th century in the developed world, only lower respiratory tract infections still ranked in the top 10 causes of mortality. More specifically, for the eight decades spanning 1900 to 1980, infectious disease mortality in the developed world fell from 797/100,000 to 36/100,000, a tribute to improved public health and the impact of antimicrobial therapeutics. But the 15-year interval from 1981 to 1995 saw a rise in mortality rates from that 36/100,000 to 63/100,000 (life expectancy had increased to 76 years), reflecting changes in the patterns of infectious diseases (Cohen, 2000). The developing world had no such success story, with 13 million infectious disease-related deaths in 1998, almost a quarter of the global total deaths. The big three bacterial diseases—pneumonia, tuberculosis, and diarrheal disease—remained prevalent in the developing world.

The widespread and often inappropriate use of antibiotics has consequences for antibiotic resistance

In addition to the examples listed above and elsewhere in this book, Wenzel and Edmond (2000) caution that epidemiologic studies indicate that the incidence of pneumococcal pneumonia went up in young children, over a 15-year period ending in 1998 in West Virginia, from 21/100,000 to 45/100,000. This increase was not restricted to the pediatric population. The geriatric group, aged 70 to 79 years, also saw a more than doubling of incidence, from 15/100,0000 to 39/100,000. Further, human immunodeficiency virus-infected patients with invasive pneumonia had an almost eight-fold higher mortality rate if the *Streptococcus pneumoniae* was penicillin resistant, reinforcing the deadly interactions between new and old pathogens. Wenzel and Edmond also note that nosocomial infections of the bloodstream have high rates of mortality: 21% in coagulase-negative staphylococcal infections, 25% in *Staphylococcus aureus* infections, and 25% in enterococcal infections. The high incidences of antibiotic resistance in these three deadly pathogens (with 80% being methicillin resistant, 30% methicillin resistant, and 20% vancomycin resistant, respectively) contribute to diminished therapeutic options and bad outcomes. Among the U.S. population of 275 million people, there are 160 million prescriptions and 23 million kilograms of antibiotics (Wenzel and Edmond, 2000) prescribed annually. In 1992, 18% of all the antibacterial prescriptions in the United States were for respiratory tract infections. One outcome was strong selective pressure for drug-resistant *S. pneumoniae*.

Humans have recently been characterized as the world's greatest evolutionary force (Palumbi, 2001), with dramatic alterations in global ecology and the global biosphere as a consequence of human activities and interventions. Among the human-induced acceleration of evolutionary changes are pressures to drive low-frequency antibiotic resistance in natural bacterial populations to high prevalence and rapid acquisition of new resistance traits. Table 1.1 in chapter 1 shows the first year of deployment of antibiotics that have been of major importance in human therapy in the past 70 years and the dates of detection of clinically significant resistance, ranging from a short 1 to 3 years for several generations of β-lactams to 5 years for tetracycline to 30+ years for vancomycin. While the enormous tonnage of antibiotic production is probably the primary human role in priming the evolutionary engine of microbial genetic resistance, Palumbi notes evolutionary pressure from widespread prophylactic use of antibiotics in livestock, accounting for 25 to 50% of all antibiotic production. He also lists suboptimal dosing and failure of patients to complete treatment courses as accelerating evolution, as well as the report (Nyquist et al., 1998) that up to one-third of the antibiotic prescriptions written by U.S. pediatricians are for childhood viral illnesses where no antibacterial response is mechanistically possible. From the perspective of slowing the pace of evolutionary change, Palumbi lists several approaches that fall into three categories: (i) reducing variation in a fitness-related trait; (ii) reducing directional selection; and (iii) reducing heritability of a fitness-related trait. In the first category he recommends combination therapy (e.g., sulfonamide-trimethoprim) and direct observation by the medical system to ensure full dosage, as is the standard in multiple-drug treatment for tuberculosis. For reducing directional selection, he argues that varying the choice of antibiotics, limiting exposure to selection (e.g., withholding the last-resort drugs such as vancomycin from general use), and avoiding broad-spectrum antibiotics will slow microbial evolution. We take up several of these issues below, including the argument for antibiotic combinations and rotations, the mistake of using vancomycin analogs in animal feed, and the liability from widespread use of the very safe, broad-spectrum cephalosporins.

Multidrug resistant pathogens and the challenges for antibacterial therapy

Emerging bacterial diseases

Among the constant challenges in managing bacterial infections are the outbreak of new infectious diseases and the evolution of known commensal and pathogenic bacteria to problem status by acquisition of new resistance determinants. A National Academy of Sciences report, "Emerging and Re-emerging Diseases: Global Microbial Threats in the 1990s," listed infectious diseases that have become recognized since 1973 (Davis and Lederberg, 2000). The bacterial diseases in that category are excerpted in **Table 17.1** and include the toxic shock syndrome forms of *S. aureus*, *Legionella pneumophila*, and peptic ulcer-causing *Helicobacter pylori*. In a world of global travel and change of habitats, new diseases emerge. Once identified, most are currently treatable with existing antibiotics, but that will start the accelerated path to evolution of drug resistance. In companion, for newly emerging viral diseases there may be no available therapies. Cohen (2000) notes that changes in societal patterns contribute to the changing patterns of infectious disease, with a huge increase in the pool of immunocompromised patients arising from organ transplant medicine and the human immunodeficiency virus epidemic. This permits second-rate pathogens (e.g., enterococci and *Pseudomonas aeruginosa*) to cause life-threatening disease. The emergence of huge population centers, with 10 to 20 million inhabitants in large cities without adequate hygiene and sanitation, has been described as a time

Table 17.1 New bacterial diseases since 1973

Year	Agent	Comment
1977	*Legionella pneumophila*	Legionnaires' disease
1977	*Campylobacter jejuni*	Enteric pathogen, global distribution
1981	Toxin-producing strains of *Staphylococcus aureus*	Toxic shock syndrome
1982	*Borrelia burgdorferi*	Lyme disease
1983	*Helicobacter pylori*	Peptic ulcer disease
1989	*Ehrlichia chafeensis*	Human erlichiosis
1992	*Vibrio cholerae* O139	New strain, epidemic cholera
1992	*Bartonella henselae*	Cat-scratch disease; bacillary angiomatosis

bomb for emergence of new infectious diseases (Garrett, 1995). Food-borne disease is likely to be even more prevalent, with more ready-to-eat foods and meals outside the home. We note in sections below transmission of zoonotic pathogens such as *Salmonella enterica* serovar Typhimurium DT104 and *Escherichia coli* O157:H7 through contaminated meat products.

Drug-resistant pathogenic bacteria for the 21st century

As a counterpoint to newly emerging bacterial pathogens is the increase in known pathogens with new arsenals of drug resistance. Some recent outbreaks of drug-resistant bacteria and issues for antibiotic control strategies are raised below. Also, Cohen (2000) has listed the following hospital-acquired and community-acquired infections as key treatment challenges in the first decades of this century (Table 17.2).

MRSA and VRSA

Methicillin-resistant *S. aureus* (MRSA) has been a problematic bacterial pathogen in hospital settings since its widespread dissemination in the 1970s (Hiramatsu et al., 2001). The genome sequence of an MRSA strain (Kuroda et al., 2001) (see chapter 7) has confirmed that an antibiotic resistance island of 21 to 67 kb, SCC_{mec}, produces the phenotype. This SCC has evolved over the four decades since MRSA was first detected in 1961 to capture additional antibiotic resistance genes on stranded plasmids and provide multiple-antibiotic resistance (Hiramatsu et al., 2001). Evolution of pre-MRSA strains to full methicillin resistance has often involved mutation of the MecI repressor or its operator DNA sequence to derepress transcription of the PBP2A (penicillin-binding protein 2A) transpeptidase (chapter 10), which has such low affinity for methicillin and other β-lactams that PBP2A saturation by penicillins is not achievable at clinical drug concentrations.

Even more ominous has been the evolution of *S. aureus* strains to vancomycin resistance (VRSA). MRSA strains were isolated in 1996 in Japan that were also nonresponsive to vancomycin therapy (see Hiramatsu, 1998). Subsequently, other VRSA strains have been isolated from many countries (Hiramatsu et al., 2001), indicating global spread. The genome sequence of the VRSA strain Mu50 has been reported (Kuroda et al., 2001), but the exact mechanism of resistance has not yet been determined. It is not the standard five-gene resistance mechanism of vancomycin-resistant enterococci (VRE) (noted in chapter 10), where D-Ala-D-Lactate peptidoglycan termini with lower affinity to vancomycin are

Table 17.2 Hospital- and community-based problem bacteria

Hospital-acquired infections	Methicillin-resistant *Staphylococcus aureus* Vancomycin-resistant enterococci Vancomycin-resistant staphylococci Cephalosporin-resistant gram-negative bacteria
Community-acquired infections	Multidrug-resistant pneumococci Multidrug-resistant *Salmonella* Multidrug-resistant *Shigella* Fluoroquinolone-resistant gonococci Multidrug-resistant tuberculosis

produced. Instead, VRSA strains appear to elaborate a thickened cell wall and titrate higher amounts of vancomycin by providing excess binding sites for drug (Davies, 1994). There are no good treatments for *S. aureus* strains that are both MRSA and VRSA in phenotype. Hiramatsu et al. (2001) note that MRSA may become the ultimate flora of humans: "It is clear that MRSA has conquered all the available antibiotics and established itself as the ultimate hospital pathogen. Given the genetic flexibility it has demonstrated in the past, it is also clear that it will acquire resistance to any novel antibiotics developed in the future." They concluded that the only path forward is better hospital infection-control procedures.

Pathogenic *E. coli*

Community-acquired urinary tract infections are usually caused by uropathogenic *E. coli*, moving from colonization of GI epithelia into the urinary tract with expression of the surface adhesion molecules (see chapter 9) necessary for attachment to the uroepithelium. Widespread use of the combination trimethoprim-sulfamethoxazole in the United States may have engendered problematic levels of clinical resistance (Manges et al., 2001; Stamm, 2001), with the proportion of organisms that are resistant approaching 20%. This has been foreshadowed by 30 to 50% resistance in parts of Europe, Israel, and Bangladesh (Stamm, 2001). Outbreaks in women in California, Michigan, and Minnesota arose from a single clone (Manges et al., 2001), suggesting widespread distribution of a virulent strain, perhaps through contaminated food sources. An option for subsequent therapy for uropathogenic *E. coli* infections that are also resistant to penicillins and oral cephalosporins as well as tetracycline, conferred by a single plasmid (Sahm et al., 2001; Stamm, 2001), remains the fluoroquinolones, but will perhaps be outflanked by the reports of fluoroquinolone-resistant *E. coli* strains in urinary tract infections.

Multiple factors are probably involved in this resistance, including widespread use of the two-drug combination for many years and its recent use as a prophylactic agent for *Pneumocystis carinii*-induced pneumonia in immunocompromised patients. Use of trimethoprim-sulfonamide combinations in animal feeds also seems likely to have generated drug-resistant pathogenic reservoirs of *E. coli* in animals.

The persistence of drug resistance determinants has been investigated in the sulfonamide-trimethoprim context in United Kingdom, where restrictions were placed on the combination in 1995 and a switch to trimethoprim alone ensued. Prescriptions dropped from 320,000 per year to 77,000 per year between 1991 and 1999 (Enne et al., 2001). In 1999 the prevalence of sulfonamide resistance in clinical isolates in general practice in the United Kingdom were at 46%, compared to 40% in 1991, with acquisition of the genes for drug-insensitive dihydropteroate synthase (chapter 6) on mobile elements as the cause. It is not yet clear whether additional time will lead to a decrease in the prevalence of resistance or whether widespread dissemination of resistance in many genetic contexts of *E. coli* will make the determinants difficult to displace. Enne et al. (2001) noted the continuing sale of 80 tons per year of sulfonamide-trimethoprim in food animals for 1998 as a potential reservoir for maintenance of resistant strains.

This contrasts with the decrease in erythromycin resistance in *Streptococcus pyogenes* in Finland (Seppala et al., 1997), but those were recently evolved clones of *S. pyogenes*, not multidrug resistant, and may not have had time to become fully optimized for survival.

Salmonella serovar Typhimurium DT104

Salmonella serovar Typhimurium DT104 has spread dramatically as a multidrug-resistant pathogen in patients in Western Europe and North America (Threlfall, 2000). This strain was first detected in gulls in the 1980s, became widely distributed in cattle in the United Kingdom in the early 1990s, and spread into humans through the food chain. It has been implicated in human infections throughout the European Union, Canada, and the United States. This pathogen is typically resistant to ampicillin, chloramphenicol, streptomycin, sulfonamides, and tetracycline, via a gene cassette containing genes encoding the ANT (3″)-1a aminoglycoside nucleotidyltransferase and the CARB-2 (PSE-1) β-lactamase that flank chloramphenicol acetyltransferase and tetracycline-resistance genes (Briggs and Fratamico, 1999). Isolates with additional resistance to trimethoprim (a drug-resistant dihydrofolate reductase mutant) and ciprofloxacin (Asp87 mutants in GyrB subunit) have been reported for DT104 strains (see Threlfall, 2000) (**Fig. 17.1**), making these strains particularly problematic with their full arsenal of antibiotic resistance. Four of 11 patients hospitalized with such infections in Denmark in 1998 did not respond to ciprofloxacin, with two fatalities (Molbak et al., 1999). This case is emblematic of drug resistance in zoonotic pathogens, where the use of antibacterial drugs in livestock and food animals ensures a shortened lifetime for such antibiotic use in humans. Threlfall (2000) has noted that the acquisition of ciprofloxacin resistance in serovar Typhimurium DT104 infections of humans in the United Kingdom followed the licensing of a ciprofloxacin analog, enterofloxacin, for veterinary use in late 1993, where it has gained widespread use as a veterinary prophylactic agent. He noted that enterofloxacin has recently been approved by the U.S. Food and Drug Administration for use in pigs and cattle. This may presage the zoonotic fluoroquinolone-resistant spread of this pathogen in humans in the United States and calls out forcefully for a different approach to both surveillance and licensing of analogs of life-saving categories of human antibiotics. The genomic sequence of two *Salmonella enterica* serovars has been determined: for serovar Typhimurium LT2 (McClelland et al., 2001) and for serovar Typhimurium CT18 (Parkhill et al., 2001), the former causing gastroenteritis, the latter causing typhoid fever.

Figure 17.1 Antibiotic resistance phenotypes of multidrug-resistant *Salmonella enterica* serovar typhimurium DT104.

Ampicillin	Trimethoprim
Chloramphenicol	Tetracycline
Streptomycin	Kanamycin
Sulfonamide	Ciprofloxacin

Medical consequences of antibiotic use in agriculture

While hospitals are clearly fertile arenas for selection of antibiotic-resistant pathogenic bacteria, a complementary arena that has been understood for decades is the use of antibiotics in animal feed, for growth promotion and infectious disease prophylaxis (see Witte, 1998). The spread of resistance genes on transposons and plasmids (Davis and Lederberg, 2000; Levy, 1998) means that food animals are significant reservoirs for transmission of zoonotic pathogens, as detailed above for the spread of multidrug-resistant *Salmonella* serovar Typhimurium DT 104 in meat products and sulfonamide-trimethoprim-resistant strains of *E. coli*.

Three other examples serve to generalize the point. The first deals with an analog of the glycopeptide antibiotic vancomycin, avoparcin, used widely in animal feed. In 1994, 1,000 times as much avoparcin (24,000 kg) was used in Denmark for agricultural feedstock as vancomycin (24 kg) in human therapeutics. The same kind of five-gene *vanRSHAX* (see chapter 10) resistance to avoparcin occurs in animals and can be transmitted zoonotically. In Australia in 1992 to 1996 there was a similar 1,000-fold excess of avoparcin use for animal husbandry compared with vancomycin use for human disease (Witte, 1998). This seems like a tremendously risky policy and one that virtually ensures the selection and maintenance of resistance to a particularly consequential class of life-saving antibiotic. Indeed, the European Union went on to ban avoparcin use in animal feed.

For life-threatening enterococcal infections that are thus resistant to vancomycin, the pristinamycin combination (chapter 4) has recently been approved. These are members of the streptogramin family, and resistance showed up immediately in some patients in Germany (see Witte, 1998), most probably reflecting a significant resistance gene reservoir in animals due to 20 years of prior use of the related streptogramin virginiamycin (chapter 11) in animal feed. The use of important classes of human antibiotics, or potential human antibiotics, in animal feed can place severe constraints on the subsequent lifetime and utility of the class in human therapeutics. They compromise the future.

The third example arises from fluoroquinolone use in infectious disease prophylaxis (120 tons in animals, 800 tons in humans annually) in the poultry industry (Falkow and Kennedy, 2001; Gaunt and Piddock, 1996), which has selected for fluoroquinolone-resistant strains of *Campylobacter jejuni*. Zoonotic transfers are the suspected source of diarrheal disease in humans caused by *C. jejuni* (2.4 million cases in the United States yearly [Engberg et al., 2001]), paralleling the fluoroquinolone-resistant *Salmonella* disease. Prior to use of quinolones in poultry farming, such drug-resistant *Campylobacter* were not seen in humans without prior fluoroquinolone exposure (Gaunt and Piddock, 1996; Witte, 1998). But from 1991 to 1998 ciprofloxacin resistance in *Campylobacter* went from 0 to 13.6% (Cohen, 2000).

This is not exactly a new problem. The Swann Committee in the United Kingdom in 1969 clearly recommended that antibiotics used in human therapy not be used as growth promoters in animals. This recommendation includes classes of drugs, not just specific molecules, or else the avoparcin/vancomycin loopholes get continuously recreated. A World Health Organization workshop

28 years later in 1997 reiterated these recommendations forcefully (see Witte, 1998). The conclusions were not new, but three decades of harm had ensued. Nor is the situation conclusively resolved yet in the developed world, as indicated by the Food and Drug Administration's approval of enterofloxacin use in animal feed, as noted above. Indeed, two reports on food-borne antibiotic-resistant *Salmonella* and enterococci in the United States have recently appeared (McDonald et al., 2001; White et al., 2001), along with a scorching companion editorial in the *New England Journal of Medicine* (Gorbach, 2001) titled "Antimicrobial Use in Animal Feed—Time to Stop."

Since antibiotic resistance is clearly a global problem, the lack of policies in the developing world, which is responsible for 25% of world meat production (Witte, 1998), is acutely problematic. A policy of avoidance of any subtherapeutic doses of antimicrobial agents (and forgoing the 4 to 5% improvement in body weight that the drug provides, or else implementing better hygiene to increase livestock health and weight) would seem the most sensible and prudent route to ensure that there will be effective antibiotics left for life-threatening bacterial infections of humans (e.g., see Falkow and Kennedy, 2001). Finally, the problem goes beyond animal husbandry; it is also in the practice of agriculture and horticulture that vast quantities of major classes of human antibiotics, albeit older ones, are sprayed into the environment. In the United States in 1996, 300,000 pounds of streptomycin and oxytetracycline were sprayed on apples and pears as prophylaxis against infections (NAS Workshop on Emerging Infectious Diseases [Davis and Lederberg, 2000]).

Cephalosporins: widepread success leads to overgrowth of resistant organisms with pathogenic potential

It is accepted that antibiotic use will engender resistance in a bacterial population, as examined extensively throughout this book. The widespread use of cephalosporins, as the most widely prescribed, safe, broad-spectrum antibiotics, may paradoxically have contributed not only to the emergence of β-lactam-resistant organisms but also to the selection, propagation, and overgrowth of many problem microbes (Dancer, 2001). Cephalosporin therapy selects for overgrowth both of commensal microbes such as coagulase-negative staphylococci, *P. aeruginosa*, and various enterococci, as well as more aggressive pathogens, such as *Clostridium difficile*, MRSA, penicillin-resistant streptococci, and multidrug-resistant forms of *E. coli* and *Salmonella*.

In hospitals where cephalosporins are the main drug given for antibacterial prophylaxis before surgery, patients may acquire coagulase-negative staphylococci (Dancer, 2001) within hours of admission. These methicillin-resistant bacteria proliferate on and within patients receiving cephalosporins and are prevalent in infections of patients with catheters and prostheses. Analogously, use of cephalosporins in hospitals is associated with overgrowth of and recovery of *P. aeruginosa*, with inherent low sensitivity to β-lactams. They can mutate in the face of continuing therapy to lactam resistance. We noted in chapter 7 that enterococci overgrowth is associated with cephalosporin use, as they colonize GI sites previously populated by drug-sensitive bacteria, now wiped out by the antibiotic. The same argument applies to *C. difficile*, a causative agent for antibiotic-associated diarrhea, as the clostridia take over the niches formerly occupied by drug-sensitive organisms. Dancer (2001) notes that *C. difficile* overgrowth has led to restrictions on cephalosporin use in certain geriatric populations and that extensive use of cephalosporins in the 1980s played a significant part in the emergence and spread of MRSA in London and in Tokyo hospitals as well as the selection for *E. coli* and *Enterobacter cloacae* strains with many mutational variants of the plasmid-encoded β-lactamases. He concludes with the observation: "It is unlikely, however, that we would have seen the prolific rise of multiply-resistant organisms if the cephalosporins had never been introduced. This is because few of the existing agents offered such broad-spectrum activity, with such low toxicity, and consequently would not have been universally prescribed. A greater range of antibiotics would have been utilized, diffusing the selection potential."

These are just the properties one would have wanted ab initio for new antibiotics and raises the clear caution that now and in the future, even with the most promising of antibiotics, low usage of the antibiotic, enforced through physician and patient education, and strictly followed practice guidelines will not only enhance the useful life of that particular antibiotic but also lower the rates of overgrowth of microbes with natural and acquired resistance capabilities. The greater the frequency of antibiotic-resistant strains, the slower will be the re-establishment of sensitive strains as predominant flora on antibiotic withdrawal (Levy, 2001).

Strategies for control of antimicrobial drug resistance

Over the past few years there has been an increase in the understanding of the need for revised antibiotic policies to control antibiotic resistance (Gould, 1999; Kunin, 1997; Levy, 1992; McGowan and Tenover, 1997; Shlaes et al., 1997a, 1997b). This has involved both clinical and epidemiologic approaches to evaluate the main routes and causes for appearance and spread of antimicrobial resistance in hospital organisms and in community settings, with appreciation of population dynamics. Clinical infectious disease specialists have come up with guidelines (Shlaes et al., 1997a) that argue for the four principles of Table 17.3.

The optimal use recommendation needs to integrate all of the observations noted in this chapter and may point toward narrow-spectrum rather than broad-spectrum drugs to treat bacterial infections. To do this effectively will require progression from current empiric therapy where the causative agents are not

Table 17.3 Guidelines for extending the useful life of antimicrobial drugs

1. Optimal use of all antibacterial drugs
2. Selective removal, control, or restriction of classes of antibacterial agents
3. Use of antibacterial drugs in rotation or cyclic patterns
4. Use of combination antibacterial therapy to slow the emergence of resistance

From Shlaes et al. (1997a), with permission.

known until one to two days after the start of treatment. In the near future it may be that multiplexed real-time (e.g., 30 min or less time) PCR analysis will provide definitive diagnosis of pathogenic bacteria and their inventory of known resistance genes to provide an optimized choice of narrow-spectrum antibiotics with minimized risk of resistance induction in the bacterial flora of the patient.

The selective removal and control recommendation requires that patients and physicians change their prescription patterns and expectations to more effectively balance individual patient need with public health requirements that arise from the antibiotic burden in the environment. Again, this will have to be coupled with much better real-time diagnosis of pathogen to guide treatment strategies, including viral versus bacterial etiology in respiratory tract infections.

The recommendation for rotation of antibiotics, particularly in hospital settings, is part of infection control strategy and pathogen surveillance. Gould (1999) summarizes a scheme for antibiotic cycling in sepsis units (**Fig. 17.2**). First-line therapy would be to start with one of the three main β-lactam categories, for example, a β-lactam plus lactamase inhibitor (e.g., the amoxicillin-clavulanate combination). After 2 months the unit would cycle to carbapenem antibiotics as front-line therapy. At the end of the next 2 months, a third- or fourth-generation (expanded-spectrum and higher) cephalosporin would become the front-line choice. Then, one would cycle back to the initial combination choice, completing a three-drug traverse in the 6-month period.

The combination-therapy recommendation, in which two drugs are administered simultaneously to reduce the probability of mutation to clinically significant resistance, is exemplified in the above scheme by the amoxicillin-clavulanate combination. It is in practice in the sulfonamide-trimethoprim combination and in the recently introduced Synercid pair of pristinamycins. Models that evaluate treatment protocols to prevent antibiotic resistance (Bonhoeffer et al., 1997) support combination therapy as the optimal treatment strategy. It is the norm in the treatment of tuberculosis around the world. Drlica (2001) has argued that antibiotic doses should be high enough to block the selective enrichment of resistant mutants. Even though resistant mutants will be generated, if they can be kept as a minuscule fraction of the population by keeping therapeutic concentrations above the mutant selection window, then mutant population expansion will be blocked.

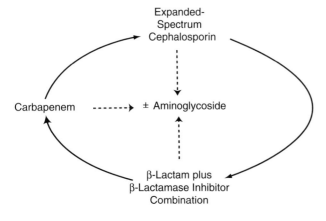

Figure 17.2 Suggestion for antibiotic cycling to treat bacterial sepsis in hospitals. (From Gould [1999], with permission.)

Implementation of successful control measures is ultimately transnational and global. Countries will need to implement the World Health Organization and Centers for Disease Control and Prevention recommendations for an international surveillance system (Williams and Heymann, 1998) for resistant bacterial strains to make rational decisions about what antibiotics to use. These include (i) enhanced surveillance and response to new pathogens; (ii) more applied research; (iii) strengthening of the public health infrastructure; and (iv) provision of training to develop, implement, and evaluate strategies for prevention and control.

In conclusion, increased molecular knowledge about essential bacterial genes and the ability to screen such validated targets with libraries of new synthetic and natural products are likely to turn up new antibiotics against nontraditional bacterial targets. But new antibiotic molecules by themselves will not alter the kinetics of the cycles of resistance development. In fact, wider and more indiscriminate use of new antibiotics could actually shorten the cycle time and push evolution of more aggressive and deadly bacterial pathogens unless the behavioral changes described in Table 17.3 occur and result in the proper valuation of antibiotics as finite resources.

References

Achari, A., D. O. Somers, J. N. Champness, P. K. Bryant, J. Rosemond, and D. K. Stammers. 1997. Crystal structure of the anti-bacterial sulfonamide drug target dihydropteroate synthase. *Nat. Struct. Biol.* **4:**490–497.

Admiraal, S. J., C. T. Walsh, and C. Khosla. 2001. The loading module of rifamycin synthetase is an adenylation-thiolation didomain with substrate tolerance for substituted benzoates. *Biochemistry* **40:**6116–6123.

Allen, N. E. 1985. Nonclassical targets for antibacterial agents. *Annu. Rep. Med. Chem.* **20:**155–162.

Amyes, S. G. B. 2001. *Magic Bullets, Lost Horizons: the Rise and Fall of Antibiotics.* Taylor and Francis, New York, N.Y.

Anborgh, P. H., and A. Parmeggiani. 1991. New antibiotic that acts specifically on the GTP-bound form of elongation factor Tu. *EMBO J.* **10:**779–784.

Andres, C. J., J. J. Bronson, S. V. D'Andrea, M. S. Deshpande, P. J. Falk, K. A. Grant-Young, W. E. Harte, H. T. Ho, P. F. Misco, J. G. Robertson, D. Stock, Y. Sun, and A. W. Walsh. 2000. 4-Thiazolidinones: novel inhibitors of the bacterial enzyme MurB. *Bioorg. Med. Chem. Lett.* **10:**715–717.

Anonymous. 1999. The choice of antibacterial drugs. *Med. Lett.* **41:**95–104.

Anonymous. 2001. The choice of antibacterial drugs. *Med. Lett.* **43:**69–78.

Apfel, C. M., H. Locher, S. Evers, B. Takacs, C. Hubschwerlen, W. Pirson, M. G. Page, and W. Keck. 2001. Peptide deformylase as an antibacterial drug target: target validation and resistance development. *Antimicrob. Agents Chemother.* **45:**1058–1064.

Araoz, R., E. Anhalt, L. Rene, M. A. Badet-Denisot, P. Courvalin, and B. Badet. 2000. Mechanism-based inactivation of VanX, a D-alanyl-D-alanine dipeptidase necessary for vancomycin resistance. *Biochemistry* **39:**15971–15979.

Arthur, M., and P. Courvalin. 1993. Genetics and mechanisms of glycopeptide resistance in enterococci. *Antimicrob. Agents Chemother.* **37:**1563–1571.

Arya, P., D. T. H. Chou, and M. G. Baek. 2001. Diversity-based organic synthesis in the era of genomics and proteomics. *Angew. Chem. Int. Ed.* **40:**339–346.

Arya, P., R. Joseph, and D. T. Chou. 2002. Toward high-throughput synthesis of complex natural product-like compounds in the genomics and proteomics age. *Chem. Biol.* **9:**145–156.

Asahi, Y., Y. Takeuchi, and K. Ubukata. 1999. Diversity of substitutions within or adjacent to conserved amino acid motifs of penicillin-binding protein 2X in cephalosporin-resistant *Streptococcus pneumoniae* isolates. *Antimicrob. Agents Chemother.* **43:**1252–1255.

Bachmann, B. O., R. Li, and C. A. Townsend. 1998. β-lactam synthetase: a new biosynthetic enzyme. *Proc. Natl. Acad. Sci. USA* **95:**9082–9086.

Baizman, E. R., A. A. Branstrom, C. B. Longley, N. Allanson, M. J. Sofia, D. Gange, and R. C. Goldman. 2000. Antibacterial activity of synthetic analogues based on the disaccharide structure of moenomycin, an inhibitor of bacterial transglycosylase. *Microbiology* **146**(Pt. 12)**:**3129–3140.

Baltz, R. H. 1997. Lipopeptide antibiotics produced by *Streptomyces roseosporus* and *Streptomyces fradiae*, p. 415–430. *In* W. R. Strohl (ed.), *Biotechnology of Antibiotics*, 2nd ed. Marcel Dekker Inc., New York, N.Y.

Ban, C., and W. Yang. 1998. Crystal structure and ATPase activity of MutL: implications for DNA repair and mutagenesis. *Cell* **95:**541–552.

Ban, N., P. Nissen, J. Hansen, P. B. Moore, and T. A. Steitz. 2000. The complete atomic structure of the large ribosomal subunit at 2.4 Å resolution. *Science* **289:** 905–920.

Barrett, J. F., and J. A. Hoch. 1998. Two-component signal transduction as a target for microbial anti-infective therapy. *Antimicrob. Agents Chemother.* **42:**1529–1536.

Barriere, J. C., N. Berthaud, D. Beyer, S. Dutka-Malen, J. M. Paris, and J. F. Desnottes. 1998. Recent developments in streptogramin research. *Curr. Pharm. Des.* **4:**155–180.

Barton, D., Sir, K. Nakanishi, O. Meth-Cohn, and U. Sankawa. 1999. *Comprehensive Natural Products Chemistry*. Pergamon, New York, N.Y.

Bayles, K. W. 2000. The bactericidal action of penicillin: new clues to an unsolved mystery. *Trends Microbiol.* **8:**274–278.

Beadle, B. M., I. Trehan, P. J. Focia, and B. K. Shoichet. 2002. Structural milestones in the reaction pathway of an amide hydrolase: substrate, acyl, and product complexes of cephalothin with AmpC beta-lactamase. *Structure* (Cambridge) **10:**413–424.

Belova, L., T. Tenson, L. Xiong, P. M. McNicholas, and A. S. Mankin. 2001. A novel site of antibiotic action in the ribosome: interaction of everninomicin with the large ribosomal subunit. *Proc. Natl. Acad. Sci. USA* **98:**3726–3731.

Benson, T. E., D. J. Filman, C. T. Walsh, and J. M. Hogle. 1995. An enzyme-substrate complex involved in bacterial cell wall biosynthesis. *Nat. Struct. Biol.* **2:**644–653.

Benson, T. E., J. L. Marquardt, A. C. Marquardt, F. A. Etzkorn, and C. T. Walsh. 1993. Overexpression, purification, and mechanistic study of UDP-*N*-acetylenolpyruvylglucosamine reductase. *Biochemistry* **32:**2024–2030.

Bentley, S. D., K. F. Chater, A. M. Cerdeno-Tarraga, G. L. Challis, N. R. Thomson, K. D. James, D. E. Harris, M. A. Quail, H. Kieser, D. Harper, A. Bateman, S. Brown, G. Chandra, C. W. Chen, M. Collins, A. Cronin, A. Fraser, A. Goble, J. Hidalgo,

T. Hornsby, S. Howarth, C. H. Huang, T. Kieser, L. Larke, L. Murphy, K. Oliver, S. O'Neil, E. Rabbinowitsch, M. A. Rajandream, K. Rutherford, S. Rutter, K. Seeger, D. Saunders, S. Sharp, R. Squares, S. Squares, K. Taylor, T. Warren, A. Wietzorrek, J. Woodward, B. G. Barrell, J. Parkhill, and D. A. Hopwood. 2002. Complete genome sequence of the model actinomycete *Streptomyces coelicolor* A3(2). *Nature* **417:** 141–147.

Berger, J. M., S. J. Gamblin, S. C. Harrison, and J. C. Wang. 1996. Structure and mechanism of DNA topoisomerase II. *Nature* **379:**225–232.

Berger-Bachi, B., and M. Tschierske. 1998. Role of Fem factors in methicillin resistance. *Drug Resist. Update* **2:**310–324.

Bernat, B. A., L. T. Laughlin, and R. N. Armstrong. 1997. Fosfomycin resistance protein (FosA) is a manganese metalloglutathione transferase related to glyoxalase I and the extradiol dioxygenases. *Biochemistry* **36:**3050–3055.

Besra, G. S., K. H. Khoo, M. R. McNeil, A. Dell, H. R. Morris, and P. J. Brennan. 1995. A new interpretation of the structure of the mycolyl-arabinogalactan complex of *Mycobacterium tuberculosis* as revealed through characterization of oligoglycosylalditol fragments by fast-atom bombardment mass spectrometry and 1H nuclear magnetic resonance spectroscopy. *Biochemistry* **34:**4257–4266.

Bibb, M. 1996. 1995 Colworth Prize Lecture. The regulation of antibiotic production in *Streptomyces coelicolor* A3(2). *Microbiology* **142**(Pt. 6)**:**1335–1344.

Bibb, M. J., V. Molle, and M. J. Buttner. 2000. Sigma(BldN), an extracytoplasmic function RNA polymerase Sigma factor required for aerial mycelium formation in *Streptomyces coelicolor* A3(2). *J. Bacteriol.* **182:**4606–4616.

Bischoff, D., S. Pelzer, A. Holtzel, G. J. Nicholson, S. Stockert, W. Wohlleben, G. Jung, and R. D. Sussmuth. 2001. The biosynthesis of vancomycin-type glycopeptide antibiotics—new insights into the cyclization steps. *Angew. Chem. Int. Ed.* **40:**1693–1696.

Bonhoeffer, S., M. Lipsitch, and B. R. Levin. 1997. Evaluating treatment protocols to prevent antibiotic resistance. *Proc. Natl. Acad. Sci. USA* **94:**12106–12111.

Borges-Walmsley, M. I., and A. R. Walmsley. 2001. The structure and function of drug pumps. *Trends Microbiol.* **9:**71–79.

Borisova, S. A., L. Zhao, D. H. Sherman, and H. W. Liu. 1999. Biosynthesis of desosamine: construction of a new macrolide carrying a genetically designed sugar moiety. *Org. Lett.* **1:**133–136.

Born, T. L., and J. S. Blanchard. 1999. Structure/function studies on enzymes in the diaminopimelate pathway of bacterial cell wall biosynthesis. *Curr. Opin. Chem. Biol.* **3:**607–613.

Bozdogan, B., and R. Leclercq. 1999. Effects of genes encoding resistance to streptogramins A and B on the activity of quinupristin-dalfopristin against *Enterococcus faecium*. *Antimicrob. Agents Chemother.* **43:**2720–2725.

Braun, V., and K. Hantke. 1974. Biochemistry of bacterial cell envelopes. *Annu. Rev. Biochem.* **43:**89–121.

Breukink, E., I. Wiedemann, C. van Kraaij, O. P. Kuipers, H. Sahl, and B. de Kruijff. 1999. Use of the cell wall precursor lipid II by a pore-forming peptide antibiotic. *Science* **286:**2361–2364.

Briggs, C. E., and P. M. Fratamico. 1999. Molecular characterization of an antibiotic resistance gene cluster of *Salmonella typhimurium* DT104. *Antimicrob. Agents Chemother.* **43:**846–849.

Brock, T. D., M. T. Madigan, J. M. Martinko, and J. Parker. 1994. *Biology of Microorganisms*, 7th ed. Prentice-Hall, Inc., Englewood Cliffs, N.J.

Bronson, J. J., and J. F. Barrett. 2001a. Recent developments in antibacterial research. *Annu. Rep. Med. Chem.* **36:**89–98.

Bronson, J. J., and J. F. Barrett. 2001b. Quinolone, everninomycin, glycylcycline, carbapenem, lipopeptide and cephem antibacterials in clinical development. *Curr. Med. Chem.* **8:**1775–1793.

Brotz, H., G. Bierbaum, K. Leopold, P. E. Reynolds, and H. G. Sahl. 1998. The lantibiotic mersacidin inhibits peptidoglycan synthesis by targeting lipid II. *Antimicrob. Agents Chemother.* **42:**154–160.

Brotz, H., and H. G. Sahl. 2000. New insights into the mechanism of action of lantibiotics-diverse biological effects by binding to the same molecular target. *J. Antimicrob. Chemother.* **46:**1–6.

Bugg, T. D., G. D. Wright, S. Dutka-Malen, M. Arthur, P. Courvalin, and C. T. Walsh. 1991. Molecular basis for vancomycin resistance in *Enterococcus faecium* BM4147: biosynthesis of a depsipeptide peptidoglycan precursor by vancomycin resistance proteins VanH and VanA. *Biochemistry* **30:**10408–10415.

Bugg, T. D., and C. T. Walsh. 1992. Intracellular steps of bacterial cell wall peptidoglycan biosynthesis: enzymology, antibiotics, and antibiotic resistance. *Nat. Prod. Rep.* **9:**199–215.

Bugg, T. D., and P. E. Brandish. 1994. From peptidoglycan to glycoproteins: common features of lipid-linked oligosaccharide biosynthesis. *FEMS Microbiol. Lett.* **119:** 255–262.

Bush, K., and S. Mobashery. 1998. How beta-lactamases have driven pharmaceutical drug discovery. From mechanistic knowledge to clinical circumvention. *Adv. Exp. Med. Biol.* **456:**71–98.

Bush, K., and M. Macielag. 2000. New approaches in the treatment of bacterial infections. *Curr. Opin. Chem. Biol.* **4:**433–439.

Bussiere, D. E., S. W. Muchmore, C. G. Dealwis, G. Schluckebier, V. L. Nienaber, R. P. Edalji, K. A. Walter, U. S. Ladror, T. F. Holzman, and C. Abad-Zapatero. 1998. Crystal structure of ErmC', an rRNA methyltransferase which mediates antibiotic resistance in bacteria. *Biochemistry* **37:**7103–7112.

Bycroft, B. W., C. Maslen, S. J. Box, A. Brown, and J. W. Tyler. 1988. The biosynthetic implications of acetate and glutamate incorporation into (3R,5R)-carbapenam-3-carboxylic acid and (5R)-carbapen-2-em-3-carboxylic acid by *Serratia* sp. *J. Antibiot.* (Tokyo) **41:**1231–1242.

Calfee, M. W., J. P. Coleman, and E. C. Pesci. 2001. Interference with *Pseudomonas* quinolone signal synthesis inhibits virulence factor expression by *Pseudomonas aeruginosa*. *Proc. Natl. Acad. Sci. USA* **98:**11633–11637.

Campbell, E. A., N. Korzheva, A. Mustaev, K. Murakami, S. Nair, A. Goldfarb, and S. A. Darst. 2001. Structural mechanism for rifampicin inhibition of bacterial RNA polymerase. *Cell* **104:**901–912.

Capobianco, J. O., Z. Cao, V. D. Shortridge, Z. Ma, R. K. Flamm, and P. Zhong. 2000. Studies of the novel ketolide ABT-773: transport, binding to ribosomes, and inhibition of protein synthesis in *Streptococcus pneumoniae*. *Antimicrob. Agents Chemother.* **44:**1562–1567.

Carter, A. P., W. M. Clemons, D. E. Brodersen, R. J. Morgan-Warren, B. T. Wimberly, and V. Ramakrishnan. 2000. Functional insights from the structure of the 30S ribosomal subunit and its interactions with antibiotics. *Nature* **407:**340–348.

Cassidy, P. J., and F. M. Kahan. 1973. A stable enzyme-phosphoenolpyruvate intermediate in the synthesis of uridine-5′-diphospho-*N*-acetyl-2-amino-2-deoxy-glucose 3-*O*-enolpyruvyl ether. *Biochemistry* **12:**1364–1374.

Cetinkaya, Y., P. Falk, and C. G. Mayhall. 2000. Vancomycin-resistant enterococci. *Clin. Microbiol. Rev.* **13:**686–707.

Chakraburtty, R., and M. Bibb. 1997. The ppGpp synthetase gene (relA) of *Streptomyces coelicolor* A3(2) plays a conditional role in antibiotic production and morphological differentiation. *J. Bacteriol.* **179:**5854–5861.

Champness, W. C. 2000. *Prokaryotic Development*. ASM Press, Washington, D.C.

Chang, G., and C. B. Roth. 2001. Structure of MsbA from *E. coli*: a homolog of the multidrug resistance ATP binding cassette (ABC) transporters. *Science* **293:**1793–1800.

Chang, H. M., M. Y. Chen, Y. T. Shieh, M. J. Bibb, and C. W. Chen. 1996. The cutRS signal transduction system of *Streptomyces lividans* represses the biosynthesis of the polyketide antibiotic actinorhodin. *Mol. Microbiol.* **21:**1075–1085.

Chang, Y. T., N. S. Gray, G. R. Rosania, D. P. Sutherlin, S. Kwon, T. C. Norman, R. Sarohia, M. Leost, L. Meijer, and P. G. Schultz. 1999. Synthesis and application of functionally diverse 2,6,9-trisubstituted purine libraries as CDK inhibitors. *Chem. Biol.* **6:**361–375.

Chen, H., M. G. Thomas, B. K. Hubbard, H. C. Losey, C. T. Walsh, and M. D. Burkart. 2000. Deoxysugars in glycopeptide antibiotics: enzymatic synthesis of TDP-L-epivancosamine in chloroeremomycin biosynthesis. *Proc. Natl. Acad. Sci. USA* **97:** 11942–11947.

Chen, H., and C. T. Walsh. 2001. Coumarin formation in novobiocin biosynthesis: beta-hydroxylation of the aminoacyl enzyme tyrosyl-*S*-NovH by a cytochrome P450 NovI. *Chem. Biol.* **8:**301–312.

Chen, X., S. Schauder, N. Potier, A. Van Dorsselaer, I. Pelczer, B. L. Bassler, and F. M. Hughson. 2002. Structural identification of a bacterial quorum-sensing signal containing boron. *Nature* **415:**545–549.

Chirgadze, N. Y., S. L. Briggs, K. A. McAllister, A. S. Fischl, and G. Zhao. 2000. Crystal structure of *Streptococcus pneumoniae* acyl carrier protein synthase: an essential enzyme in bacterial fatty acid biosynthesis. *EMBO J.* **19:**5281–5287.

Chopra, I., J. Hodgson, B. Metcalf, and G. Poste. 1997. The search for antimicrobial agents effective against bacteria resistant to multiple antibiotics. *Antimicrob. Agents Chemother.* **41:**497–503.

Chopra, I., and M. Roberts. 2001. Tetracycline antibiotics: mode of action, applications, molecular biology, and epidemiology of bacterial resistance. *Microbiol. Mol. Biol. Rev.* **65:**232–260.

Chu, D. T. 1999. Recent progress in novel macrolides, quinolones, and 2-pyridones to overcome bacterial resistance. *Med. Res. Rev.* **19:**497–520.

Chu, D. T., J. J. Plattner, and L. Katz. 1996. New directions in antibacterial research. *J. Med. Chem.* **39:**3853–3874.

Chuanchuen, R., K. Beinlich, T. T. Hoang, A. Becher, R. R. Karkhoff-Schweizer, and H. P. Schweizer. 2001. Cross-resistance between triclosan and antibiotics in *Pseudomonas aeruginosa* is mediated by multidrug efflux pumps: exposure of a susceptible mutant strain to triclosan selects nfxB mutants overexpressing MexCD-OprJ. *Antimicrob. Agents Chemother.* **45:**428–432.

Clements, J. M., F. Coignard, I. Johnson, S. Chandler, S. Palan, A. Waller, J. Wijkmans, and M. G. Hunter. 2002. Antibacterial activities and characterization of novel inhibitors of LpxC. *Antimicrob. Agents Chemother.* **46:**1793–1799.

Cockerill, F. R., III. 1999. Genetic methods for assessing antimicrobial resistance. *Antimicrob. Agents Chemother.* **43:**199–212.

Cohen, M. L. 2000. Changing patterns of infectious disease. *Nature* **406:**762–767.

Coote, J. G. 1992. Structural and functional relationships among the RTX toxin determinants of gram-negative bacteria. *FEMS Microbiol. Rev.* **8:**137–161.

Cortes, J., S. F. Haydock, G. A. Roberts, D. J. Bevitt, and P. F. Leadlay. 1990. An unusually large multifunctional polypeptide in the erythromycin-producing polyketide synthase of *Saccharopolyspora erythraea*. *Nature* **348:**176–178.

Couturier, M., M. el Bahassi, and L. Van Melderen. 1998. Bacterial death by DNA gyrase poisoning. *Trends Microbiol.* **6:**269–275.

Cozzarelli, N. R. 1980. DNA gyrase and the supercoiling of DNA. *Science* **207:**953–960.

Crump, M. P., J. Crosby, C. E. Dempsey, J. A. Parkinson, M. Murray, D. A. Hopwood, and T. J. Simpson. 1997. Solution structure of the actinorhodin polyketide synthase acyl carrier protein from *Streptomyces coelicolor* A3(2). *Biochemistry* **36:**6000–6008.

Cubbon, M. D., and R. G. Masterton. 2000. New quinolones—a fresh answer to the pneumococcus. *J. Antimicrob. Chemother.* **46:**869–872.

Cudic, M., and L. Otvos, Jr. 2002. Intracellular targets of antibacterial peptides. *Curr. Drug Targets* **3:**101–106.

Cudic, P., J. K. Kranz, D. C. Behenna, R. G. Kruger, H. Tadesse, A. J. Wand, Y. I. Veklich, J. W. Weisel, and D. G. McCafferty. 2002. Complexation of peptidoglycan intermediates by the lipoglycodepsipeptide antibiotic ramoplanin: minimal structural requirements for intermolecular complexation and fibril formation. *Proc. Natl. Acad. Sci. USA* **99:**7384–7389.

Culver, G. M. 2001. Meanderings of the mRNA through the ribosome. *Structure* (Cambridge) **9:**751–758.

Dancer, S. J. 2001. The problem with cephalosporins. *J. Antimicrob. Chemother.* **48:**463–478.

Datta, N., and P. Kontomichalou. 1965. Penicillinase synthesis controlled by infectious R factors in Enterobacteriaceae. *Nature* **208:**239–41.

Davies, J. 1994. Inactivation of antibiotics and the dissemination of resistance genes. *Science* **264:**375–382.

Davis, J. R., and J. Lederberg. 2000. *NAS Workshop Report: Emerging Infectious Diseases from the Global to the Local Perspective.* National Academy of Sciences, Washington, D.C.

Decicco, C. P., D. J. Nelson, Y. Luo, L. Shen, K. Y. Horiuchi, K. M. Amsler, L. A. Foster, S. M. Spitz, J. J. Merrill, C. F. Sizemore, K. C. Rogers, R. A. Copeland, and M. R. Harpel. 2001. Glutamyl-gamma-boronate inhibitors of bacterial GlutRNA(Gln) amidotransferase. *Bioorg. Med. Chem. Lett.* **11:**2561–2564.

Denome, S. A., P. K. Elf, T. A. Henderson, D. E. Nelson, and K. D. Young. 1999. *Escherichia coli* mutants lacking all possible combinations of eight penicillin binding proteins: viability, characteristics, and implications for peptidoglycan synthesis. *J. Bacteriol.* **181:**3981–3993.

DeVito, J. A., J. A. Mills, V. G. Liu, A. Agarwal, C. F. Sizemore, Z. Yao, D. M. Stoughton, M. G. Cappiello, M. D. Barbosa, L. A. Foster, and D. L. Pompliano. 2002. An array of target-specific screening strains for antibacterial discovery. *Nat. Biotechnol.* **20:**478–483.

Diederichs, K., J. Diez, G. Greller, C. Muller, J. Breed, C. Schnell, C. Vonrhein, W. Boos, and W. Welte. 2000. Crystal structure of MalK, the ATPase subunit of the trehalose/maltose ABC transporter of the archaeon Thermococcus litoralis. *EMBO J.* **19:**5951–5961.

Dinos, G. P., and D. L. Kalpaxis. 2000. Kinetic studies on the interaction between a ribosomal complex active in peptide bond formation and the macrolide antibiotics tylosin and erythromycin. *Biochemistry* **39:**11621–11628.

Doekel, S., and M. A. Marahiel. 2001. Biosynthesis of natural products on modular peptide synthetases. *Metab. Eng.* **3:**64–77.

Dolle, R. E. 2000. Comprehensive survey of combinatorial library synthesis: 1999. *J. Comb. Chem.* **2:**383–433.

Donadio, S., M. J. Staver, J. B. McAlpine, S. J. Swanson, and L. Katz. 1991. Modular organization of genes required for complex polyketide biosynthesis. *Science* **252:**675–679.

Dong, Y. H., J. L. Xu, X. Z. Li, and L. H. Zhang. 2000. AiiA, an enzyme that inactivates the acylhomoserine lactone quorum-sensing signal and attenuates the virulence of *Erwinia carotovora. Proc. Natl. Acad. Sci. USA* **97:**3526–3531.

Dougherty, T. J., K. Kennedy, R. E. Kessler, and M. J. Pucci. 1996. Direct quantitation of the number of individual penicillin-binding proteins per cell in *Escherichia coli. J. Bacteriol.* **178:**6110–6115.

Douthwaite, S., L. H. Hansen, and P. Mauvais. 2000. Macrolide-ketolide inhibition of MLS-resistant ribosomes is improved by alternative drug interaction with domain II of 23S rRNA. *Mol. Microbiol.* **36:**183–193.

Drenkard, E., and F. M. Ausubel. 2002. Pseudomonas biofilm formation and antibiotic resistance are linked to phenotypic variation. *Nature* **416:**740–743.

Drlica, K. 2001. Antibiotic resistance: can we beat the bugs? *Drug Discov. Today* **6:**714–715.

Du, L., C. Sanchez, and B. Shen. 2001. Hybrid peptide-polyketide natural products: biosynthesis and prospects toward engineering novel molecules. *Metab. Eng.* **3:**78–95.

Duitman, E. H., L. W. Hamoen, M. Rembold, G. Venema, H. Seitz, W. Saenger, F. Bernhard, R. Reinhardt, M. Schmidt, C. Ullrich, T. Stein, F. Leenders, and J. Vater. 1999. The mycosubtilin synthetase of *Bacillus subtilis* ATCC6633: a multifunctional hybrid between a peptide synthetase, an amino transferase, and a fatty acid synthase. *Proc. Natl. Acad. Sci. USA* **96**:13294–13299.

Eggert, U. S., N. Ruiz, B. V. Falcone, A. A. Branstrom, R. C. Goldman, T. J. Silhavy, and D. Kahne. 2001. Genetic basis for activity differences between vancomycin and glycolipid derivatives of vancomycin. *Science* **294**:361–364.

Elliot, T. S., J. G. M. Hastings, and U. Desselberger. 1997. *Lecture Notes on Medical Microbiology*, 3rd ed. Blackwell Scientific Publications, Ltd., Oxford, United Kingdom.

Engberg, J., F. M. Aarestrup, D. E. Taylor, P. Gerner-Smidt, and I. Nachamkin. 2001. Quinolone and macrolide resistance in *Campylobacter jejuni* and *C. coli*: resistance mechanisms and trends in human isolates. *Emerg. Infect. Dis.* **7**:24–34.

Enne, V. I., D. M. Livermore, P. Stephens, and L. M. Hall. 2001. Persistence of sulphonamide resistance in *Escherichia coli* in the UK despite national prescribing restriction. *Lancet* **357**:1325–1328.

Erlandsen, H., E. E. Abola, and R. C. Stevens. 2000. Combining structural genomics and enzymology: completing the picture in metabolic pathways and enzyme active sites. *Curr. Opin. Struct. Biol.* **10**:719–730.

Falkow, S., and D. Kennedy. 2001. Antibiotics, animals, and people—again! *Science* **291**:397.

Fan, C., P. C. Moews, C. T. Walsh, and J. R. Knox. 1994. Vancomycin resistance: structure of D-alanine:D-alanine ligase at 2.3 Å resolution. *Science* **266**:439–443.

Fernandez-Lopez, S., H. S. Kim, E. C. Choi, M. Delgado, J. R. Granja, A. Khasanov, K. Kraehenbuehl, G. Long, D. A. Weinberger, K. M. Wilcoxen, and M. R. Ghadiri. 2001. Antibacterial agents based on the cyclic D,L-alpha-peptide architecture. *Nature* **412**:452–455.

Fierro, J. F., C. Hardisson, and J. A. Salas. 1987. Resistance to oleandomycin in *Streptomyces antibioticus*, the producer organism. *J. Gen. Microbiol.* **133**(Pt. 7):1931–1939.

Filipe, S. R., M. G. Pinho, and A. Tomasz. 2000. Characterization of the murMN operon involved in the synthesis of branched peptidoglycan peptides in *Streptococcus pneumoniae*. *J. Biol. Chem.* **275**:27768–27774.

Fisher, J., J. G. Belasco, S. Khosla, and J. R. Knowles. 1980. β-lactamase proceeds via an acyl-enzyme intermediate. Interaction of the *Escherichia coli* RTEM enzyme with cefoxitin. *Biochemistry* **19**:2895–2901.

Fralick, J. A. 1996. Evidence that TolC is required for functioning of the Mar/AcrAB efflux pump of *Escherichia coli*. *J. Bacteriol.* **178**:5803–5805.

Fuchs, P. C., A. L. Barry, and S. D. Brown. 2001. In vitro activities of ertapenem (MK-0826) against clinical bacterial isolates from 11 North American medical centers. *Antimicrob. Agents Chemother.* **45**:1915–1918.

Fujihashi, M., Y. W. Zhang, Y. Higuchi, X. Y. Li, T. Koyama, and K. Miki. 2001. Crystal structure of cis-prenyl chain elongating enzyme, undecaprenyl diphosphate synthase. *Proc. Natl. Acad. Sci. USA* **98**:4337–4342.

Galan, J. E., and A. Collmer. 1999. Type III secretion machines: bacterial devices for protein delivery into host cells. *Science* **284:**1322–1328.

Gale, E. F., E. Cundliffe, P. E. Reynolds, M. H. Richmond, and M. J. Waring. 1981. *The Molecular Basis of Antibiotic Action*, 2nd ed. Wiley, London, United Kingdom.

Garrett, L. 1995. *The Coming Plague: Newly Emerging Diseases in a World out of Balance*. Virago, London, United Kingdom.

Gaunt, P. N., and L. J. Piddock. 1996. Ciprofloxacin resistant *Campylobacter* spp. in humans: an epidemiological and laboratory study. *J. Antimicrob. Chemother.* **37:**747–757.

Ge, M., Z. Chen, H. R. Onishi, J. Kohler, L. L. Silver, R. Kerns, S. Fukuzawa, C. Thompson, and D. Kahne. 1999. Vancomycin derivatives that inhibit peptidoglycan biosynthesis without binding D-Ala-D-Ala. *Science* **284:**507–511.

Gegnas, L. D., S. T. Waddell, R. M. Chabin, S. Reddy, and K. K. Wong. 1998. Inhibitors of the bacterial cell wall biosynthesis enzyme MurD. *Bioorg. Med. Chem. Lett.* **8:**1643–1618.

Gehring, A. M., W. J. Lees, D. J. Mindiola, C. T. Walsh, and E. D. Brown. 1996. Acetyltransfer precedes uridylyltransfer in the formation of UDP-*N*-acetylglucosamine in separable active sites of the bifunctional GlmU protein of Escherichia coli. *Biochemistry* **35:**579–585.

Ghuysen, J. M. 1991. Serine beta-lactamases and penicillin-binding proteins. *Annu. Rev. Microbiol.* **45:**37–67.

Gokhale, R. S., S. Y. Tsuji, D. E. Cane, and C. Khosla. 1999. Dissecting and exploiting intermodular communication in polyketide synthases. *Science* **284:**482–485.

Goldman, R. C., S. W. Fesik, and C. C. Doran. 1990. Role of protonated and neutral forms of macrolides in binding to ribosomes from gram-positive and gram-negative bacteria. *Antimicrob. Agents Chemother.* **34:**426–431.

Gorbach, S. L. 2001. Antimicrobial use in animal feed—time to stop. *N. Engl. J. Med.* **345:**1202–1203.

Gould, I. M. 1999. A review of the role of antibiotic policies in the control of antibiotic resistance. *J. Antimicrob. Chemother.* **43:**459–465.

Goussard, S., and P. Courvalin. 1999. Updated sequence information for TEM beta-lactamase genes. *Antimicrob. Agents Chemother.* **43:**367–370.

Greenwood, D., and F. O'Grady. 1969. A comparison of the effects of ampicillin on Escherichia coli and Proteus mirabilis. *J. Med. Microbiol.* **2:**435–441.

Greenwood, D. 2000. *Antimicrobial Chemotherapy*, 4th ed. Oxford University Press, Oxford, United Kingdom.

Greenwood, D., and F. O'Grady. 1973. The two sites of penicillin action in Escherichia coli. *J. Infect. Dis.* **128:**791–794.

Groisman, E. A. 2001. *Principles of Bacterial Pathogenesis*. Academic Press Inc., San Diego, Calif.

Guan, K. L., and J. E. Dixon. 1990. Protein tyrosine phosphatase activity of an essential virulence determinant in Yersinia. *Science* **249:**553–556.

Guo, L., K. B. Lim, J. S. Gunn, B. Bainbridge, R. P. Darveau, M. Hackett, and S. I. Miller. 1997. Regulation of lipid A modifications by Salmonella typhimurium virulence genes phoP-phoQ. *Science* **276:**250–253.

Guo, L., K. B. Lim, C. M. Poduje, M. Daniel, J. S. Gunn, M. Hackett, and S. I. Miller. 1998. Lipid A acylation and bacterial resistance against vertebrate antimicrobial peptides. *Cell* **95:**189–198.

Ha, S., E. Chang, M.-C. Lo., H. Men, P. Park, M. Ge, and S. Walker. 1999. The kinetic characterization of *Escherichia coli* MurG using synthetic substrate analogues. *J. Am. Chem. Soc.* **121:**8415–8426.

Ha, S., D. Walker, Y. Shi, and S. Walker. 2000. The 1.9 Å crystal structure of Escherichia coli MurG, a membrane-associated glycosyltransferase involved in peptidoglycan biosynthesis. *Protein Sci.* **9:**1045–1052.

Hakenbeck, R. 1998. Mosaic genes and their role in penicillin-resistant *Streptococcus pneumoniae. Electrophoresis* **19:**597–601.

Hakenbeck, R., T. Grebe, D. Zahner, and J. B. Stock. 1999. Beta-lactam resistance in *Streptococcus pneumoniae*: penicillin-binding proteins and non-penicillin-binding proteins. *Mol. Microbiol.* **33:**673–678.

Hall, D. G., S. Manku, and F. Wang. 2001. Solution- and solid-phase strategies for the design, synthesis, and screening of libraries based on natural product templates: a comprehensive survey. *J. Comb. Chem.* **3:**125–150.

Hancock, R. E., and D. S. Chapple. 1999. Peptide antibiotics. *Antimicrob. Agents Chemother.* **43:**1317–1323.

Hansen, J. N. 1997. Nisin and related antimicrobial peptides, p. 437–470. *In* W. R. Strohl (ed.), Biotechnology of Antibiotics, 2nd ed. Marcel Dekker Inc., New York, N.Y.

Hansen, J. L., J. A. Ippolito, N. Ban, P. Nissen, P. B. Moore, and T. A. Steitz. 2002. The structures of four macrolide antibiotics bound to the large ribosomal subunit. *Mol. Cell* **10:**117–128.

Hanzelka, B. L., M. R. Parsek, D. L. Val, P. V. Dunlap, J. E. Cronan, Jr., and E. P. Greenberg. 1999. Acylhomoserine lactone synthase activity of the *Vibrio fischeri* AinS protein. *J. Bacteriol.* **181:**5766–5770.

Hecht, S., W. Eisenreich, P. Adam, S. Amslinger, K. Kis, A. Bacher, D. Arigoni, and F. Rohdich. 2001. Studies on the nonmevalonate pathway to terpenes: the role of the GcpE (IspG) protein. *Proc. Natl. Acad. Sci. USA* **98:**14837–14842.

Heddle, J. G., S. J. Blance, D. B. Zamble, F. Hollfelder, D. A. Miller, L. M. Wentzell, C. T. Walsh, and A. Maxwell. 2001. The antibiotic microcin B17 is a DNA gyrase poison: characterisation of the mode of inhibition. *J. Mol. Biol.* **307:**1223–1234.

Hedl, M., A. Sutherlin, E. I. Wilding, M. Mazzulla, D. McDevitt, P. Lane, J. W. Burgner, 2nd, K. R. Lehnbeuter, C. V. Stauffacher, M. N. Gwynn, and V. W. Rodwell. 2002. *Enterococcus faecalis* acetoacetyl-coenzyme A thiolase/3-hydroxy-3-methylglutaryl-coenzyme A reductase, a dual-function protein of isopentenyl diphosphate biosynthesis. *J. Bacteriol.* **184:**2116–2122.

Heep, M., U. Rieger, D. Beck, and N. Lehn. 2000. Mutations in the beginning of the rpoB gene can induce resistance to rifamycins in both *Helicobacter pylori* and *Mycobacterium tuberculosis. Antimicrob. Agents Chemother.* **44:**1075–1077.

Heerding, D. A., G. Chan, W. E. DeWolf, A. P. Fosberry, C. A. Janson, D. D. Jaworski, E. McManus, W. H. Miller, T. D. Moore, D. J. Payne, X. Qiu, S. F. Rittenhouse, C. Slater-Radosti, W. Smith, D. T. Takata, K. S. Vaidya, C. C. Yuan, and W. F. Huffman. 2001. 1,4-Disubstituted imidazoles are potential antibacterial agents functioning as inhibitors of enoyl acyl carrier protein reductase. *Bioorg. Med. Chem. Lett.* **11**:2061–2065.

Heffron, S. E., and F. Jurnak. 2000. Structure of an EF-Tu complex with a thiazolyl peptide determined at 2.35 Å resolution: atomic basis for GE2270A inhibition of EF-Tu. *Biochemistry* **39**:37–45.

Hensel, M., J. E. Shea, C. Gleeson, M. D. Jones, E. Dalton, and D. W. Holden. 1995. Simultaneous identification of bacterial virulence genes by negative selection. *Science* **269**:400–403.

Hilliard, J. J., R. M. Goldschmidt, L. Licata, E. Z. Baum, and K. Bush. 1999. Multiple mechanisms of action for inhibitors of histidine protein kinases from bacterial two-component systems. *Antimicrob. Agents Chemother.* **43**:1693–1699.

Hiramatsu, K. 1998. The emergence of *Staphylococcus aureus* with reduced susceptibility to vancomycin in Japan. *Am. J. Med.* **104**:7S–10S.

Hiramatsu, K., L. Cui, M. Kuroda, and T. Ito. 2001. The emergence and evolution of methicillin-resistant Staphylococcus aureus. *Trends Microbiol.* **9**:486–493.

Holdgate, G. A., A. Tunnicliffe, W. H. Ward, S. A. Weston, G. Rosenbrock, P. T. Barth, I. W. Taylor, R. A. Pauptit, and D. Timms. 1997. The entropic penalty of ordered water accounts for weaker binding of the antibiotic novobiocin to a resistant mutant of DNA gyrase: a thermodynamic and crystallographic study. *Biochemistry* **36**:9663–9673.

Holtje, J. V. 1998. Growth of the stress-bearing and shape-maintaining murein sacculus of *Escherichia coli*. *Microbiol. Mol. Biol. Rev.* **62**:181–203.

Hon, W. C., G. A. McKay, P. R. Thompson, R. M. Sweet, D. S. Yang, G. D. Wright, and A. M. Berghuis. 1997. Structure of an enzyme required for aminoglycoside antibiotic resistance reveals homology to eukaryotic protein kinases. *Cell* **89**:887–895.

Hopwood, D. A. 1997. Genetic contributions to understanding polyketide synthases. *Chem. Rev.* **97**:2465–2498.

Hu, H., Q. Zhang, and K. Ochi. 2002. Activation of antibiotic biosynthesis by specified mutations in the *rpoB* gene (encoding the RNA polymerase beta subunit) of *Streptomyces lividans*. *J. Bacteriol.* **184**:3984–3991.

Hubbard, B. K., M. G. Thomas, and C. T. Walsh. 2000. Biosynthesis of L-p-hydroxyphenylglycine, a non-proteinogenic amino acid constituent of peptide antibiotics. *Chem. Biol.* **7**:931–942.

Hubbard, B. K., and C. T. Walsh. Vancomycin assembly; Nature's way. *Angew. Chem. Int. Ed. Engl.*, in press.

Hughes, J. M., and F. C. Tenover. 1997. Approaches to limiting emergence of antimicrobial resistance in bacteria in human populations. *Clin. Infect. Dis.* **24**(Suppl. 1):S131–S135.

Hung, L. W., I. X. Wang, K. Nikaido, P. Q. Liu, G. F. Ames, and S. H. Kim. 1998. Crystal structure of the ATP-binding subunit of an ABC transporter. *Nature* **396**:703–707.

Huntington, K. M., T. Yi, Y. Wei, and D. Pei. 2000. Synthesis and antibacterial activity of peptide deformylase inhibitors. *Biochemistry* **39**:4543–4551.

Hutchinson, C. R. 1997. Antibiotics from genetically engineered microorganisms, p. 683–702. *In* W. R. Strohl (ed.), *Biotechnology of Antibiotics,* 2nd ed. Marcel Dekker Inc., New York, N.Y.

Hutchinson, C. R., and I. Fujii. 1995. Polyketide synthase gene manipulation: a structure-function approach in engineering novel antibiotics. *Annu. Rev. Microbiol.* **49:**201–238.

Ilangovan, U., H. Ton-That, J. Iwahara, O. Schneewind, and R. T. Clubb. 2001. Structure of sortase, the transpeptidase that anchors proteins to the cell wall of *Staphylococcus aureus. Proc. Natl. Acad. Sci. USA* **98:**6056–6061.

Isberg, R. R., and J. M. Leong. 1990. Multiple beta 1 chain integrins are receptors for invasin, a protein that promotes bacterial penetration into mammalian cells. *Cell* **60:**861–871.

Jack, R., G. Bierbaum, C. Heidrich, and H. G. Sahl. 1995. The genetics of lantibiotic biosynthesis. *Bioessays* **17:**793–802.

Jackman, J. E., C. R. Raetz, and C. A. Fierke. 1999. UDP-3-*O*-(R-3-hydroxy-myristoyl)-*N*-acetylglucosamine deacetylase of *Escherichia coli* is a zinc metallo-enzyme. *Biochemistry* **38:**1902–1911.

Jacobs, C., J. M. Frere, and S. Normark. 1997. Cytosolic intermediates for cell wall biosynthesis and degradation control inducible beta-lactam resistance in gram-negative bacteria. *Cell* **88:**823–832.

Jain, R., M. C. Rivera, and J. A. Lake. 1999. Horizontal gene transfer among genomes: the complexity hypothesis. *Proc. Natl. Acad. Sci. USA* **96:**3801–3806.

Jarvest, R. L., J. M. Berge, C. S. Houge-Frydrych, L. M. Mensah, P. J. O'Hanlon, and A. J. Pope. 2001. Inhibitors of bacterial tyrosyl tRNA synthetase: synthesis of carbocyclic analogues of the natural product SB-219383. *Bioorg. Med. Chem. Lett.* **11:**2499–2502.

Ji, Y., B. Zhang, S. F. Van Horn, P. Warren, G. Woodnutt, M. K. Burnham, and M. Rosenberg. 2001. Identification of critical staphylococcal genes using conditional phenotypes generated by antisense RNA. *Science* **293:**2266–2269.

Jiang, W., J. Wanner, R. J. Lee, P. Y. Bounaud, and D. L. Boger. 2002. Total synthesis of the ramoplanin A2 and ramoplanose aglycon. *J. Am. Chem. Soc.* **124:**5288–5290.

Kahan, J. S., F. M. Kahan, R. Goegelman, S. A. Currie, M. Jackson, E. O. Stapley, T. W. Miller, A. K. Miller, D. Hendlin, S. Mochales, S. Hernandez, H. B. Woodruff, and J. Birnbaum. 1979. Thienamycin, a new beta-lactam antibiotic. I. Discovery, taxonomy, isolation and physical properties. *J. Antibiot.* (Tokyo) **32:**1–12.

Kaper, J. B., and A. D. O'Brien. 1998. Escherichia coli *O157:H7 and other Shiga toxin-producing* E. coli *strains.* ASM Press, Washington, D.C.

Karmali, M. A. 1989. Infection by verocytotoxin-producing *Escherichia coli. Clin. Microbiol. Rev.* **2:**15–38.

Katz, L. 1997. Manipulation of modular polyketide synthases. *Chem. Rev.* **97:**2557–2576.

Kawachi, R., U. Wangchaisoonthorn, T. Nihira, and Y. Yamada. 2000. Identification by gene deletion analysis of a regulator, VmsR, that controls virginiamycin biosynthesis in *Streptomyces virginiae. J. Bacteriol.* **182:**6259–6263.

Keating, T. A., and C. T. Walsh. 1999. Initiation, elongation, and termination strategies in polyketide and polypeptide antibiotic biosynthesis. *Curr. Opin. Chem. Biol.* **3:**598–606.

Kemp, L. E., C. S. Bond, and W. N. Hunter. 2002. Structure of 2C-methyl-D-erythritol 2,4-cyclodiphosphate synthase: an essential enzyme for isoprenoid biosynthesis and target for antimicrobial drug development. *Proc. Natl. Acad. Sci. USA* **99:**6591–6596.

Khaleeli, N., R. W. Busby, and C. A. Townsend. 2000. Site-directed mutagenesis and biochemical analysis of the endogenous ligands in the ferrous active site of clavaminate synthase: the His-3 variant of the 2-His-1-carboxylate mold. *Biochemistry* **39:**8666–8673.

Khosla, C. 1997. Harnessing the biosynthetic potential of modular polyketide synthases. *Chem. Rev.* **97:**2577–2590.

Kieser, T., K. F. Chater, M. Bibb, M. J. Buttner, and D. A. Hopwood. 2000. *Practical* Streptomyces *Genetics.* The John Innes Foundation, Norwich.

Kinoshita, K., P. G. Willard, C. Khosla, and D. E. Cane. 2001. Precursor-directed biosynthesis of 16-membered macrolides by the erythromycin polyketide synthase. *J. Am. Chem. Soc.* **123:**2495–2502.

Kleerebezem, M., L. E. Quadri, O. P. Kuipers, and W. M. de Vos. 1997. Quorum sensing by peptide pheromones and two-component signal-transduction systems in gram-positive bacteria. *Mol. Microbiol.* **24:**895–904.

Kloss, P., L. Xiong, D. L. Shinabarger, and A. S. Mankin. 1999. Resistance mutations in 23S rRNA identify the site of action of the protein synthesis inhibitor linezolid in the ribosomal peptidyl transferase center. *J. Mol. Biol.* **294:**93–101.

Knowles, J. R. 1985. Penicillin resistance: the chemistry of β-lactamase inhibition. *Acc. Chem. Res.* 18:97–104.

Knox, J. R. 1995. Extended-spectrum and inhibitor-resistant TEM-type beta-lactamases: mutations, specificity, and three-dimensional structure. *Antimicrob. Agents Chemother.* **39:**2593–2601.

Knox, J. R., P. C. Moews, and J. M. Frere. 1996. Molecular evolution of bacterial beta-lactam resistance. *Chem. Biol.* **3:**937–947.

Kobayashi, K., M. Ogura, H. Yamaguchi, K. Yoshida, N. Ogasawara, T. Tanaka, and Y. Fujita. 2001. Comprehensive DNA microarray analysis of *Bacillus subtilis* two-component regulatory systems. *J. Bacteriol.* **183:**7365–7370.

Koebnik, R., K. P. Locher, and P. Van Gelder. 2000. Structure and function of bacterial outer membrane proteins: barrels in a nutshell. *Mol. Microbiol.* **37:**239–253.

Konz, D., and M. A. Marahiel. 1999. How do peptide synthetases generate structural diversity? *Chem. Biol.* **6:**R39–R48.

Koppisch, A. T., D. T. Fox, B. S. Blagg, and C. D. Poulter. 2002. *E. coli* MEP synthase: steady-state kinetic analysis and substrate binding. *Biochemistry* **41:**236–243.

Koronakis, V., A. Sharff, E. Koronakis, B. Luisi, and C. Hughes. 2000. Crystal structure of the bacterial membrane protein TolC central to multidrug efflux and protein export. *Nature* **405:**914–919.

Kostrewa, D., A. D'Arcy, B. Takacs, and M. Kamber. 2001. Crystal structures of *Streptococcus pneumoniae* N-acetylglucosamine-1-phosphate uridyltransferase, GlmU, in apo form at 2.33 Å resolution and in complex with UDP-N-acetylglucosamine and Mg(2+) at 1.96 Å resolution. *J. Mol. Biol.* **305**:279–289.

Kotra, L. P., J. Haddad, and S. Mobashery. 2000. Aminoglycosides: perspectives on mechanisms of action and resistance and strategies to counter resistance. *Antimicrob. Agents Chemother.* **44**:3249–3256.

Kragol, G., S. Lovas, G. Varadi, B. A. Condie, R. Hoffmann, and L. Otvos, Jr. 2001. The antibacterial peptide pyrrhocoricin inhibits the ATPase actions of DnaK and prevents chaperone-assisted protein folding. *Biochemistry* **40**:3016–3026.

Kunin, C. M. 1997. Antibiotic armageddon. *Clin. Infect. Dis.* **25**:240–241.

Kuroda, M., T. Ohta, I. Uchiyama, T. Baba, H. Yuzawa, I. Kobayashi, L. Cui, A. Oguchi, K. Aoki, Y. Nagai, J. Lian, T. Ito, M. Kanamori, H. Matsumaru, A. Maruyama, H. Murakami, A. Hosoyama, Y. Mizutani-Ui, N. K. Takahashi, T. Sawano, R. Inoue, C. Kaito, K. Sekimizu, H. Hirakawa, S. Kuhara, S. Goto, J. Yabuzaki, M. Kanehisa, A. Yamashita, K. Oshima, K. Furuya, C. Yoshino, T. Shiba, M. Hattori, N. Ogasawara, H. Hayashi, and K. Hiramatsu. 2001. Whole genome sequencing of methicillin-resistant *Staphylococcus aureus*. *Lancet* **357**:1225–1240.

Kurokawa, H., T. Yagi, N. Shibata, K. Shibayama, and Y. Arakawa. 1999. Worldwide proliferation of carbapenem-resistant gram-negative bacteria. *Lancet* **354**:955.

Kurz, M., and W. Guba. 1996. 3D structure of ramoplanin: a potent inhibitor of bacterial cell wall synthesis. *Biochemistry* **35**:12570–12575.

Kurz, M., W. Guba, and L. Vertesy. 1998. Three-dimensional structure of moenomycin A—a potent inhibitor of penicillin-binding protein 1b. *Eur. J. Biochem.* **252**:500–507.

Kuzin, A. P., T. Sun, J. Jorczak-Baillass, V. L. Healy, C. T. Walsh, and J. R. Knox. 2000. Enzymes of vancomycin resistance: the structure of D-alanine-D-lactate ligase of naturally resistant *Leuconostoc mesenteroides*. *Structure* **8**:463–470.

Lambalot, R. H., A. M. Gehring, R. S. Flugel, P. Zuber, M. LaCelle, M. A. Marahiel, R. Reid, C. Khosla, and C. T. Walsh. 1996. A new enzyme superfamily—the phosphopantetheinyl transferases. *Chem. Biol.* **3**:923–936.

Lancini, G. 1983. Ansamycins, p. 231–254. *In* L. C. Vining (ed.), *Biochemistry and Genetic Regulation of Commercially Important Antibiotics.* Addison-Wesley Publishing Co., Inc., Reading, Mass.

Lee, D., J. K. Sello, and S. L. Schreiber. 1999. A strategy for macrocyclic ring closure and functionalization aimed toward split-pool syntheses. *J. Am. Chem. Soc.* **121**:10648–10649.

Lee, J., S. U. Kang, S. Y. Kim, S. E. Kim, Y. J. Job, and S. Kim. 2001. Vanilloid and isovanilloid analogues as inhibitors of methionyl-tRNA and isoleucyl-tRNA synthetases. *Bioorg. Med. Chem. Lett.* **11**:965–968.

Lee, V. J., and S. J. Hecker. 1999. Antibiotic resistance versus small molecules, the chemical evolution. *Med. Res. Rev.* **19**:521–542.

Lee, V. T., and O. Schneewind. 2001. Protein secretion and the pathogenesis of bacterial infections. *Genes Dev.* **15**:1725–1752.

Lessard, I. A., V. L. Healy, I. S. Park, and C. T. Walsh. 1999. Determinants for differential effects on D-Ala-D-lactate vs D-Ala-D-Ala formation by the VanA ligase from vancomycin-resistant enterococci. *Biochemistry* **38**:14006–14022.

Lessard, I. A., and C. T. Walsh. 1999. Mutational analysis of active-site residues of the enterococcal D-Ala-D-Ala dipeptidase VanX and comparison with *Escherichia coli* D-Ala-D-Ala ligase and D-Ala-D-Ala carboxypeptidase VanY. *Chem. Biol.* **6:**177–187.

Levy, S. B. 1992. *The Antibiotic Paradox: How Miracle Drugs are Destroying the Miracle.* Plenum Press, New York, N.Y.

Levy, S. B. 1998. The challenge of antibiotic resistance. *Sci. Am.* **278:**46–53.

Levy, S. B. 2001. Antimicrobial resistance potential. *Lancet* **358:**1100–1101.

Lewis, H. A., E. B. Furlong, B. Laubert, G. A. Eroshkina, Y. Batiyenko, J. M. Adams, M. G. Bergseid, C. D. Marsh, T. S. Peat, W. E. Sanderson, J. M. Sauder, and S. G. Buchanan. 2001. A structural genomics approach to the study of quorum sensing: crystal structures of three LuxS orthologs. *Structure* **9:**527–537.

Lewis, R. J., O. M. Singh, C. V. Smith, T. Skarzynski, A. Maxwell, A. J. Wonacott, and D. B. Wigley. 1996. The nature of inhibition of DNA gyrase by the coumarins and the cyclothialidines revealed by X-ray crystallography. *EMBO J.* **15:**1412–1420.

Li, R., N. Khaleeli, and C. A. Townsend. 2000. Expansion of the clavulanic acid gene cluster: identification and in vivo functional analysis of three new genes required for biosynthesis of clavulanic acid by *Streptomyces clavuligerus*. *J. Bacteriol.* **182:**4087–4095.

Lim, D., H. U. Park, L. De Castro, S. G. Kang, H. S. Lee, S. Jensen, K. J. Lee, and N. C. Strynadka. 2001. Crystal structure and kinetic analysis of beta-lactamase inhibitor protein-II in complex with TEM-1 beta-lactamase. *Nat. Struct. Biol.* **8:**848–852.

Lindsley, C. W., L. K. Chan, B. C. Goess, R. Joseph, and M. D. Shair. 2000. Solid-phase biomimetic synthesis of carpanone-like molecules. *J. Am. Chem. Soc.* **122:**422–423.

Liu, H., R. Sadamoto, P. S. Sears, and C. H. Wong. 2001. An efficient chemo-enzymatic strategy for the synthesis of wild-type and vancomycin-resistant bacterial cell-wall precursors: UDP-*N*-acetylmuramyl-peptides. *J. Am. Chem. Soc.* **123:**9916–9917.

Liu, H. W., and J. S. Thorson. 1994. Pathways and mechanisms in the biogenesis of novel deoxysugars by bacteria. *Annu. Rev. Microbiol.* **48:**223–256.

Livermore, D. M. 2000. Quinupristin/dalfopristin and linezolid: where, when, which and whether to use? *J. Antimicrob. Chemother.* **46:**347–350.

Livermore, D. M., and N. Woodford. 2000. Carbapenemases: a problem in waiting? *Curr. Opin. Microbiol.* **3:**489–495.

Lo, M.-C., H. Men, A. Branstrom, J. Helm, N. Yao, R. Goldman, and S. Walker. 2000. A new mechanism of action proposed for ramoplanin. *J. Am. Chem. Soc.* **122:**3540–3541.

Locher, K. P., A. T. Lee, and D. C. Rees. 2002. The E. coli BtuCD structure: a framework for ABC transporter architecture and mechanism. *Science* **296:**1091–1098.

Lomovskaya, O., M. S. Warren, A. Lee, J. Galazzo, R. Fronko, M. Lee, J. Blais, D. Cho, S. Chamberland, T. Renau, R. Leger, S. Hecker, W. Watkins, K. Hoshino, H. Ishida, and V. J. Lee. 2001. Identification and characterization of inhibitors of multidrug resistance efflux pumps in *Pseudomonas aeruginosa*: novel agents for combination therapy. *Antimicrob. Agents Chemother.* **45:**105–116.

Lorenz, M. C., and G. R. Fink. 2001. The glyoxylate cycle is required for fungal virulence. *Nature* **412**:83–86.

Lorian, V., and F. Fernandes. 1997. The effect of vancomycin on the structure of vancomycin-susceptible and -resistant *Enterococcus faecium* strains. *Antimicrob. Agents Chemother.* **41**:1410–1411.

Losey, H. C., M. W. Peczuh, Z. Chen, U. S. Eggert, S. D. Dong, I. Pelczer, D. Kahne, and C. T. Walsh. 2001. Tandem action of glycosyltransferases in the maturation of vancomycin and teicoplanin aglycones: novel glycopeptides. *Biochemistry* **40**:4745–4755.

Lowy, F. D. 1998. *Staphylococcus aureus* infections. *N. Engl. J. Med.* **339**:520–532.

Lyon, G. J., P. Mayville, T. W. Muir, and R. P. Novick. 2000. Rational design of a global inhibitor of the virulence response in *Staphylococcus aureus*, based in part on localization of the site of inhibition to the receptor-histidine kinase, AgrC. *Proc. Natl. Acad. Sci. USA* **97**:13330–13335.

Ma, Y., F. Pan, and M. McNeil. 2002. Formation of dTDP-rhamnose is essential for growth of mycobacteria. *J. Bacteriol.* **184**:3392–3395.

Mahan, M. J., J. M. Slauch, and J. J. Mekalanos. 1993. Selection of bacterial virulence genes that are specifically induced in host tissues. *Science* **259**:686–688.

Mahan, M. J., J. W. Tobias, J. M. Slauch, P. C. Hanna, R. J. Collier, and J. J. Mekalanos. 1995. Antibiotic-based selection for bacterial genes that are specifically induced during infection of a host. *Proc. Natl. Acad. Sci. USA* **92**:669–673.

Maiti, S. N., O. A. Phillips, R. G. Micetich, and D. M. Livermore. 1998. Beta-lactamase inhibitors: agents to overcome bacterial resistance. *Curr. Med. Chem.* **5**:441–456.

Malik, V. S. 1972. Chloramphenicol. *Adv. Appl. Microbiol.* **15**:297–336.

Manges, A. R., J. R. Johnson, B. Foxman, T. T. O'Bryan, K. E. Fullerton, and L. W. Riley. 2001. Widespread distribution of urinary tract infections caused by a multidrug-resistant *Escherichia coli* clonal group. *N. Engl. J. Med.* **345**:1007–1013.

Marahiel, M. A., T. Stachelhaus, and H. D. Mootz. 1997. Modular peptide synthetases involved in nonribosomal peptide synthesis. *Chem. Rev.* **97**:2651–2674.

Marmor, S., C. P. Petersen, F. Reck, W. Yang, N. Gao, and S. L. Fisher. 2001. Biochemical characterization of a phosphinate inhibitor of *Escherichia coli* MurC. *Biochemistry* **40**:12207–12214.

Marshall, C. G., G. Broadhead, B. K. Leskiw, and G. D. Wright. 1997. D-Ala-D-Ala ligases from glycopeptide antibiotic-producing organisms are highly homologous to the enterococcal vancomycin-resistance ligases VanA and VanB. *Proc. Natl. Acad. Sci. USA* **94**:6480–6483.

Marshall, C. G., I. A. Lessard, I. Park, and G. D. Wright. 1998. Glycopeptide antibiotic resistance genes in glycopeptide-producing organisms. *Antimicrob. Agents Chemother.* **42**:2215–2220.

Martinez, M. B., M. Flickinger, L. Higgins, T. Krick, and G. L. Nelsestuen. 2001. Reduced outer membrane permeability of *Escherichia coli* O157:H7: suggested role of modified outer membrane porins and theoretical function in resistance to antimicrobial agents. *Biochemistry* **40**:11965–11974.

Martinez-Hackert, E., S. Harlocker, M. Inouye, H. M. Berman, and A. M. Stock. 1996. Crystallization, X-ray studies, and site-directed cysteine mutagenesis of the DNA-binding domain of OmpR. *Protein Sci.* **5:**1429–1433.

Martinez-Hackert, E., and A. M. Stock. 1997. The DNA-binding domain of OmpR: crystal structures of a winged helix transcription factor. *Structure* **5:**109–124.

Massova, I., and S. Mobashery. 1998. Kinship and diversification of bacterial penicillin-binding proteins and beta-lactamases. *Antimicrob. Agents Chemother.* **42:**1–17.

Matsushita, M., and K. D. Janda. 2002. Histidine kinases as targets for new antimicrobial agents. *Bioorg. Med. Chem.* **10:**855–867.

Maxwell, A. 1997. DNA gyrase as a drug target. *Trends Microbiol.* **5:**102–109.

Mazmanian, S. K., G. Liu, H. Ton-That, and O. Schneewind. 1999. *Staphylococcus aureus* sortase, an enzyme that anchors surface proteins to the cell wall. *Science* **285:**760–763.

Mazmanian, S. K., H. Ton-That, and O. Schneewind. 2001. Sortase-catalysed anchoring of surface proteins to the cell wall of Staphylococcus aureus. *Mol. Microbiol.* **40:**1049–1057.

McCafferty, D. G., P. Cudic, M. K. Yu, D. C. Behenna, and R. Kruger. 1999. Synergy and duality in peptide antibiotic mechanisms. *Curr. Opin. Chem. Biol.* **3:**672–680.

McClelland, M., K. E. Sanderson, J. Spieth, S. W. Clifton, P. Latreille, L. Courtney, S. Porwollik, J. Ali, M. Dante, F. Du, S. Hou, D. Layman, S. Leonard, C. Nguyen, K. Scott, A. Holmes, N. Grewal, E. Mulvaney, E. Ryan, H. Sun, L. Florea, W. Miller, T. Stoneking, M. Nhan, R. Waterston, and R. K. Wilson. 2001. Complete genome sequence of *Salmonella enterica* serovar Typhimurium LT2. *Nature* **413:**852–856.

McDaniel, R., A. Thamchaipenet, C. Gustafsson, H. Fu, M. Betlach, and G. Ashley. 1999. Multiple genetic modifications of the erythromycin polyketide synthase to produce a library of novel "unnatural" natural products. *Proc. Natl. Acad. Sci. USA* **96:**1846–1851.

McDevitt, D., and M. Rosenberg. 2001. Exploiting genomics to discover new antibiotics. *Trends Microbiol.* **9:**611–617.

McDonald, L. C., S. Rossiter, C. Mackinson, Y. Y. Wang, S. Johnson, M. Sullivan, R. Sokolow, E. DeBess, L. Gilbert, J. A. Benson, B. Hill, and F. J. Angulo. 2001. Quinupristin-dalfopristin-resistant *Enterococcus faecium* on chicken and in human stool specimens. *N. Engl. J. Med.* **345:**1155–1160.

McDowell, P., Z. Affas, C. Reynolds, M. T. Holden, S. J. Wood, S. Saint, A. Cockayne, P. J. Hill, C. E. Dodd, B. W. Bycroft, W. C. Chan, and P. Williams. 2001. Structure, activity and evolution of the group I thiolactone peptide quorum-sensing system of *Staphylococcus aureus*. *Mol. Microbiol.* **41:**503–512.

McGowan, J. E., Jr., and F. C. Tenover. 1997. Control of antimicrobial resistance in the health care system. *Infect. Dis. Clin. North. Am.* **11:**297–311.

McKinney, J. D., K. Honer zu Bentrup, E. J. Munoz-Elias, A. Miczak, B. Chen, W. T. Chan, D. Swenson, J. C. Sacchettini, W. R. Jacobs, Jr., and D. G. Russell. 2000. Persistence of *Mycobacterium tuberculosis* in macrophages and mice requires the glyoxylate shunt enzyme isocitrate lyase. *Nature* **406:**735–738.

McKinney, T. K., V. K. Sharma, W. A. Craig, and G. L. Archer. 2001. Transcription of the gene mediating methicillin resistance in *Staphylococcus aureus* (*mecA*) is corepressed but not coinduced by cognate *mecA* and beta-lactamase regulators. *J. Bacteriol.* **183:**6862–6868.

McMahon, G., L. Su, C. Liang, and C. Tang. 1998. Protein kinase inhibitors: structural determinants for target specificity. *Curr. Opin. Drug Discov.* **1:**131–146.

McMurry, L. M., M. Oethinger, and S. B. Levy. 1998. Triclosan targets lipid synthesis. *Nature* **394:**531–532.

Mead, P. S., L. Slutsker, V. Dietz, L. F. McCaig, J. S. Bresee, C. Shapiro, P. M. Griffin, and R. V. Tauxe. 1999. Food-related illness and death in the United States. *Emerg. Infect. Dis.* **5:**607–625.

Men, H., P. Park, M. Ge, and S. Walker. 1998. Substrate synthesis and activity assay for MurG. *J. Am. Chem. Soc.* **120:**2484–2485.

Mengin-Lecreulx, D., and J. van Heijenoort. 1994. Copurification of glucosamine-1-phosphate acetyltransferase and *N*-acetylglucosamine-1-phosphate uridyltransferase activities of *Escherichia coli*: characterization of the glmU gene product as a bifunctional enzyme catalyzing two subsequent steps in the pathway for UDP-*N*-acetylglucosamine synthesis. *J. Bacteriol.* **176:**5788–5795.

Miller, D. A., L. Luo, N. Hillson, T. A. Keating, and C. T. Walsh. 2002. Yersiniabactin synthetase. A four-protein assembly line producing the nonribosomal peptide/polyketide hybrid siderophore of *Yersinia pestis*. *Chem. Biol.* **9:**333–344.

Miller, D. J., S. M. Hammond, D. Anderluzzi, and T. D. H. Bugg. 1998. Aminoalkylphosphinate inhibitors of D-Ala-D-Ala adding enzyme. *J. Chem. Soc., Perkin Trans.* **1:**131–142.

Miller, M. B., and B. L. Bassler. 2001. Quorum sensing in bacteria. *Annu. Rev. Microbiol.* **55:**165–199.

Miller, M. T., B. O. Bachmann, C. A. Townsend, and A. L. Rosenzweig. 2001. Structure of β-lactam synthetase reveals how to synthesize antibiotics instead of asparagine. *Nat. Struct. Biol.* **8:**684–689.

Mitscher, L. A., S. P. Pillai, E. J. Gentry, and D. M. Shankel. 1999. Multiple drug resistance. *Med. Res. Rev.* **19:**477–496.

Mittl, P. R., and M. G. Grutter. 2001. Structural genomics: opportunities and challenges. *Curr. Opin. Chem. Biol.* **5:**402–408.

Miyadoh, S., N. Tsuchizaki, J. Ishikawa, and K. Hotta. 1997. *Atlas of Actinomycetes*. Asakura Publishing Co., Ltd., Tokyo, Japan.

Molbak, K., D. L. Baggesen, F. M. Aarestrup, J. M. Ebbesen, J. Engberg, K. Frydendahl, P. Gerner-Smidt, A. M. Petersen, and H. C. Wegener. 1999. An outbreak of multidrug-resistant, quinolone-resistant *Salmonella enterica* serotype Typhimurium DT104. *N. Engl. J. Med.* **341:**1420–1425.

Murray, B. E. 2000. Problems and perils of vancomycin resistant enterococci. *Braz. J. Infect. Dis.* **4:**9–14.

Nagai, K., T. A. Davies, M. R. Jacobs, and P. C. Appelbaum. 2002. Effects of amino acid alterations in penicillin-binding proteins (PBPs) 1a, 2b, and 2x on PBP affinities of penicillin, ampicillin, amoxicillin, cefditoren, cefuroxime, cefprozil, and cefaclor in 18 clinical isolates of penicillin-susceptible, -intermediate, and -resistant pneumococci. *Antimicrob. Agents Chemother.* **46:**1273–1280.

Nataro, J. P., and J. B. Kaper. 1998. Diarrheagenic *Escherichia coli. Clin. Microbiol. Rev.* **11:**142–201.

Navarre, W. W., and O. Schneewind. 1999. Surface proteins of gram-positive bacteria and mechanisms of their targeting to the cell wall envelope. *Microbiol. Mol. Biol. Rev.* **63:**174–229.

Navarro, F., and P. Courvalin. 1994. Analysis of genes encoding D-alanine-D-alanine ligase-related enzymes in *Enterococcus casseliflavus* and *Enterococcus flavescens. Antimicrob. Agents Chemother.* **38:**1788–1793.

Neuhaus, F. C., and W. P. Hammes. 1981. Inhibition of cell wall biosynthesis by analogues and alanine. *Pharmacol. Ther.* **14:**265–319.

Ng, E. Y., M. Trucksis, and D. C. Hooper. 1996. Quinolone resistance mutations in topoisomerase IV: relationship to the flqA locus and genetic evidence that topoisomerase IV is the primary target and DNA gyrase is the secondary target of fluoroquinolones in *Staphylococcus aureus. Antimicrob. Agents Chemother.* **40:**1881–1888.

Nicholson, T. P., B. A. Rudd, M. Dawson, C. M. Lazarus, T. J. Simpson, and R. J. Cox. 2001. Design and utility of oligonucleotide gene probes for fungal polyketide synthases. *Chem. Biol.* **8:**157–178.

Nicolaou, K. C., J. A. Pfefferkorn, A. J. Roecker, G.-Q. Cao, S. Barluenga, and H. J. Mitchell. 2000a. Natural product-like combinatorial libraries based on privileged structures. 1. General principles and solid-phase synthesis of benzopyrans. *J. Am. Chem. Soc.* **122:**9939–9953.

Nicolaou, K. C., J. A. Pfefferkorn, H. J. Mitchell, A. J. Roecker, S. Barluenga, G.-Q. Cao, R. L. Affleck, and J. E. Lillig. 2000b. Natural product-like combinatorial libraries based on privileged structures. 2. Construction of a 10,000-membered benzopyran library by directed split-and-pool chemistry using NanoKans and optical encoding. *J. Am. Chem. Soc.* **122:**9954–9967.

Nicolaou, K. C., J. A. Pfefferkorn, S. Barluenga, H. J. Mitchell, A. J. Roecker, and G.-Q. Cao. 2000c. Natural product-like combinatorial libraries based on privileged structures. 3. The "libraries from libraries" principle for diversity enhancement of benzopyran libraries. *J. Am. Chem. Soc.* **122:**9968–9976.

Nikaido, H. 1994. Prevention of drug access to bacterial targets: permeability barriers and active efflux. *Science* **264:**382–388.

Nikaido, H. 1998. Antibiotic resistance caused by gram negative multidrug efflux pumps. *Clin. Infect. Dis.* **27**(Suppl. 1):S32–S41.

Nishino, K., and A. Yamaguchi. 2001. Analysis of a complete library of putative drug transporter genes in Escherichia coli. *J. Bacteriol.* **183:**5803–5812.

Nissen, P., J. Hansen, N. Ban, P. B. Moore, and T. A. Steitz. 2000. The structural basis of ribosome activity in peptide bond synthesis. *Science* **289:**920–930.

Nouwen, N., N. Ranson, H. Saibil, B. Wolpensinger, A. Engel, A. Ghazi, and A. P. Pugsley. 1999. Secretin PulD: association with pilot PulS, structure, and ion-conducting channel formation. *Proc. Natl. Acad. Sci. USA* **96:**8173–8177.

Novak, R., E. Charpentier, J. S. Braun, and E. Tuomanen. 2000. Signal transduction by a death signal peptide: uncovering the mechanism of bacterial killing by penicillin. *Mol. Cell* **5:**49–57.

Novick, R. P. 1962. Staphylococcal penicillinase and new penicillins. *J. Bacteriol.* **83:** 229–234.

Nyquist, A. C., R. Gonzales, J. F. Steiner, and M. A. Sande. 1998. Antibiotic prescribing for children with colds, upper respiratory tract infections, and bronchitis. *JAMA* **279:**875–877.

Onishi, H. R., B. A. Pelak, L. S. Gerckens, L. L. Silver, F. M. Kahan, M. H. Chen, A. A. Patchett, S. M. Galloway, S. A. Hyland, M. S. Anderson, and C. R. Raetz. 1996. Antibacterial agents that inhibit lipid A biosynthesis. *Science* **274:**980–982.

Onodera, Y., Y. Uchida, M. Tanaka, and K. Sato. 1999. Dual inhibitory activity of sitafloxacin (DU-6859a) against DNA gyrase and topoisomerase IV of *Streptococcus pneumoniae*. *J. Antimicrob. Chemother.* **44:**533–536.

Orth, P., D. Schnappinger, W. Hillen, W. Saenger, and W. Hinrichs. 2000. Structural basis of gene regulation by the tetracycline inducible Tet repressor-operator system. *Nat. Struct. Biol.* **7:**215–219.

O'Sullivan, J., and C. Ball. 1983. β-lactams, p. 73–94. *In* L. C. Vining (ed.), *Biochemistry and Genetic Regulation of Commercially Important Antibiotics.* Addison-Wesley Publishing Co., Inc., Reading, Mass.

Paik, J., I. Kern, R. Lurz, and R. Hakenbeck. 1999. Mutational analysis of the *Streptococcus pneumoniae* bimodular class A penicillin-binding proteins. *J. Bacteriol.* **181:**3852–3856.

Pallen, M. J., A. C. Lam, M. Antonio, and K. Dunbar. 2001. An embarrassment of sortases—a richness of substrates? *Trends Microbiol.* **9:**97–102.

Palumbi, S. R. 2001. Humans as the world's greatest evolutionary force. *Science* **293:**1786–1790.

Pan, X. S., and M. Fisher. 1997. Targeting of DNA gyrase in *Streptococcus pneumoniae* by sparfloxacin: selective targeting of gyrase or topoisomerase IV by quinolones. *Antimicrob. Agents Chemother.* **41:**471–474.

Pares, S., N. Mouz, Y. Petillot, R. Hakenbeck, and O. Dideberg. 1996. X-ray structure of *Streptococcus pneumoniae* PBP2x, a primary penicillin target enzyme. *Nat. Struct. Biol.* **3:**284–289.

Park, I. S., C. H. Lin, and C. T. Walsh. 1997. Bacterial resistance to vancomycin: overproduction, purification, and characterization of VanC2 from *Enterococcus casseliflavus* as a D-Ala-D-Ser ligase. *Proc. Natl. Acad. Sci. USA* **94:**10040–10044.

Parkhill, J., G. Dougan, K. D. James, N. R. Thomson, D. Pickard, J. Wain, C. Churcher, K. L. Mungall, S. D. Bentley, M. T. Holden, M. Sebaihia, S. Baker, D. Basham, K. Brooks, T. Chillingworth, P. Connerton, A. Cronin, P. Davis, R. M. Davies, L. Dowd, N. White, J. Farrar, T. Feltwell, N. Hamlin, A. Haque, T. T. Hien, S. Holroyd, K. Jagels, A. Krogh, T. S. Larsen, S. Leather, S. Moule, P. O'Gaora, C. Parry, M. Quail, K. Rutherford, M. Simmonds, J. Skelton, K. Stevens, S. Whitehead, and B. G. Barrell. 2001. Complete genome sequence of a multiple drug resistant *Salmonella enterica* serovar Typhi CT18. *Nature* **413:**848–852.

Parris, K. D., L. Lin, A. Tam, R. Mathew, J. Hixon, M. Stahl, C. C. Fritz, J. Seehra, and W. S. Somers. 2000. Crystal structures of substrate binding to *Bacillus subtilis* holo-(acyl carrier protein) synthase reveal a novel trimeric arrangement of molecules resulting in three active sites. *Structure Fold. Des.* **8:**883–895.

Patel, H. M., and C. T. Walsh. 2001. In vitro reconstitution of the *Pseudomonas aeruginosa* nonribosomal peptide synthesis of pyochelin: characterization of backbone tailoring thiazoline reductase and *N*-methyltransferase activities. *Biochemistry* **40:**9023–9031.

Patel, U., Y. P. Yan, F. W. Hobbs, Jr., J. Kaczmarczyk, A. M. Slee, D. L. Pompliano, M. G. Kurilla, and E. V. Bobkova. 2001. Oxazolidinones mechanism of action: inhibition of the first peptide bond formation. *J. Biol. Chem.* **276:**37199–37205.

Paulsen, I. T., M. H. Brown, and R. A. Skurray. 1996. Proton-dependent multidrug efflux systems. *Microbiol. Rev.* **60:**575–608.

Payne, D. J., J. A. Hueso-Rodriguez, H. Boyd, N. O. Concha, C. A. Janson, M. Gilpin, J. H. Bateson, C. Cheever, N. L. Niconovich, S. Pearson, S. Rittenhouse, D. Tew, E. Diez, P. Perez, J. De La Fuente, M. Rees, and A. Rivera-Sagredo. 2002. Identification of a series of tricyclic natural products as potent broad-spectrum inhibitors of metallo-beta-lactamases. *Antimicrob. Agents Chemother.* **46:**1880–1886.

Perego, M., and J. A. Hoch. 2001. Functional Genomics of Gram-Positive Microorganisms: review of the meeting, San Diego, California, 24 to 28 June 2001. *J. Bacteriol.* **183:**6973–6978.

Perna, N. T., G. Plunkett III, V. Burland, B. Mau, J. D. Glasner, D. J. Rose, G. F. Mayhew, P. S. Evans, J. Gregor, H. A. Kirkpatrick, G. Posfai, J. Hackett, S. Klink, A. Boutin, Y. Shao, L. Miller, E. J. Grotbeck, N. W. Davis, A. Lim, E. T. Dimalanta, K. D. Potamousis, J. Apodaca, T. S. Anantharaman, J. Lin, G. Yen, D. C. Schwartz, R. A. Welch, and F. R. Blattner. 2001. Genome sequence of enterohaemorrhagic *Escherichia coli* O157:H7. *Nature* **409:**529–533.

Perry, R. D., and J. D. Fetherston. 1997. Yersinia pestis—etiologic agent of plague. *Clin. Microbiol. Rev.* **10:**35–66.

Persson, C., N. Carballeira, H. Wolf-Watz, and M. Fallman. 1997. The PTPase YopH inhibits uptake of Yersinia, tyrosine phosphorylation of p130Cas and FAK, and the associated accumulation of these proteins in peripheral focal adhesions. *EMBO J.* **16:**2307–2318.

Petkovic, H., A. Thamchaipenet, L. H. Zhou, D. Hranueli, P. Raspor, P. G. Waterman, and I. S. Hunter. 1999. Disruption of an aromatase/cyclase from the oxytetracycline gene cluster of *Streptomyces rimosus* results in production of novel polyketides with shorter chain lengths. *J. Biol. Chem.* **274:**32829–32834.

Piepersberg, W. 1997. Molecular biology, biochemistry and fermentation of aminoglycoside antibiotics, p. 842. *In* W. R. Strohl (ed.), *Biotechnology of Antibiotics*, 2nd ed. Marcel Dekker Inc., New York, N.Y.

Pioletti, M., F. Schlunzen, J. Harms, R. Zarivach, M. Gluhmann, H. Avila, A. Bashan, H. Bartels, T. Auerbach, C. Jacobi, T. Hartsch, A. Yonath, and F. Franceschi. 2001. Crystal structures of complexes of the small ribosomal subunit with tetracycline, edeine and IF3. *EMBO J.* **20:**1829–1839.

Poole, K. 2001. Overcoming antimicrobial resistance by targeting resistance mechanisms. *J. Pharm. Pharmacol.* **53:**283–294.

Pootoolal, J., M. G. Thomas, C. G. Marshall, J. M. Neu, B. K. Hubbard, C. T. Walsh, and G. D. Wright. 2002. Assembling the glycopeptide antibiotic scaffold: the biosynthesis of A47934 from *Streptomyces topocaensis* NRRL15009. *Proc. Natl. Acad. Sci. USA* **99:**8962–8967.

Poulsen, S. M., C. Kofoed, and B. Vester. 2000. Inhibition of the ribosomal peptidyl transferase reaction by the mycarose moiety of the antibiotics carbomycin, spiramycin and tylosin. *J. Mol. Biol.* **304:**471–481.

Poulsen, S. M., M. Karlsson, L. B. Johansson, and B. Vester. 2001. The pleuromutilin drugs tiamulin and valnemulin bind to the RNA at the peptidyl transferase centre on the ribosome. *Mol. Microbiol.* **41:**1091–1099.

Prasch, T., T. Naumann, R. L. Markert, M. Sattler, W. Schubert, S. Schaal, M. Bauch, H. Kogler, and C. Griesinger. 1997. Constitution and solution conformation of the antibiotic mersacidin determined by NMR and molecular dynamics. *Eur. J. Biochem.* **244:**501–512.

Prente, J. L., and B. B. Finlay. 2001. Pathogenic *E. coli*, p. 388–422. *In* E. A. Groisman (ed.), *Principles of Bacterial Pathogenesis*. Academic Press Inc., San Diego, Calif.

Pucci, M. J., and T. J. Dougherty. 2002. Direct quantitation of the numbers of individual penicillin-binding proteins per cell in *Staphylococcus aureus. J. Bacteriol.* **184:**588–591.

Puech, V., N. Bayan, K. Salim, G. Leblon, and M. Daffe. 2000. Characterization of the in vivo acceptors of the mycoloyl residues transferred by the corynebacterial PS1 and the related mycobacterial antigens 85. *Mol. Microbiol.* **35:**1026–1041.

Putman, M., H. W. van Veen, and W. N. Konings. 2000. Molecular properties of bacterial multidrug transporters. *Microbiol. Mol. Biol. Rev.* **64:**672–693.

Qiu, X., C. A. Janson, W. W. Smith, S. M. Green, P. McDevitt, K. Johanson, P. Carter, M. Hibbs, C. Lewis, A. Chalker, A. Fosberry, J. Lalonde, J. Berge, P. Brown, C. S. Houge-Frydrych, and R. L. Jarvest. 2001. Crystal structure of *Staphylococcus aureus* tyrosyl-tRNA synthetase in complex with a class of potent and specific inhibitors. *Protein Sci.* **10:**2008–2016.

Que, L., Jr. 2000. One motif—many different reactions. *Nat. Struct. Biol.* **7:**182–184.

Quiros, L. M., I. Aguirrezabalaga, C. Olano, C. Mendez, and J. A. Salas. 1998. Two glycosyltransferases and a glycosidase are involved in oleandomycin modification during its biosynthesis by Streptomyces antibioticus. *Mol. Microbiol.* **28:**1177–1185.

Raetz, C. 1987. Structure and biosynthesis of lipid A in *E. coli*, p. 498–503. *In* F. C. Neidhart (ed.), Escherichia coli *and* Salmonella typhimurium: *Cellular and Molecular Biology*. ASM Press, Washington, D.C.

Rajagopalan, P. T., A. Datta, and D. Pei. 1997. Purification, characterization, and inhibition of peptide deformylase from *Escherichia coli. Biochemistry* **36:**13910–13918.

Rasmussen, B. A., and K. Bush. 1997. Carbapenem-hydrolyzing beta-lactamases. *Antimicrob. Agents Chemother.* **41:**223–232.

Raviv, Y., H. B. Pollard, E. P. Bruggemann, I. Pastan, and M. M. Gottesman. 1990. Photosensitized labeling of a functional multidrug transporter in living drug-resistant tumor cells. *J. Biol. Chem.* **265:**3975–3980.

Rawlings, B. J. 1999. Biosynthesis of polyketides (other than actinomycete macrolides). *Nat. Prod. Rep.* **16:**425–484.

Rawlings, B. J. 2001a. Type I polyketide biosynthesis in bacteria (part A—erythromycin biosynthesis). *Nat. Prod. Rep.* **18:**190–227.

Rawlings, B. J. 2001b. Type I polyketide biosynthesis in bacteria (part B). *Nat. Prod. Rep.* **18:**231–281.

Reid, S. D., N. M. Green, J. K. Buss, B. Lei, and J. M. Musser. 2001. Multilocus analysis of extracellular putative virulence proteins made by group A streptococcus: population genetics, human serologic response, and gene transcription. *Proc. Natl. Acad. Sci. USA* **98:**7552–7557.

Reuter, K., M. R. Mofid, M. A. Marahiel, and R. Ficner. 1999. Crystal structure of the surfactin synthetase-activating enzyme sfp: a prototype of the 4′-phospho-pantetheinyl transferase superfamily. *EMBO J.* **18:**6823–6831.

Ritter, T. K., and C. H. Wong. 2001. Carbohydrate-based antibiotics: a new approach to tackling the problem of resistance. *Angew. Chem. Int. Ed. Engl.* **40:**3508–3533.

Roach, P. L., I. J. Clifton, C. M. Hensgens, N. Shibata, C. J. Schofield, J. Hajdu, and J. E. Baldwin. 1997. Structure of isopenicillin N synthase complexed with substrate and the mechanism of penicillin formation. *Nature* **387:**827–830.

Robinson, V. L., and A. M. Stock. 1999. High energy exchange: proteins that make or break phosphoramidate bonds. *Structure Fold. Des.* **7:**R47–R53.

Rodnina, M. V., and W. Wintermeyer. 2001. Ribosome fidelity: tRNA discrimination, proofreading and induced fit. *Trends Biochem. Sci.* **26:**124–130.

Rodrigue, A., Y. Quentin, A. Lazdunski, V. Mejean, and M. Foglino. 2000. Two-component systems in *Pseudomonas aeruginosa*: why so many? *Trends Microbiol.* **8:** 498–504.

Rodriguez, E., and R. McDaniel. 2001. Combinatorial biosynthesis of antimicrobials and other natural products. *Curr. Opin. Microbiol.* **4:**526–534.

Roestamadji, J., I. Grapsas, and S. Mobashery. 1995. Mechanism-based inactivation of bacterial aminoglycoside 3′-phosphotransferases. *J. Am. Chem. Soc.* **117:**80–84.

Rohdich, F., K. Kis, A. Bacher, and W. Eisenreich. 2001. The non-mevalonate pathway of isoprenoids: genes, enzymes and intermediates. *Curr. Opin. Chem. Biol.* **5:** 535–540.

Roper, D. I., T. Huyton, A. Vagin, and G. Dodson. 2000. The molecular basis of vancomycin resistance in clinically relevant enterococci: crystal structure of D-alanyl-D-lactate ligase (VanA). *Proc. Natl. Acad. Sci. USA* **97:**8921–8925.

Rosamond, J., and A. Allsop. 2000. Harnessing the power of the genome in the search for new antibiotics. *Science* **287:**1973–1976.

Rosen, H., R. Hajdu, L. Silver, H. Kropp, K. Dorso, J. Kohler, J. G. Sundelof, J. Huber, G. G. Hammond, J. J. Jackson, C. J. Gill, R. Thompson, B. A. Pelak, J. H. Epstein-Toney, G. Lankas, R. R. Wilkening, K. J. Wildonger, T. A. Blizzard, F. P. DiNinno, R. W. Ratcliffe, J. V. Heck, J. W. Kozarich, and M. L. Hammond. 1999. Reduced immunotoxicity and preservation of antibacterial activity in a releasable side-chain carbapenem antibiotic. *Science* **283:**703–706.

Rowe, C. J., I. U. Bohm, I. P. Thomas, B. Wilkinson, B. A. Rudd, G. Foster, A. P. Blackaby, P. J. Sidebottom, Y. Roddis, A. D. Buss, J. Staunton, and P. F. Leadlay. 2001. Engineering a polyketide with a longer chain by insertion of an extra module into the erythromycin-producing polyketide synthase. *Chem. Biol.* **8:**475–485.

Rozwarski, D. A., G. A. Grant, D. H. Barton, W. R. Jacobs, Jr., and J. C. Sacchettini. 1998. Modification of the NADH of the isoniazid target (InhA) from *Mycobacterium tuberculosis. Science* **279:**98–102.

Rudgers, G. W., W. Huang, and T. Palzkill. 2001. Binding properties of a peptide derived from beta-lactamase inhibitory protein. *Antimicrob. Agents Chemother.* **45:** 3279–3286.

Russel, M. 1998. Macromolecular assembly and secretion across the bacterial cell envelope: type II protein secretion systems. *J. Mol. Biol.* **279:**485–499.

Russell, A. D., and I. Chopra. 1996. *Understanding Antibacterial Action and Resistance,* 2nd ed. Ellis Horwood, New York, N.Y.

Sahl, H. G., and G. Bierbaum. 1998. Lantibiotics: biosynthesis and biological activities of uniquely modified peptides from gram-positive bacteria. *Annu. Rev. Microbiol.* **52:**41–79.

Sahm, D. F., C. Thornsberry, D. C. Mayfield, M. E. Jones, and J. A. Karlowsky. 2001. Multidrug-resistant urinary tract isolates of *Escherichia coli*: prevalence and patient demographics in the United States in 2000. *Antimicrob. Agents Chemother.* **45:**1402–1406.

Saier, M. H., Jr., I. T. Paulsen, M. K. Sliwinski, S. S. Pao, R. A. Skurray, and H. Nikaido. 1998. Evolutionary origins of multidrug and drug-specific efflux pumps in bacteria. *FASEB J.* **12:**265–274.

Sanders, D. A., A. G. Staines, S. A. McMahon, M. R. McNeil, C. Whitfield, and J. H. Naismith. 2001. UDP-galactopyranose mutase has a novel structure and mechanism. *Nat. Struct. Biol.* **8:**858–863.

Sansonetti, P., C. Egile, and C. Wenneras. 2001. Shigellosis: from disease symptoms to molecular and cellular pathogenesis, p. 336–387. *In* E. A. Groisman (ed.), *Principles of Bacterial Pathogenesis.* Academic Press Inc., San Diego, Calif.

Sathyamoorthy, N., and K. Takayama. 1987. Purification and characterization of a novel mycolic acid exchange enzyme from *Mycobacterium smegmatis. J. Biol. Chem.* **262:**13417–13423.

Schauder, S., and B. L. Bassler. 2001. The languages of bacteria. *Genes Dev.* **15:** 1468–1480.

Schauder, S., K. Shokat, M. G. Surette, and B. L. Bassler. 2001. The LuxS family of bacterial autoinducers: biosynthesis of a novel quorum-sensing signal molecule. *Mol. Microbiol.* **41:**463–476.

Schentag, J. J., J. M. Hyatt, J. R. Carr, J. A. Paladino, M. C. Birmingham, G. S. Zimmer, and T. J. Cumbo. 1998. Genesis of methicillin-resistant *Staphylococcus aureus* (MRSA), how treatment of MRSA infections has selected for vancomycin-resistant *Enterococcus faecium*, and the importance of antibiotic management and infection control. *Clin. Infect. Dis.* **26:**1204–1214.

Schiffer, G., and J. V. Holtje. 1999. Cloning and characterization of PBP 1C, a third member of the multimodular class A penicillin-binding proteins of *Escherichia coli. J. Biol. Chem.* **274:**32031–32039.

Schlunzen, F., R. Zarivach, J. Harms, A. Bashan, A. Tocilj, R. Albrecht, A. Yonath, and F. Franceschi. 2001. Structural basis for the interaction of antibiotics with the peptidyl transferase centre in eubacteria. *Nature* **413:**814–821.

Schmitz, F. J., A. C. Fluit, D. Milatovic, J. Verhoef, H. P. Heinz, and S. Brisse. 2000. In vitro potency of moxifloxacin, clinafloxacin and sitafloxacin against 248 genetically defined clinical isolates of *Staphylococcus aureus. J. Antimicrob. Chemother.* **46:**109–113.

Scholar, E. M., and W. B. Pratt. 2000. *The Antimicrobial Drugs*, 2nd ed. Oxford University Press, New York, N.Y.

Schonbrunn, E., S. Sack, S. Eschenburg, A. Perrakis, F. Krekel, N. Amrhein, and E. Mandelkow. 1996. Crystal structure of UDP-*N*-acetylglucosamine enolpyruvyltransferase, the target of the antibiotic fosfomycin. *Structure* **4:**1065–1075.

Schreiber, S. L. 2000. Target-oriented and diversity-oriented organic synthesis in drug discovery. *Science* **287:**1964–1969.

Schwartz, B., J. A. Markwalder, and Y. Wang. 2001. Lipid II: total synthesis of the bacterial cell wall precursor and utilization as a substrate for glycosyltransfer and transpeptidation by penicillin binding protein (PBP) 1b of *Escherichia coli. J. Am. Chem. Soc.* **123:**11638–11643.

Selinsky, B. S., K. Gupta, C. T. Sharkey, and P. J. Loll. 2001. Structural analysis of NSAID binding by prostaglandin H2 synthase: time-dependent and time-independent inhibitors elicit identical enzyme conformations. *Biochemistry* **40:**5172–5180.

Seppala, H., T. Klaukka, J. Vuopio-Varkila, A. Muotiala, H. Helenius, K. Lager, and P. Huovinen. 1997. The effect of changes in the consumption of macrolide antibiotics on erythromycin resistance in group A streptococci in Finland. Finnish Study Group for Antimicrobial Resistance. *N. Engl. J. Med.* **337:**441–446.

Seto, H. 1999. Biosynthesis of the natural C-P compounds, Bialaphos and fosfomycin, p. 865–880. *In* D. Barton, K. Nakanishi, and O. Meth-Cohn (ed.), *Comprehensive Natural Products Chemistry*, vol. 1. Pergamon Press, Inc., Elmsford, N.Y.

Shaw, J. P., G. A. Petsko, and D. Ringe. 1997. Determination of the structure of alanine racemase from *Bacillus stearothermophilus* at 1.9-Å resolution. *Biochemistry* **36:**1329–1342.

Sheldon, P. J., D. A. Johnson, P. R. August, H. W. Liu, and D. H. Sherman. 1997. Characterization of a mitomycin-binding drug resistance mechanism from the producing organism, *Streptomyces lavendulae. J. Bacteriol.* **179:**1796–1804.

Shen, B. 2000. Biosynthesis of aromatic polyketides. *Top. Curr. Chem.* **209:**1–51.

Shi, Y., and C. T. Walsh. 1995. Active site mapping of Escherichia coli D-Ala-D-Ala ligase by structure-based mutagenesis. *Biochemistry* **34:**2768–2776.

Shlaes, D. M., D. N. Gerding, J. F. John, Jr., W. A. Craig, D. L. Bornstein, R. A. Duncan, M. R. Eckman, W. E. Farrer, W. H. Greene, V. Lorian, S. Levy, J. E. McGowan, Jr., S. M. Paul, J. Ruskin, F. C. Tenover, and C. Watanakunakorn. 1997a. Society for Healthcare Epidemiology of America and Infectious Diseases Society of America Joint Committee on the Prevention of Antimicrobial Resistance: guidelines for the prevention of antimicrobial resistance in hospitals. *Clin. Infect. Dis.* **25:**584–599.

Shlaes, D. M., D. N. Gerding, J. F. John, Jr., W. A. Craig, D. L. Bornstein, R. A. Duncan, M. R. Eckman, W. E. Farrer, W. H. Greene, V. Lorian, S. Levy, J. E. McGowan, Jr., S. M. Paul, J. Ruskin, F. C. Tenover, and C. Watanakunakorn. 1997b. Society for Healthcare Epidemiology of America and Infectious Diseases Society of America Joint Committee on the Prevention of Antimicrobial Resistance: guidelines for the prevention of antimicrobial resistance in hospitals. *Infect. Control Hosp. Epidemiol.* **18:**275–291.

Silvian, L. F., J. Wang, and T. A. Steitz. 1999. Insights into editing from an Ile-tRNA synthetase structure with tRNAile and mupirocin. *Science* **285:**1074–1077.

Sinha Roy, R., A. M. Gehring, J. C. Milne, P. J. Belshaw, and C. T. Walsh. 1999. Thiazole and oxazole peptides: biosynthesis and molecular machinery. *Nat. Prod. Rep.* **16:**249–263.

Sinha Roy, R., P. Yang, S. Kodali, Y. Xiong, R. M. Kim, P. R. Griffin, H. R. Onishi, J. Kohler, L. L. Silver, and K. Chapman. 2001. Direct interaction of a vancomycin derivative with bacterial enzymes involved in cell wall biosynthesis. *Chem. Biol.* **8:** 1095–1106.

Skarzynski, T., A. Mistry, A. Wonacott, S. E. Hutchinson, V. A. Kelly, and K. Duncan. 1996. Structure of UDP-N-acetylglucosamine enolpyruvyl transferase, an enzyme essential for the synthesis of bacterial peptidoglycan, complexed with substrate UDP-N-acetylglucosamine and the drug fosfomycin. *Structure* **4:**1465–1474.

Skarzynski, T., D. H. Kim, W. J. Lees, C. T. Walsh, and K. Duncan. 1998. Stereochemical course of enzymatic enolpyruvyl transfer and catalytic conformation of the active site revealed by the crystal structure of the fluorinated analogue of the reaction tetrahedral intermediate bound to the active site of the C115A mutant of MurA. *Biochemistry* **37:**2572–2577.

Solenberg, P. J., P. Matsushima, D. R. Stack, S. C. Wilkie, R. C. Thompson, and R. H. Baltz. 1997. Production of hybrid glycopeptide antibiotics in vitro and in *Streptomyces toyocaensis. Chem. Biol.* **4:**195–202.

Soltani, M., D. Beighton, J. Philpott-Howard, and N. Woodford. 2001. Identification of vat(E-3), a novel gene encoding resistance to quinupristin-dalfopristin in a strain of *Enterococcus faecium* from a hospital patient in the United Kingdom. *Antimicrob. Agents Chemother.* **45:**645–646.

Sosio, M., A. Bianchi, E. Bossi, and S. Donadio. 2000. Teicoplanin biosynthesis genes in *Actinoplanes teichomyceticus. Antonie Leeuwenhoek* **78:**379–384.

Spahn, C. M., G. Blaha, R. K. Agrawal, P. Penczek, R. A. Grassucci, C. A. Trieber, S. R. Connell, D. E. Taylor, K. H. Nierhaus, and J. Frank. 2001. Localization of the ribosomal protection protein Tet(O) on the ribosome and the mechanism of tetracycline resistance. *Mol. Cell* **7:**1037–1045.

Spratt, B. G. 1977. Properties of the penicillin-binding proteins of Escherichia coli K12. *Eur. J. Biochem.* **72:**341–352.

Spratt, B. G. 1994. Resistance to antibiotics mediated by target alterations. *Science* **264:**388–393.

Stachelhaus, T., H. D. Mootz, and M. A. Marahiel. 1999. The specificity-conferring code of adenylation domains in nonribosomal peptide synthetases. *Chem. Biol.* **6:** 493–505.

Stamm, W. E. 2001. An epidemic of urinary tract infections? *N. Engl. J. Med.* **345:** 1055–1057.

Stebbins, C. E., and J. E. Galan. 2000. Modulation of host signaling by a bacterial mimic: structure of the Salmonella effector SptP bound to Rac1. *Mol. Cell* **6:**1449–1460.

Stein, T., S. Borchert, P. Kiesau, S. Heinzmann, S. Kloss, C. Klein, M. Helfrich, and K. D. Entian. 2002. Dual control of subtilin biosynthesis and immunity in Bacillus subtilis. *Mol. Microbiol.* **44:**403–416.

Stephenson, K., Y. Yamaguchi, and J. A. Hoch. 2000. The mechanism of action of inhibitors of bacterial two-component signal transduction systems. *J. Biol. Chem.* **275:**38900–38904.

Stermitz, F. R., P. Lorenz, J. N. Tawara, L. A. Zenewicz, and K. Lewis. 2000. Synergy in a medicinal plant: antimicrobial action of berberine potentiated by 5′-methoxyhydnocarpin, a multidrug pump inhibitor. *Proc. Natl. Acad. Sci. USA* **97:** 1433–1437.

Stover, C. K., X. Q. Pham, A. L. Erwin, S. D. Mizoguchi, P. Warrener, M. J. Hickey, F. S. Brinkman, W. O. Hufnagle, D. J. Kowalik, M. Lagrou, R. L. Garber, L. Goltry, E. Tolentino, S. Westbrock-Wadman, Y. Yuan, L. L. Brody, S. N. Coulter, K. R. Folger, A. Kas, K. Larbig, R. Lim, K. Smith, D. Spencer, G. K. Wong, Z. Wu, I. T. Paulsen, J. Reizer, M. H. Saier, R. E. Hancock, S. Lory, and M. V. Olson. 2000. Complete genome sequence of *Pseudomonas aeruginosa* PA01, an opportunistic pathogen. *Nature* **406:**959–964.

Stratigopoulos, G., and E. Cundliffe. 2002. Expression analysis of the tylosin-biosynthetic gene cluster. Pivotal regulatory role of the tylQ product. *Chem. Biol.* **9:** 71–78.

Strohl, W. R. 2001. Biochemical engineering of natural product biosynthesis pathways. *Metab. Eng.* **3:**4–14.

Strynadka, N. C., S. E. Jensen, P. M. Alzari, and M. N. James. 1996. A potent new mode of beta-lactamase inhibition revealed by the 1.7 Å X-ray crystallographic structure of the TEM-1-BLIP complex. *Nat. Struct. Biol.* **3:**290–297.

Sucheck, S. J., A. L. Wong, K. M. Koeller, D. D. Boehr, K. Draker, P. Sears, G. D. Wright, and C. H. Wong. 2000. Design of bifunctional antibiotics that target bacterial rRNA and inhibit resistance-causing enzymes. *J. Am. Chem. Soc.* **122:**5230–5231.

Sucheck, S. J., and C. H. Wong. 2000. RNA as a target for small molecules. *Curr. Opin. Chem. Biol.* **4:**678–686.

Sugantino, M., and S. L. Roderick. 2002. Crystal structure of Vat(D): an acetyltransferase that inactivates streptogramin group A antibiotics. *Biochemistry* **41:**2209–2216.

Sun, B., Z. Chen, U. S. Eggert, S. J. Shaw, J. V. LaTour, and D. Kahne. 2001. Hybrid glycopeptide antibiotics. *J. Am. Chem. Soc.* **123:**12722–12723.

Sutcliffe, J. A. 1988. Novel approaches toward discovery of antibacterial agents. *Annu. Rep. Med. Chem.* **23:**141–150.

Swift, S., J. P. Throup, P. Williams, G. P. Salmond, and G. S. Stewart. 1996. Quorum sensing: a population-density component in the determination of bacterial phenotype. *Trends Biochem. Sci.* **21:**214–219.

Takano, E., T. Nihira, Y. Hara, J. J. Jones, C. J. Gershater, Y. Yamada, and M. Bibb. 2000. Purification and structural determination of SCB1, a gamma-butyrolactone that elicits antibiotic production in *Streptomyces coelicolor* A3(2). *J. Biol. Chem.* **275:** 11010–11016.

Takei, M., H. Fukuda, R. Kishii, and M. Hosaka. 2001. Target preference of 15 quinolones against *Staphylococcus aureus*, based on antibacterial activities and target inhibition. *Antimicrob. Agents Chemother.* **45:**3544–3547.

Tally, F. P., and M. F. DeBruin. 2000. Development of daptomycin for gram-positive infections. *J. Antimicrob. Chemother.* **46:**523–526.

Tan, D. S., M. A. Foley, M. D. Shair, and S. L. Schreiber. 1998. Stereoselective synthesis of over two million compounds having structural features both reminiscent of natural products and compatible with miniaturized cell-based assays. *J. Am. Chem. Soc.* **120:**8565–8566.

Tan, D. S., M. A. Foley, B. R. Stockwell, M. D. Shair, and S. L. Schreiber. 1999. Synthesis and preliminary evaluation of a library of polycyclic small molecules for use in chemical genetic assays. *J. Am. Chem. Soc.* **121:**9073–9087.

Tang, L., and R. McDaniel. 2001. Construction of desosamine containing polyketide libraries using a glycosyltransferase with broad substrate specificity. *Chem. Biol.* **8:** 547–555.

Tanner, N. K., and P. Linder. 2001. DExD/H box RNA helicases: from generic motors to specific dissociation functions. *Mol. Cell* **8:**251–262.

Teichmann, S. A., A. G. Murzin, and C. Chothia. 2001. Determination of protein function, evolution and interactions by structural genomics. *Curr. Opin. Struct. Biol.* **11:**354–363.

Tettelin, H., K. E. Nelson, I. T. Paulsen, J. A. Eisen, T. D. Read, S. Peterson, J. Heidelberg, R. T. DeBoy, D. H. Haft, R. J. Dodson, A. S. Durkin, M. Gwinn, J. F. Kolonay, W. C. Nelson, J. D. Peterson, L. A. Umayam, O. White, S. L. Salzberg, M. R. Lewis, D. Radune, E. Holtzapple, H. Khouri, A. M. Wolf, T. R. Utterback, C. L. Hansen, L. A. McDonald, T. V. Feldblyum, S. Angiuoli, T. Dickinson, E. K. Hickey, I. E. Holt, B. J. Loftus, F. Yang, H. O. Smith, J. C. Venter, B. A. Dougherty, D. A. Morrison, S. K. Hollingshead, and C. M. Fraser. 2001. Complete genome sequence of a virulent isolate of *Streptococcus pneumoniae. Science* **293:**498–506.

Thomas, M. G., M. D. Burkart, and C. T. Walsh. 2002. Conversion of L-proline to pyrrolyl-2-carboxyl-S-PCP during undecylprodigiosin and pyoluteorin biosynthesis. *Chem. Biol.* **9:**171–184.

Thomson, K. S., and E. S. Moland. 2000. Version 2000: the new beta-lactamases of gram-negative bacteria at the dawn of the new millennium. *Microbes Infect.* **2:**1225–1235.

Thorson, J. S., T. J. Hosted, J. Q. Jiang, J. B. Biggins, and J. Ahlert. 2001. Nature's carbohydrate chemists: the enzymatic glycosylation of bioactive bacterial metabolites. *Curr. Org. Chem.* **5:**139–167.

Threlfall, E. J. 2000. Epidemic *Salmonella typhimurium* DT 104—a truly international multiresistant clone. *J. Antimicrob. Chemother.* **46:**7–10.

Throup, J. P., K. K. Koretke, A. P. Bryant, K. A. Ingraham, A. F. Chalker, Y. Ge, A. Marra, N. G. Wallis, J. R. Brown, D. J. Holmes, M. Rosenberg, and M. K. Burnham. 2000. A genomic analysis of two-component signal transduction in *Streptococcus pneumoniae. Mol. Microbiol.* **35:**566–576.

Throup, J. P., F. Zappacosta, R. D. Lunsford, R. S. Annan, S. A. Carr, J. T. Lonsdale, A. P. Bryant, D. McDevitt, M. Rosenberg, and M. K. Burnham. 2001. The srhSR gene pair from *Staphylococcus aureus:* genomic and proteomic approaches to the identification and characterization of gene function. *Biochemistry* **40:**10392–10401.

Toney, J. H., P. M. Fitzgerald, N. Grover-Sharma, S. H. Olson, W. J. May, J. G. Sundelof, D. E. Vanderwall, K. A. Cleary, S. K. Grant, J. K. Wu, J. W. Kozarich, D. L. Pompliano, and G. G. Hammond. 1998. Antibiotic sensitization using biphenyl tetrazoles as potent inhibitors of *Bacteroides fragilis* metallo-beta-lactamase. *Chem. Biol.* **5**:185–196.

Ton-That, H., G. Liu, S. K. Mazmanian, K. F. Faull, and O. Schneewind. 1999. Purification and characterization of sortase, the transpeptidase that cleaves surface proteins of *Staphylococcus aureus* at the LPXTG motif. *Proc. Natl. Acad. Sci. USA* **96**:12424–12429.

Trauger, J. W., R. M. Kohli, H. D. Mootz, M. A. Marahiel, and C. T. Walsh. 2000. Peptide cyclization catalysed by the thioesterase domain of tyrocidine synthetase. *Nature* **407**:215–218.

Trauger, J. W., and C. T. Walsh. 2000. Heterologous expression in *Escherichia coli* of the first module of the nonribosomal peptide synthetase for chloroeremomycin, a vancomycin-type glycopeptide antibiotic. *Proc. Natl. Acad. Sci. USA* **97**:3112–3117.

Trias, J. 2001. The role of combichem in antibiotic discovery. *Curr. Opin. Microbiol.* **4**:520–525.

Trias, J., and Z. Yuan. 1999. Mining bacterial cell wall biosynthesis with new tools: multitarget screens. *Drug Resist. Update* **2**:358–362.

Tsai, F. T., O. M. Singh, T. Skarzynski, A. J. Wonacott, S. Weston, A. Tucker, R. A. Pauptit, A. L. Breeze, J. P. Poyser, R. O'Brien, J. E. Ladbury, and D. B. Wigley. 1997. The high-resolution crystal structure of a 24-kDa gyrase B fragment from E. coli complexed with one of the most potent coumarin inhibitors, clorobiocin. *Proteins* **28**:41–52.

Valegard, K., A. C. van Scheltinga, M. D. Lloyd, T. Hara, S. Ramaswamy, A. Perrakis, A. Thompson, H. J. Lee, J. E. Baldwin, C. J. Schofield, J. Hajdu, and I. Andersson. 1998. Structure of a cephalosporin synthase. *Nature* **394**:805–809.

van Asselt, E. J., K. H. Kalk, and B. W. Dijkstra. 2000. Crystallographic studies of the interactions of *Escherichia coli* lytic transglycosylase Slt35 with peptidoglycan. *Biochemistry* **39**:1924–1934.

van Heijenoort, J. 2001a. Formation of the glycan chains in the synthesis of bacterial peptidoglycan. *Glycobiology* **11**:25R–36R.

van Heijenoort, J. 2001b. Recent advances in the formation of the bacterial peptidoglycan monomer unit. *Nat. Prod. Rep.* **18**:503–519.

VanNieuwenhze, M. S., S. C. Mauldin, M. Zia-Ebrahimi, B. E. Winger, W. J. Hornback, S. L. Saha, J. A. Aikins, and L. C. Blaszczak. 2002. The first total synthesis of lipid II: the final monomeric intermediate in bacterial cell wall biosynthesis. *J. Am. Chem. Soc.* **124**:3656–3660.

van Wageningen, A. M., P. N. Kirkpatrick, D. H. Williams, B. R. Harris, J. K. Kershaw, N. J. Lennard, M. Jones, S. J. Jones, and P. J. Solenberg. 1998. Sequencing and analysis of genes involved in the biosynthesis of a vancomycin group antibiotic. *Chem. Biol.* **5**:155–162.

Vester, B., and S. Douthwaite. 2001. Macrolide resistance conferred by base substitutions in 23S rRNA. *Antimicrob. Agents Chemother.* **45**:1–12.

Vining, L. C., and C. Stuttard. 1995. Chloramphenicol. *Biotechnology* **28**:505–530.

Vollmer, W., and J. V. Holtje. 2000. A simple screen for murein transglycosylase inhibitors. *Antimicrob. Agents Chemother.* **44**:1181–1185.

von Dohren, H., U. Keller, J. Vater, and R. Zocher. 1997. Multifunctional peptide synthetases. *Chem. Rev.* **97**:2675–2706.

Walsh, C. 1979. *Enzymatic Reaction Mechanisms.* W. H. Freeman & Co., San Francisco, Calif.

Walsh, C. T. 1988. Enzymes in the D-alanine branch of bacterial cell wall peptidoglycan assembly. *J. Biol. Chem.* **264**:2393–2396.

Walsh, C. T., T. E. Benson, D. H. Kim, and W. J. Lees. 1996a. The versatility of phosphoenolpyruvate and its vinyl ether products in biosynthesis. *Chem. Biol.* **3**:83–91.

Walsh, C. T., S. L. Fisher, I. S. Park, M. Prahalad, and Z. Wu. 1996b. Bacterial resistance to vancomycin: five genes and one missing hydrogen bond tell the story. *Chem. Biol.* **3**:21–28.

Wang, J. C. 1996. DNA topoisomerases. *Annu. Rev. Biochem.* **65**:635–692.

Wang, Z., W. Fast, A. M. Valentine, and S. J. Benkovic. 1999. Metallo-beta-lactamase: structure and mechanism. *Curr. Opin. Chem. Biol.* **3**:614–622.

Watson, W. T., T. D. Minogue, D. L. Val, S. B. von Bodman, and M. E. Churchill. 2002. Structural basis and specificity of acyl-homoserine lactone signal production in bacterial quorum sensing. *Mol. Cell* **9**:685–694.

Wenzel, R. P., and M. B. Edmond. 2000. Managing antibiotic resistance. *N. Engl. J. Med.* **343**:1961–1963.

Wess, G., M. Urmann, and B. Sickenberger. 2001. Medicinal chemistry: challenges and opportunities. *Angew. Chem. Int. Ed. Engl.* **40**:3341–3350.

White, D. G., S. Zhao, R. Sudler, S. Ayers, S. Friedman, S. Chen, P. F. McDermott, S. McDermott, D. W. Wagner, and J. Meng. 2001. The isolation of antibiotic-resistant Salmonella from retail ground meats. *N. Engl. J. Med.* **345**:1147–1154.

Whittle, G., B. D. Hund, N. B. Shoemaker, and A. A. Salyers. 2001. Characterization of the 13-kilobase ermF region of the Bacteroides conjugative transposon CTnDOT. *Appl. Environ. Microbiol.* **67**:3488–3495.

Wiedemann, B., C. Kliebe, and M. Kresken. 1989. The epidemiology of beta-lactamases. *J. Antimicrob. Chemother.* **24**(Suppl. B):1–22.

Wilkinson, B., G. Foster, B. A. Rudd, N. L. Taylor, A. P. Blackaby, P. J. Sidebottom, D. J. Cooper, M. J. Dawson, A. D. Buss, S. Gaisser, I. U. Bohm, C. J. Rowe, J. Cortes, P. F. Leadlay, and J. Staunton. 2000. Novel octaketide macrolides related to 6-deoxyerythronolide B provide evidence for iterative operation of the erythromycin polyketide synthase. *Chem. Biol.* **7**:111–117.

Williams, D. H. 1996. The glycopeptide story—how to kill the deadly "superbugs." *Nat. Prod. Rep.* **13**:469–477.

Williams, D. H., and B. Bardsley. 1999. The vancomycin group of antibiotics and the fight against resistant bacteria. *Angew. Chem. Int. Ed. Engl.* **38**:1172–1193.

Williams, R. J., and D. L. Heymann. 1998. Containment of antibiotic resistance. *Science* **279**:1153–1154.

Wilson, M., J. DeRisi, H. H. Kristensen, P. Imboden, S. Rane, P. O. Brown, and G. K. Schoolnik. 1999. Exploring drug-induced alterations in gene expression in *Mycobacterium tuberculosis* by microarray hybridization. *Proc. Natl. Acad. Sci. USA* **96**:12833–12838.

Wimberly, B. T., D. E. Brodersen, W. M. Clemons, Jr., R. J. Morgan-Warren, A. P. Carter, C. Vonrhein, T. Hartsch, and V. Ramakrishnan. 2000. Structure of the 30S ribosomal subunit. *Nature* **407:**327–339.

Winzer, K., C. Falconer, N. C. Garber, S. P. Diggle, M. Camara, and P. Williams. 2000. The *Pseudomonas aeruginosa* lectins PA-IL and PA-IIL are controlled by quorum sensing and by RpoS. *J. Bacteriol.* **182:**6401–6411.

Witte, W. 1998. Medical consequences of antibiotic use in agriculture. *Science* **279:** 996–997.

Wolfson, J. S., and D. C. Hooper. 1989. *Quinolone Antimicrobial Agents.* ASM Press, Washington, D.C.

Wright, G. E. 1999. Aminoglycoside-modifying enzymes. *Curr. Opin. Microbiol.* **2:** 499–503.

Xu, G. Y., A. Tam, L. Lin, J. Hixon, C. C. Fritz, and R. Powers. 2001. Solution structure of *B. subtilis* acyl carrier protein. *Structure* **9:**277–287.

Xue, Y., and D. A. Sherman. 2001. Biosynthesis and combinatorial biosynthesis of pikromycin-related macrolides in *Streptomyces venezuelae. Metab. Eng.* **3:**15–26.

Yamada, Y., and T. Nihara. 1999. Microbial hormones and microbial chemical ecology, p. 377–413. *In* D. Barton, K. Nakanishi, and O. Meth-Cohn (ed.), *Comprehensive Natural Products Chemistry,* vol. 8. Elsevier, Oxford, United Kingdom.

Yano, H., A. Kuga, K. Irinoda, R. Okamoto, T. Kobayashi, and M. Inoue. 1999. Presence of genes for beta-lactamases of two different classes on a single plasmid from a clinical isolate of *Serratia marcescens. J. Antibiot.* **52:**1135–1139.

Ye, X. Y., M. C. Lo, L. Brunner, D. Walker, D. Kahne, and S. Walker. 2001. Better substrates for bacterial transglycosylases. *J. Am. Chem. Soc.* **123:**3155–3156.

Yin, C. C., M. L. Aldema-Ramos, M. I. Borges-Walmsley, R. W. Taylor, A. R. Walmsley, S. B. Levy, and P. A. Bullough. 2000. The quarternary molecular architecture of TetA, a secondary tetracycline transporter from *Escherichia coli. Mol. Microbiol.* **38:**482–492.

Young, R., I. N. Wang, and W. D. Roof. 2000. Phages will out: strategies of host cell lysis. *Trends Microbiol.* **8:**120–128.

Yusupov, M. M., G. Z. Yusupova, A. Baucom, K. Lieberman, T. N. Earnest, J. H. Cate, and H. F. Noller. 2001. Crystal structure of the ribosome at 5.5 Å resolution. *Science* **292:**883–896.

Yusupova, G. Z., M. M. Yusupov, J. H. D. Cate, and H. F. Noller. 2001. The path of messenger RNA through the ribosome. *Cell* **106:**233–241.

Zasloff, M. 2002. Antimicrobial peptides of multicellular organisms. *Nature* **415:** 389–395.

Zhang, H. Z., C. J. Hackbarth, K. M. Chansky, and H. F. Chambers. 2001. A proteolytic transmembrane signaling pathway and resistance to beta-lactams in staphylococci. *Science* **291:**1962–1965.

Zhang, Y. X., K. Perry, V. A. Vinci, K. Powell, W. P. Stemmer, and S. B. del Cardayre. 2002. Genome shuffling leads to rapid phenotypic improvement in bacteria. *Nature* **415:**644–646.

Zhang, Z., J. Ren, D. K. Stammers, J. E. Baldwin, K. Harlos, and C. J. Schofield. 2000. Structural origins of the selectivity of the trifunctional oxygenase clavaminic acid synthase. *Nat. Struct. Biol.* **7:**127–133.

Zhao, L. S., J. Ahlert, Y. Q. Xue, J. S. Thorson, D. H. Sherman, and H. W. Liu. 1999. Engineering a methymycin/pikromycin-calicheamicin hybrid: construction of two new macrolides carrying a designed sugar moiety. *J. Am. Chem. Soc.* **121:**9881–9882.

Zheleznova, E. E., P. N. Markham, A. A. Neyfakh, and R. G. Brennan. 1999. Structural basis of multidrug recognition by BmrR, a transcription activator of a multidrug transporter. *Cell* **96:**353–362.

Zheleznova, E. E., P. Markham, R. Edgar, E. Bibi, A. A. Neyfakh, and R. G. Brennan. 2000. A structure-based mechanism for drug binding by multidrug transporters. *Trends Biochem. Sci.* **25:**39–43.

Zimmermann, N., and G. Jung. 1997. The three-dimensional solution structure of the lantibiotic murein-biosynthesis-inhibitor actagardine determined by NMR. *Eur. J. Biochem.* **246:**809–819.

Index

A

A47934 (glycopeptide), structure of, 100

Abs proteins, *Streptomyces coelicolor*, in antibiotic biosynthesis regulation, 162–164

ABT-773 (ketolide), structure of, 148

Acetyl-CoA, in ketide synthesis, 175

Acetylation, in aminoglycoside deactivation, 120–122

Actinonin, structure of, 253

Actinoplanes, vancomycin producing, self-protection against, 99

Actinorhodin, biosynthesis of, 161–164

Acyl carrier protein, in ketide synthesis, 176–181

Acylhomoserine lactones, as antibiotic targets, 266–267

Adenylylation, in aminoglycoside deactivation, 120–122

AfsQ proteins, *Streptomyces coelicolor*, in antibiotic biosynthesis regulation, 162–164

Agr proteins, *Staphylococcus aureus*, 265–266

Agriculture, antibiotic use in, resistance development in, 291–292

AI-2 quorum autoinducers, as antibiotic targets, 267

Alanine racemase, in peptidoglycan assembly, 30–32

D-Alanyl-D-alanine ligase, in cell wall biosynthesis, 30–32, 149–153

L-Aminoadipyl-L-cysteinyl-L-valine (ACV), in peptide antibiotic biosynthesis, 195
- bacitracin, 204–206
- cephalosporins, 206–211
- chloreremomycin, 202–204
- penicillins, 206–211
- teicoplanin, 211–214
- tyrocidine, 204–206
- vancomycin, 202–204, 211–214

L-Aminoadipyl-L-cysteinyl-D-valine (ACV) synthase, 195–197, 200–201

Aminocoumarins
- bacteria producing, self-protection against, 99
- biosynthesis of, 226–228

Aminoglycosides
- biosynthesis of, 222–226
- protein biosynthesis effects of, 66–67, 249
- resistance to, enzymes causing, 120–122

Amoxicillin, structure of, 12

Amoxicillin-clavulanate, mechanism of action of, 113–114

Amoxicillin-sulbactam, mechanism of action of, 114

Amp proteins, in *Escherichia coli* resistance, 115–117

Amycolatopsis orientalis, in vancomycin biosynthesis, 158

Antibiotic(s)
- appropriate use of, 293–295

bacterial self-protection against, *see* Bacteria, self-protection in

classification of, 4–5, 13–18

definition of, 3

efflux from bacteria, *see* Efflux pumps

first-line selections of, 16–18

new, *see* Novel antibiotics

resistance to, *see* Resistance

sales of, 13

structures of, 12

targets for, *see* Bacterial targets

Antibiotic biosynthesis, 5, *see also specific antibiotics*
- nonribosomal peptide, 195–218
- novel
  - libraries for, 271–277
  - nonribosomal peptides, 278–282
  - polyketides, 274–282
- polyketides, 175–193
- regulation of, 159–173
  - in gram-negative bacteria, 171–173
  - in streptomycetes, 159–170

Arp proteins, in antibiotic biosynthesis, 168

ATP-binding cassette family, of efflux pumps, characteristics of, 126–127, 129–132

Avoparcin, for food animals, resistance development and, 291

Azithromycin
- indications for, 59
- resistance to, 147–148
- structure of, 58